ADDRESSING FOODBORNE THREATS TO HEALTH

Policies, Practices, and Global Coordination

Workshop Summary

Forum on Microbial Threats
Board on Global Health

INSTITUTE OF MEDICINE
OF THE NATIONAL ACADEMIES

THE NATIONAL ACADEMIES PRESS
Washington, D.C.
www.nap.edu

THE NATIONAL ACADEMIES PRESS 500 Fifth Street, N.W. Washington, DC 20001

NOTICE: The project that is the subject of this report was approved by the Governing Board of the National Research Council, whose members are drawn from the councils of the National Academy of Sciences, the National Academy of Engineering, and the Institute of Medicine.

This project was supported by the American Society for Microbiology; Burroughs Wellcome Fund; Defense Threat Reduction Agency; GlaxoSmithKline; Infectious Disease Society of America; Lawrence Livermore National Laboratory; Merck Company Foundation; Pfizer; Sanofi Pasteur; U.S. Department of Health and Human Services' National Institutes of Health, National Institute of Allergy and Infectious Diseases, Centers for Disease Control and Prevention, and Food and Drug Administration; U.S. Department of Defense's Global Emerging Infections Surveillance and Response System and Walter Reed Army Institute of Research; U.S. Department of Homeland Security; U.S. Department of State; and U.S. Department of Veterans Affairs. Any opinions, findings, conclusions, or recommendations expressed in this publication are those of the author(s) and do not necessarily reflect the view of the organizations or agencies that provided support for this project.

International Standard Book Number-10 0-309-10043-7 (Book)
International Standard Book Number-13 978-0-309-10043-4 (Book)
International Standard Book Number-10 0-309-65457-2 (PDF)
International Standard Book Number-13 978-0-309-65457-9 (PDF)

Additional copies of this report are available from the National Academies Press, 500 Fifth Street, N.W., Lockbox 285, Washington, DC 20055; (800) 624-6242 or (202) 334-3313 (in the Washington metropolitan area); Internet, http://www.nap.edu.

For more information about the Institute of Medicine, visit the IOM home page at: **www.iom.edu.**

Printed in the United States of America.

The serpent has been a symbol of long life, healing, and knowledge among almost all cultures and religions since the beginning of recorded history. The serpent adopted as a logotype by the Institute of Medicine is a relief carving from ancient Greece, now held by the Staatliche Museen in Berlin.

COVER: A detailed section of a stained glass window 21″ × 56″ depicting the natural history of influenza viruses and zoonotic exchange in the emergence of new strains was used to design the front cover. Based on the work done at St. Jude Children's Research Hospital supported by American Lebanese Syrian Associated Charities (ALSAC) and the National Institute of Allergy and Infectious Diseases (NIAID). Artist: Jenny Hammond, Highgreenleycleugh, Northumberland, England.

"Knowing is not enough; we must apply.
Willing is not enough; we must do."
—Goethe

INSTITUTE OF MEDICINE
OF THE NATIONAL ACADEMIES

Advising the Nation. Improving Health.

THE NATIONAL ACADEMIES

Advisers to the Nation on Science, Engineering, and Medicine

The **National Academy of Sciences** is a private, nonprofit, self-perpetuating society of distinguished scholars engaged in scientific and engineering research, dedicated to the furtherance of science and technology and to their use for the general welfare. Upon the authority of the charter granted to it by the Congress in 1863, the Academy has a mandate that requires it to advise the federal government on scientific and technical matters. Dr. Ralph J. Cicerone is president of the National Academy of Sciences.

The **National Academy of Engineering** was established in 1964, under the charter of the National Academy of Sciences, as a parallel organization of outstanding engineers. It is autonomous in its administration and in the selection of its members, sharing with the National Academy of Sciences the responsibility for advising the federal government. The National Academy of Engineering also sponsors engineering programs aimed at meeting national needs, encourages education and research, and recognizes the superior achievements of engineers. Dr. Wm. A. Wulf is president of the National Academy of Engineering.

The **Institute of Medicine** was established in 1970 by the National Academy of Sciences to secure the services of eminent members of appropriate professions in the examination of policy matters pertaining to the health of the public. The Institute acts under the responsibility given to the National Academy of Sciences by its congressional charter to be an adviser to the federal government and, upon its own initiative, to identify issues of medical care, research, and education. Dr. Harvey V. Fineberg is president of the Institute of Medicine.

The **National Research Council** was organized by the National Academy of Sciences in 1916 to associate the broad community of science and technology with the Academy's purposes of furthering knowledge and advising the federal government. Functioning in accordance with general policies determined by the Academy, the Council has become the principal operating agency of both the National Academy of Sciences and the National Academy of Engineering in providing services to the government, the public, and the scientific and engineering communities. The Council is administered jointly by both Academies and the Institute of Medicine. Dr. Ralph J. Cicerone and Dr. Wm. A. Wulf are chair and vice chair, respectively, of the National Research Council.

www.national-academies.org

FORUM ON MICROBIAL THREATS

STANLEY M. LEMON (*Chair*), School of Medicine, University of Texas Medical Branch, Galveston

MARGARET A. HAMBURG (*Vice-chair*), Nuclear Threat Initiative/Global Health & Security Initiative, Washington, D.C.

P. FREDERICK SPARLING (*Vice-chair*), University of North Carolina, Chapel Hill

DAVID W. K. ACHESON, Center for Food Safety and Applied Nutrition, Food and Drug Administration, Rockville, Maryland

RUTH L. BERKELMAN, Emory University, Center for Public Health Preparedness and Research, Rollins School of Public Health, Atlanta, Georgia

ROGER G. BREEZE, Centaur Science Group, Washington, D.C.

STEVEN J. BRICKNER, Pfizer Global Research and Development, Pfizer Inc., Groton, Connecticut

GAIL H. CASSELL, Eli Lilly & Company, Indianapolis, Indiana

RALPH L. ERICKSON, Global Emerging Infections Surveillance and Response System, Department of Defense, Silver Spring, Maryland

MARK B. FEINBERG, Merck Vaccine Division, Merck & Co., West Point, Pennsylvania

J. PATRICK FITCH, Battelle Memorial Institute, Livermore, California

DARRELL R. GALLOWAY, Medical S&T Division, Defense Threat Reduction Agency, Ft. Belvoir, Virginia

S. ELIZABETH GEORGE, Biological and Chemical Countermeasures Program, Department of Homeland Security, Washington, D.C.

JESSE L. GOODMAN, Center for Biologics Evaluation and Research, Food and Drug Administration, Rockville, Maryland

EDUARDO GOTUZZO, Instituto de Medicina Tropical–Alexander von Humbolt, Universidad Peruana Cayetano Heredia, Lima, Peru

JO HANDELSMAN, College of Agricultural and Life Sciences, University of Wisconsin, Madison

CAROLE A. HEILMAN, Division of Microbiology and Infectious Diseases, National Institute of Allergy and Infectious Diseases, National Institutes of Health, Bethesda, Maryland

DAVID L. HEYMANN, Polio Eradication, World Health Organization, Geneva, Switzerland

PHIL HOSBACH, New Products and Immunization Policy, Sanofi Pasteur, Swiftwater, Pennsylvania

JAMES M. HUGHES, Global Infectious Diseases Program, Emory University, Atlanta, Georgia

STEPHEN A. JOHNSTON, Arizona BioDesign Institute, Arizona State University, Tempe, Arizona

GERALD T. KEUSCH, Boston University School of Medicine and Boston University School of Public Health, Massachusetts

RIMA F. KHABBAZ, National Center for Preparedness, Detection and Control of Infectious Diseases, Centers for Disease Control and Prevention, Atlanta, Georgia

LONNIE J. KING, Center for Zoonotic, Vectorborne, and Enteric Diseases, Centers for Disease Control and Prevention, Atlanta, Georgia

GEORGE W. KORCH, United States Army Medical Research Institute for Infectious Diseases, Ft. Detrick, Maryland

JOSHUA LEDERBERG, The Rockefeller University, New York

LYNN G. MARKS, Medicine Development Center, GlaxoSmithKline, Collegeville, Pennsylvania

MARY McBRIDE, Science and Technology Chemical and Biological National Security Program, Lawrence Livermore National Laboratory, Livermore, California

STEPHEN S. MORSE, Center for Public Health Preparedness, Columbia University, New York

MICHAEL T. OSTERHOLM, Center for Infectious Disease Research and Policy, School of Public Health, University of Minnesota, Minneapolis

GEORGE POSTE, Arizona BioDesign Institute, Arizona State University, Tempe

DAVID A. RELMAN, Stanford University, Palo Alto, California

GARY A. ROSELLE, Central Office, Veterans Health Administration, Department of Veterans Affairs, Washington, D.C.

JANET SHOEMAKER, Office of Public Affairs, American Society for Microbiology, Washington, D.C.

BRIAN J. STASKAWICZ, Department of Plant and Microbial Biology, University of California, Berkeley

TERENCE TAYLOR, International Council for the Life Sciences, Washington, D.C.

Liaisons

ENRIQUETA C. BOND, Burroughs Wellcome Fund, Research Triangle Park, North Carolina

NANCY CARTER-FOSTER, Program for Emerging Infections and HIV/ AIDS, U.S. Department of State, Washington, D.C.

EDWARD McSWEEGAN, National Institute of Allergy and Infectious Diseases, National Institutes of Health, Bethesda, Maryland

Staff

EILEEN CHOFFNES, Forum Director

KIM LUNDBERG, Research Associate

ALISON MACK, Science Writer

KATE SKOCZDOPOLE, Research Associate

BOARD ON GLOBAL HEALTH

Margaret Hamburg (*Chair*), Consultant, Nuclear Threat Initiative, Washington, D.C.
George A.O. Alleyne, Director Emeritus, Pan American Health Organization, Washington, D.C.
Yves Bergevin, Department of Child and Adolescent Health and Development, World Health Organization, Geneva, Switzerland
Donald Berwick, Clinical Professor of Pediatrics and Health Care Policy, Harvard Medical School, and President and Chief Executive Officer, Institute of Healthcare Improvement, Boston, Massachusetts
Jo Ivey Boufford (*IOM Foreign Secretary*), Professor, Robert F. Wagner School of Public Service, New York University, New York
David R. Challoner, Vice President for Health Affairs, Emeritus, University of Florida, Gainesville
Ciro de Quadros, Director of International Programs, Sabin Vaccine Institute, Washington, D.C.
Sue Goldie, Associate Professor of Health Decision Science, Department of Health Policy and Management, Center for Risk Analysis, Harvard University School of Public Health, Boston, Massachusetts
Richard Guerrant, Thomas H. Hunter Professor of International Medicine and Director, Center for Global Health, University of Virginia School of Medicine, Charlottesville
Gerald Keusch, Assistant Provost for Global Health, Boston University School of Medicine, and Associate Dean for Global Health, Boston University School of Public Health, Massachusetts
Jeffrey Koplan, Vice President for Academic Health Affairs, Emory University, Atlanta, Georgia
Sheila Leatherman, Research Professor, University of North Carolina School of Public Health, Chapel Hill
Michael Merson, Anna M. R. Lauder Professor, Dean of Public Health, and Chair, Department of Epidemiology and Public Health, Yale University School of Medicine, New Haven, Connecticut
Mark L. Rosenberg, Executive Director, the Task Force for Child Survival and Development, Emory University, Decatur, Georgia
Philip Russell, Professor Emeritus, Bloomberg School of Public Health, Johns Hopkins University, Baltimore, Maryland

Staff

Patrick Kelley, Director
Allison Brantley, Senior Program Assistant

Reviewers

This report has been reviewed in draft form by individuals chosen for their diverse perspectives and technical expertise, in accordance with procedures approved by the NRC's Report Review Committee. The purpose of this independent review is to provide candid and critical comments that will assist the institution in making its published report as sound as possible and to ensure that the report meets institutional standards for objectivity, evidence, and responsiveness to the study charge. The review comments and draft manuscript remain confidential to protect the integrity of the deliberative process. We wish to thank the following individuals for their review of this report:

Johanna Dwyer, D.Sc., Frances Stern Nutrition Center, Tufts–New England Medical Center

Craig Hedberg, Ph.D., Division of Environmental and Occupational Health, University of Minnesota

Terence Taylor, International Council for the Life Sciences, Washington, D.C.

Mary Wilson, M.D., Department of Population and International Health, Harvard University

The review of this report was overseen by **Floyd Bloom, M.D.,** Professor Emeritus, Department of Neuropharmacology, The Scripps Research Institute, and **Melvin Worth, M.D.,** Scholar-in-Residence, National Academies, who were responsible for making certain that an independent examination of this report was carried out in accordance with institutional procedures and that all review comments were carefully considered. Responsibility for the final content of this report rests entirely with the authoring committee and the institution.

Preface

The Forum on Emerging Infections was created in 1996 in response to a request from the Centers for Disease Control and Prevention (CDC) and the National Institutes of Health (NIH). It was established by the Institute of Medicine (IOM) to provide structured opportunities for leaders from government, academia, and industry to meet and examine issues of shared concern regarding research, prevention, detection, and management of emerging or reemerging infectious diseases. In pursuing this task, the Forum provides a venue to foster the exchange of information and ideas, identify areas in need of greater attention, clarify policy issues by enhancing knowledge and identifying points of agreement, and inform decision makers about science and policy issues. The Forum seeks to illuminate issues rather than resolve them directly; for this reason, it does not provide advice or recommendations on any specific policy initiative pending before any agency or organization. Rather, its strengths are embodied in the diversity of its membership and the contributions of individual members expressed throughout the activities of the Forum. In September 2003, the Forum changed its name to the Forum on Microbial Threats.

ABOUT THE WORKSHOP

In December 2004, at a press conference called to announce his departure as Secretary of the Department of Health and Human Services (DHHS), Tommy Thompson raised both concern and controversy when he remarked that he could not understand why terrorists had not yet attacked our food supply "because it is so easy to do."[1] Three days later, the Food and Drug Administration (FDA) announced the last in a series of four food safeguards mandated under the Biopreparedness Act of 2002.[2] Although these provisions improve the FDA's ability to intercept and track the origins of food that is suspected to pose a threat to health, they cannot prevent contamination. Biological and chemical agents can be—and have been—introduced, both accidentally and deliberately, at many vulnerable points along the farm-to-table food chain.

Foodborne agents have been estimated to cause approximately 76 million illnesses, 325,000 hospitalizations, and 5,200 deaths in the United States each year.[3] More than 250 different foodborne diseases, including both infections and poisonings, have been described, according to the CDC.[4] The U.S. Department of Agriculture (USDA) estimates costs associated with medical expenses and losses in productivity due to missed work and premature deaths from five major types of foodborne illnesses (*Campylobacter, Escherichia coli* O157:H7, *Shiga* toxin-producing strains of *E. coli*, *Listeria monocytogenes*, and *Salmonella*) at $6.9 billion annually.[5] This figure likely represents the tip of the iceberg, as it does not account for the broad spectrum of foodborne illnesses or for their wide-ranging repercussions for consumers, government, and the food industry.

The potential impact on human health of deliberate adulteration of food can be estimated by extrapolation from the many documented examples of unintentional outbreaks of foodborne disease, some of which have sickened hundreds of thousands of people and killed hundreds.[6] Given the wide variety of potential chemical and biological adulterants that can be introduced at many vulnerable points along the food supply continuum, contaminating food is perhaps one of the easiest means to intentionally distribute these agents. Although the many possibilities for foodborne bioterrorism cannot be specifically prevented, strategic preparations for surveillance, diagnosis, outbreak investigation, and medical response could mitigate foodborne threats of any origin.

To examine issues critical to the protection of the nation's food supply, the Institute of Medicine's Forum on Microbial Threats hosted a public workshop on October 25 and 26, 2005, in Washington, D.C. The presentations and discussions

---

[1]Branigin W, Allen M, Mintz J. 2004 (December 3). Tommy Thompson resigns from HHS: Bush asks Defense Secretary Rumsfeld to stay. *Washington Post*. [Online]. Available: http://www.washingtonpost.com/wp-dyn/articles/A31377-2004Dec3.html [accessed May 6, 2006].

[2]Gardner A. 2004 (December 6). *U.S. Moves to Further Protect Food Supply*. [Online]. Available: http://www.healthfinder.gov/news/newsstory.asp?docID=522737 [accessed June 27, 2006].

[3]Mead PS, Slutsker L, Dietz V, McCraig LF, Bresee JS, Shapiro C, Griffin PM, Tauxe RV. 1999. Food-related illness and death in the United States. *Emerging Infectious Diseases* 5(5):607–625.

[4]CDC. 2005. *Foodborne Illness*. [Online]. Available: http://www.cdc.gov/ncidod/dbmd/diseaseinfo/foodborneinfections_g.htm#foodbornedisease [accessed June 27, 2006].

[5]Vogt DU. 2005. *Food Safety Issues in the 109th Congress*. CRS Report RL31853 Washington, D.C.: The Library of Congress.

[6]Sobel J. 2005. Food and beverage sabotage. In: Pilch RF, Zilinskas RA, Ed. *Encyclopedia of Bioterrorism Defense*. New York: Wiley-Liss, Inc. Pp. 215–220.

of the workshop were structured to explore the existing knowledge and unanswered questions indicated by (but not limited to) the following topics:

- The globalization of the U.S. food supply
- The spectrum of microbial threats to food
- Case studies of food threats
- The organization of food safety systems
- Costs and benefits of reporting foodborne threats: the case of bovine spongiform encelphalopathy (BSE)
- Surveillance for foodborne illness

ACKNOWLEDGMENTS

The Forum on Microbial Threats and the IOM wish to express their warmest appreciation to the individuals and organizations who gave their valuable time to provide information and advice to the Forum through their participation in this workshop. A full list of presenters can be found in Appendix A.

The Forum is indebted to the IOM staff who contributed during the course of the workshop and the production of this workshop summary. On behalf of the Forum, we gratefully acknowledge the efforts led by Eileen Choffnes, director of the Forum; Kim Lundberg, research associate; and Kate Skoczdopole, research associate, who dedicated much effort and time to developing this workshop's agenda, and for their thoughtful and insightful approach and skill in translating the workshop proceedings and discussion into this workshop summary. We would also like to thank our science writer, Alison Mack, for her thoughtful and insightful approach and skill in translating the workshop proceedings and discussion into this workshop summary.

Finally, the Forum also thanks the sponsors that supported this activity. Financial support for this project was provided by the U.S. Department of Health and Human Services' National Institutes of Health, National Institute of Allergy and Infectious Diseases, Centers for Disease Control and Prevention, and Food and Drug Administration; U.S. Department of Defense's Global Emerging Infections Surveillance and Response System, Walter Reed Army Institute of Research, and Defense Threat Reduction Agency; U.S. Department of State; U.S. Department of Veterans Affairs; U.S. Department of Homeland Security; Lawrence Livermore National Laboratory; American Society for Microbiology; Sanofi Pasteur; Burroughs Wellcome Fund; Pfizer; GlaxoSmithKline; Infectious Disease Society of America; and the Merck Company Foundation. The views presented in this workshop summary report are those of the editors and workshop participants and are not necessarily those of the funding organizations.

Stanley M. Lemon, *Chair*
P. Frederick Sparling, *Vice-chair*
Margaret A. Hamburg, *Vice-chair*
Forum on Microbial Threats

Contents

Tables and Figures

TABLES

FIGURES

Summary and Assessment

ADDRESSING FOODBORNE THREATS TO HEALTH: POLICIES, PRACTICES, AND GLOBAL COORDINATION

In December 2004, at a press conference called to announce his departure as Secretary of the Department of Health and Human Services (HHS), Tommy Thompson raised both concern and controversy when he remarked that he could not understand why the terrorists had not yet attacked our food supply "because it is so easy to do" (Branigin et al., 2004). Although to date the United States has been spared such a disaster, the many documented examples of unintentional outbreaks of foodborne disease—some of which have sickened hundreds of thousands of people, and killed hundreds—provide a grim basis for estimating the impact of deliberate food adulteration (Sobel, 2005). Due to the wide variety of potential chemical and biological agents that could be introduced at many vulnerable points along the food supply continuum, contaminating food is considered an especially simple, yet effective, means to threaten large populations.

Intentional adulteration is not the only reason to be concerned about the safety of the U.S. food supply, however. Accidental foodborne illness already causes an estimated 76 million illnesses, 325,000 hospitalizations, and 5,200 deaths in the United States each year (Mead et al., 1999). The U.S. Department of Agriculture (USDA) estimates costs associated with medical expenses and losses in productivity due to missed work and premature deaths from five major types of foodborne illnesses (*Campylobacter, E. coli* O157:H7, Shiga toxin-producing strains of *E. coli*, *Listeria monocytogenes*, and *Salmonella*) at $6.9 billion annually (Vogt, 2005). This figure likely represents the tip of the iceberg, as it does not account for the broad spectrum of foodborne illnesses or for their wide-ranging repercussions for consumers, government, and the food industry.

Although specific preventions cannot be mounted against the many possibilities for foodborne bioterrorism, strategic preparations to reduce vulnerability to foodborne illness—and to anticipate and address the medical, social, and economic consequences—could mitigate foodborne threats to health, whatever their origin. To explore the nature and extent of such threats, possibilities for reducing their impact, and obstacles to this goal, the Forum on Microbial Threats of the Institute of Medicine (IOM) convened the workshop *Foodborne Threats to Health: The Policies and Practice of Surveillance, Prevention, Outbreak Investigations, and International Coordination* on October 25 and 26, 2005. Workshop participants discussed the threat spectrum and burden of disease associated with foodborne illness and the role that increasing globalization of food production and distribution plays in the transmission of foodborne disease. Participants also reviewed existing research, policies, and practices concerning foodborne threats in order to identify unmet needs, challenges, and opportunities for improving food safety systems, surveillance, and emergency response.

ORGANIZATION OF THE WORKSHOP SUMMARY

This workshop summary report is prepared for the Forum membership in the name of the editors as a collection of individually authored papers and commentary. Sections of the workshop summary not specifically attributed to an individual reflect the views of the editors and not those of the Forum on Microbial Threats, its sponsors, or the IOM. The contents of the unattributed sections are based on the presentations and discussions that took place during the workshop.

The workshop summary is organized within chapters as a topic-by-topic description of the presentations and discussions. Its purpose is to present lessons from relevant experience, delineate a range of pivotal issues and their respective problems, and put forth some potential responses as described by the workshop participants.

Although this workshop summary provides an account of the individual presentations, it also reflects an important aspect of the Forum philosophy. The workshop functions as a dialogue among representatives from different sectors and presents their beliefs on which areas may merit further attention. However, the reader should be aware that the material presented here expresses the views and opinions of the individuals participating in the workshop and not the deliberations of a formally constituted IOM study committee. These proceedings summarize only what participants stated in the workshop and are not intended to be an exhaustive exploration of the subject matter or a representation of consensus evaluation.

THE SPECTRUM OF FOODBORNE THREATS

Ensuring the safety of food is a long-standing and critical objective of public health. The estimate that millions of Americans—whose food is among the safest on earth—are sickened by tainted food each year attests to the need to further safeguard our food supply, while the mounting threat of terrorism lends this mission a particular urgency. As a first step in assessing the spectrum of threats to the U.S. food supply, speakers and participants in the workshop reviewed a broad range of foodborne pathogens and poisons that are known to endanger human health. They also noted the dangers inherent in nonhuman pathogens that can harm crops or livestock, and along with them, the economic vitality of communities as small as farms and as large as nations.[1]

According to the Centers for Disease Control and Prevention (CDC), more than 250 different foodborne illnesses (including both infections and poisonings) have been described to date (CDC, 2005a). The list of major foodborne pathogens expands each year; the most recent update, presented by speaker Robert Tauxe, names 20 bacterial species, half of which have been identified within the past three decades, along with five viruses, five parasites, and prions, nearly all of which were identified after 1975 (see Chapter 3). Many of these pathogens, including most of those recently identified, have animal reservoirs—a factor that has likely contributed to their emergence, as with other zoonoses (infections or diseases transmitted from vertebrate animals to humans). These include avian influenza, severe acute respiratory syndrome (SARS), and "mad cow disease" (bovine spongiform encephalopathy or BSE; see subsequent discussion and Chapter 6).

Presenter Lonnie King observed that conditions favoring the transmission of zoonoses are at an all-time high, as are the scope, scale, and implications of such outbreaks. These include diseases that, while limited to livestock, have potentially devastating economic consequences (e.g., foot-and-mouth disease) as well as emerging infections that threaten humans (NRC, 2005). The direct and indirect economic impacts associated with the 2001 outbreak of foot-and-mouth disease among cattle and sheep in the United Kingdom has been estimated to be $25 billion, a figure that includes loss of tourism revenues, compensation to affected farmers, trade impacts, and downstream effects on associated agribusiness (e.g., slaughterhouses, auctions, transport companies, and food processors) and consumer prices (Breeze, 2004; Chalk, 2005). Crops are also currently under siege by exotic, emergent, and pesticide-resistant pathogens; workshop participants noted in passing that economically important crops represent targets for bioterrorism (NRC, 2002). Although plant pathogens do not pose a significant public health threat, their presence could trigger trade embargoes with severe

[1]It should be noted that not all foodborne illness is caused by an infection, not all foodborne disease causes diarrhea, and not all foodborne disease is acute. The cause of foodborne disease is often undefined, and, in many cases, the pathogens that cause them are not detected by routine laboratory tests.

consequences, particularly for those rural communities that depend on income from export of the affected crops (Cook, 2005).

Although discussions of food safety often focus on infectious disease threats, several workshop participants remarked that harmful chemicals represent an even greater risk to the food supply than those posed by biologic agents, given the huge number of potential chemical adulterants and the difficulty of detecting them in foods and/or eliminating them from the food chain (see Osterholm in Chapter 1 and Busta in Chapter 7). In Michigan, for example, the contamination of 200 pounds of ground beef with insecticide containing nicotine by a disgruntled supermarket employee sickened 111 people, including 40 children, in 2003 (CDC, 2003a). In 1985, approximately 1,000 people were poisoned by eating watermelon tainted with the highly toxic pesticide aldicarb, which was not registered in the United States for use on melons, and which had been linked to several prior episodes of food poisoning resulting from its intentional or inadvertent misapplication (CDC, 1986). Although such deliberate or incidental acts of adulteration are thought to account for a minute percentage of foodborne illness, they illustrate the potential for future catastrophe.

THE U.S. FOOD SYSTEM: GLOBALIZED, EFFICIENT, AND VULNERABLE

Food production and distribution for the developed world takes place across vast and intricate global networks. In the United States, thousands of different food items—many of them produced in other countries—pass quickly through an elaborate system of processors, distributors, and purveyors, to a public with increasingly broad tastes and immense purchasing power. This "farm-to-fork" continuum is an extraordinarily complicated industrial infrastructure. However, the system that has brought us increasingly cheaper food in greater variety carries increased risks associated with foodborne illness, whether accidental, incidental, or intentional (see Osterholm in Chapter 1).

Over the past decade, the annual output of the U.S. agricultural sector has consistently surpassed $1 trillion (USDA, 2006a). Agriculture accounts for 13 percent of the U.S. gross domestic product and employs 18 percent of the nation's workforce (USDA, 2005a). During fiscal year 2005, the nation's agricultural exports, at $62.4 billion, exceeded agricultural imports by $4.7 billion (USDA, 2006b). The United States is also a major importer of food, bringing in more than 75 percent of its fresh fruits and vegetables and more than 60 percent of its seafood (Hedberg et al., 1994; Khan et al., 2001). Between 2000 and 2004, the United States imported significantly greater amounts of nearly every class of commodity (Henry, 2005; see Henry in Chapter 1).

Currently more than 130,000 foreign food facilities—a number that closely approximates the number of domestic facilities—have registered with the Food and Drug Administration (FDA) as required under the Public Health Security and

Bioterrorism Preparedness and Response Act of 2002 (FDA, 2002). It cannot be assumed that domestically produced food is more "wholesome" or less vulnerable to adulteration than imported products; sanitary standards at some U.S. food production facilities may be vastly inferior to others in foreign sites (see Osterholm in Chapter 1).

Most foreign and domestic foods are transported across the country from central facilities. Meat served in American homes has typically traveled 1,000 miles from its farm of origin to the ultimate point of consumption (Chalk, 2004). If that meat happens to be a take-out hamburger, it could contain as many as 300 different ingredients, each with a distinct supply chain leading from a farm of origin to the restaurant where it was prepared (Osterholm, 2005). Food distribution systems permit the rapid delivery of perishable goods, provide just-in-time restocking of nonperishable items, and take advantage of economies of scale (Sobel, 2005). These strategies, along with improvements in production and processing, have contributed to a substantial decline in food expenditures as a percentage of disposable personal income in the United States, from more than 13.5 percent in the mid-1970s to near 10 percent by 1998. Dr. Craig W. Henry (see Chapter 1) noted that a similar trend on a global scale appears in data from the USDA's Economic Research Service, which indicates that the average percentage of income spent on major food groups had declined by approximately 3 percent between 1997 and 2003 in all but the wealthiest countries (USDA, 2005b). The efficient and widespread distribution of food permits the equally rapid transmission and propagation of foodborne illness. This situation can delay recognition of an outbreak and impede identification of adulterated food, as illustrated in recent case studies of foodborne outbreaks discussed below and detailed in Chapter 3. Even more challenging, the U.S. food supply offers countless opportunities for intentional harm (Osterholm, 2005):

- **Prefarm inputs** include cattle feed, agricultural chemicals such as fertilizers and pesticides, and water supplied for irrigation.
- **Farming practices** include intensive animal production (zoonoses), the raising of animals and crops in close proximity (fecal contamination of plant products), and corporate farming (products are widely distributed).
- **Transportation** is critical to maintaining the U.S. food supply.
- **Processing** encompasses the preparation of myriad foods in thousands of locations around the globe, any of which represent potential targets for sabotage.
- **Distribution** occurs with such rapidity and over such great distances that it resembles aerosol release. In the case of some products, a terrorist could assume overnight delivery of an adulterant to many thousands, if not millions, of people—a product that would be difficult to detect and remove from the market before considerable harm was done.
- **Retail** includes both groceries and prepared food: a huge and complex system of outlets for an equally vast array of foods, provided by a largely low-

paid and transient workforce. This is particularly the case in restaurants, which account for nearly half of all U.S. food expenditures.

As income levels in developing countries continue to rise, it is expected that global food consumption patterns—and, concomitantly, food production and distribution methods—increasingly will resemble those of developed countries (Regmi et al., 2001). Worldwide demand for high-quality animal protein continues to grow rapidly. A recent study estimates that global consumption of meat will increase by over 50 percent between 1997 and 2020 and will nearly double in developing countries during the same period. Almost all of the increased demand is expected to be met through expanded production of poultry, pork, and beef (Rosegrant et al., 2001). The globalization of the world's food supply will expose a greater proportion of its people to emerging and reemerging foodborne disease and contamination (Buzby, 2001). Meanwhile, in developed countries such as the United States, many consumers seek food that is not only appealing to the palate, but that is also safe, convenient, and produced or marketed in accord with their values (see Henry in Chapter 1). Although consumer demand may, over time, encourage the food industry to increase their investment in ensuring food safety, a number of workshop participants expressed the view that additional measures must be taken, and taken quickly, to address key vulnerabilities in the U.S. food supply.

FOOD SAFETY OVERSIGHT

The globalized food supply presents considerable difficulties to agencies charged with ensuring food safety. Conference presentations and discussions revealed opportunities and barriers to meeting these challenges in the United States, as well as at the international level, through the efforts of the World Health Organization (WHO) and other non-governmental organizations.

The U.S. Food Safety System

At least 15 federal agencies are responsible for implementing the more than 30 laws that direct food inspection in the United States (GAO, 2004, 2005a). As a reflection of their respective budgets, four agencies—USDA, FDA, Environmental Protection Agency (EPA), and the National Marine Fisheries Service (NMFS)—play central roles in overseeing the food safety "system." In 2003, these agencies combined spent about $1.7 billion and employed nearly 15,000 people (full-time equivalents) to inspect food manufacturing, processing, and storage facilities; conduct research and develop methods to reduce the prevalence of foodborne pathogens; assess risks posed by various food contaminants; and educate industry and the public on ways to mitigate or minimize foodborne illnesses (GAO, 2005b).

To coordinate food safety activities across jurisdictional boundaries, federal agencies have entered into more than 70 agreements that specify how these disparate agencies carry out their missions in a more or less "coordinated" fashion (GAO, 2005a, 2005b). In many instances, however, the agencies either do not fully implement or do not enforce these agreements, resulting in considerable waste, confusion, and inefficiencies. In recent years, the Government Accountability Office (GAO, formerly the General Accounting Office) has documented many such problems resulting from the fragmented, balkanized nature of the federal food safety system and has recommended the streamlining of relevant statutes, as well as consolidation of all food safety activities into a single agency with a single mission (GAO, 2004, 2005b). Indeed, over the past six decades, more than 21 similar proposals have advocated a reorganization of the federal food safety system (Vogt, 1998).

Such calls for reform were amplified by a 1998 report of the Institute of Medicine and National Research Council (NRC) that recommended the integration of food safety oversight into a single, independent agency (IOM/NRC, 1998). John Bailar, the chairman of the study committee that prepared this report, discussed the committee's findings at the workshop (see Chapter 2). The committee determined that no federal agency holds food safety as its primary mission and that this absence of focused leadership—which extends to the state and local level—results in inadequate surveillance, inconsistent and archaic regulations, insufficient resources, limited consumer knowledge, and poor adherence to even the minimum food safety standards now in place (Bailar, 2005).

Bailar noted that a similar set of circumstances led to the creation of the Environmental Protection Agency in 1970. Yet, despite the weight of the evidence for the food safety report's findings and the clarity of its recommendations, little progress toward implementation has been made in the seven years since its publication. Speaking from personal experience, Bailar attributed this lack of action to three possible factors: bureaucratic inertia, turf battles among agencies currently responsible for ensuring food safety, and resistance to change of any sort by the food industry. Workshop participants noted that the reorganization of food safety at the federal level could also benefit state and local food safety systems, many of which mirror the disorganization of federal jurisdictions. In discussion, some participants considered this a critical connection, because state and local officials perform many activities essential to food safety, such as the inspection of food-processing plants and surveillance for foodborne disease.

At the time of the workshop, proposals for reforming the federal food safety system were under consideration by legislators in both the House and Senate; each would create a single independent U.S. food safety agency to oversee inspections, enforcement, and standard setting (DeLauro, 2005). The Senate bill, known as the Safe Food Act of 2005 (U.S. Senate, 2005), takes into account many of the aforementioned IOM/NRC report's recommendations (Smith-DeWaal, 2005), as well as recent GAO findings describing reforms undertaken by other wealthy countries (Canada, Denmark, Ireland, Germany, the Netherlands, New Zealand, and the United Kingdom) that consolidated their food safety activities except foodborne disease surveillance (Schlundt, 2005) into a single agency (GAO, 2005a). Although these changes have proved both challenging and costly, government officials and other stakeholders in these countries report that reorganization has made their food safety systems more effective or efficient (GAO, 2005a).

Global Approaches to Ensuring Food Safety

Even the most sophisticated food safety programs cannot eliminate all risk of foodborne illness. The global nature of much of the world's food supply and the reality that safety cannot be "tested into" food necessitate the establishment of a coherent, risk-based, international system for preventing foodborne disease, according to speaker Jørgen Schlundt (see Chapter 2), director of the food safety program of the WHO. Schlundt maintained that such an international foodborne disease prevention system should focus on identifying vulnerabilities in the food chain and the most effective preventive measures that can be taken to address them.

Establishing food safety systems in resource-poor countries will be challenging, as many of them lack the basic infrastructure upon which food safety depends. Yet the achievement of this goal is increasingly urgent, not only because food exports from developing countries are on the increase, but also to address the recent introduction into developing countries of debilitating foodborne pathogens, such as *Salmonella* and *Campylobacter*, from the better-prepared industrialized world (Schlundt, 2005). WHO, in collaboration with the Food and Agriculture Organization (FAO) of the United Nations, has responded to this need by conducting risk assessments of foodborne illness and supporting training and capacity building for countries attempting to establish and meet risk-based standards for food safety (WHO, 2002a,b). This effort aims to help developing countries create efficient and appropriate food safety systems from the ground up that incorporate elements of successful systems in developed countries, Schlundt said.

WHO/FAO recommendations on the necessary elements of an effective national food safety program also served as the basis for a set of food safety guidelines developed for consumer organizations around the world by the Center for Science in the Public Interest (CSPI, 2006). As described at the workshop by CSPI food safety director Caroline Smith DeWaal, the recently published guidelines focus on eight essential elements for national food safety programs:

1. Food laws and regulations
2. Foodborne disease surveillance and investigation systems
3. Food control management
4. Inspection services

5. Recall and tracking systems
6. Food monitoring laboratories
7. Information, education, communication, and training
8. Funding and affordability of the national food safety program

Timely communication is critical to protecting the food supply, particularly at the international level. The International Food Safety Authorities Network (INFOSAN), established in 2004 by WHO and FAO, links officials responsible for food safety in 144 nations (INFOSAN, 2006). These officials receive food safety information from the network and disseminate it in their countries; they also alert the network to incidents of foodborne illness of international significance. When such emergencies occur, the WHO Global Outbreak Alert and Response Network (GOARN), which played a central role in the global response to SARS, is poised to respond (IOM, 2004; Schlundt, 2005). Under the recently revised international health regulations, due to take effect in 2007, countries with confirmed outbreaks of infectious disease that pose a threat beyond their borders are required to alert WHO. Governments of affected countries are responsible for determining whether an outbreak constitutes an international disease emergency, and in the case that such an emergency exists, for informing WHO once the problem ceases to be a threat. However, Schlundt noted, international health regulations grant WHO the right to overrule a national government that is not sharing information about a disease outbreak with any country that could potentially be affected by such an emergency.

ACCIDENTAL FOODBORNE DISEASE

Over the past two decades, cases of accidental foodborne disease reported to the CDC have outstripped incidents of intentional food adulteration by approximately 10,000 to 1, according to speaker Robert Tauxe (see Chapter 3). Although the rarity of criminal food tampering may be reassuring, this statistic also highlights the regularity—and to a certain extent the "ordinariness" of accidental foodborne illness, even in a wealthy nation. In addition to morbidity and mortality, the burden of foodborne illness borne by the industrialized world includes medical expenses, losses in productivity due to missed work and premature deaths, and trade embargoes against affected products as well as reduced profits. Consumer anxiety sparked by the contamination of a specific food brand or item can negatively affect entire agricultural sectors or industries (Tauxe, 2005). In developing countries, where food safety presents far greater challenges, foodborne disease is a fact of daily life and a significant cause of death due to diarrheal illness (WHO, 2002a,b).

The true incidence of food contamination in the United States is unknown. Epidemiologists believe that many affected people do not seek medical attention; moreover, foodborne disease is difficult to diagnose. "Unknown agents" account for 81 percent of foodborne illnesses and hospitalizations in the United States and 64 percent of such deaths (Mead et al., 1999). Detecting a foodborne outbreak is even more difficult, as illustrated by the single largest salmonella outbreak in the United States, which occurred in 1994 (Osterholm, 2005; see Osterholm in Chapter 1). In that episode, approximately 224,000 people across a large area of the United States contracted salmonellosis from ice cream that became contaminated following pasteurization (Hennessy et al., 1996; Sobel et al., 2002). Because only about 1.5 percent of the thousands of people presumed to have been infected actually reported symptoms, epidemiological analysis was necessary to determine the source of the pathogen. The following case studies presented at the workshop illustrated additional challenges inherent in the recognition and investigation of food-associated outbreaks of infectious disease.

Cyclosporiasis from Imported Produce

Speaker Barbara Herwaldt recalled that little was known about the biology or epidemiology of the coccidian parasite *Cyclospora cayetanensis* when in the mid-1990s, large, multistate outbreaks of gastroenteritis began to occur (see Chapter 3). *Cyclospora* is endemic in many tropical and subtropical countries and had previously been identified in persons with AIDS and in Western travelers to developing countries (Herwaldt, 2000, 2005). Although effective treatment for cyclosporiasis is available, most laboratories lack the tools and expertise necessary for accurate diagnosis of this foodborne parasite. Herwaldt and colleagues traced the initial U.S. outbreaks of cyclosporiasis to Guatemalan raspberries, a "stealth" food often consumed as a garnish, but rarely listed on menus. Some food safety experts initially questioned whether these outbreaks could have been caused by an obscure organism borne by a mere garnish, but Herwaldt and coworkers' conclusion was confirmed when additional outbreaks occurred much as they had predicted.

Several types of fresh produce, including mesclun (a mixture of young salad greens) and basil, have been vehicles for cyclosporiasis outbreaks. Dean Bodager described an ongoing investigation of an outbreak that occurred in Florida in early 2005 (see Chapter 3). As is typical in many foodborne outbreaks, a large number of sporadic case clusters occurred over an extended period of time (four months, in this case). The investigation, triggered by reports of an unusually large number of infections detected by a private lab, involved health departments in Florida's 67 counties and in 28 other affected states, the three different state agencies that regulate food in Florida, and two federal agencies—the CDC, and the FDA. The investigators now believe that imported basil, served in an upscale restaurant, harbored the parasite. Such investigations constitute the best method to identify foodborne pathogens and their sources, discover how they entered the food supply, and prevent similar outbreaks from occurring in the future, Herwaldt noted.

The development of preventive measures will require a better understanding of an organism Herwaldt (2005) described as "a mystery, wrapped in an enigma, served on a bed of imported produce." In the meantime, public health authorities must consider the potential of seemingly unrelated cases of cyclosporiasis (among other potentially foodborne illnesses) as indicators of outbreaks and pursue them to their sources through timely and thorough investigation.

Hepatitis A from Imported Green Onions

Although the pathogen involved is far better characterized than *Cyclospora*, investigations of foodborne illness caused by hepatitis A virus (HAV) present a similar array of challenges. Speaker Beth Bell described a series of outbreaks in late 2003, including some 600 people who ate in the same Pennsylvania restaurant over a four-day period (CDC, 2003b; Wang and Moran, 2004; see Chapter 3). This outbreak was detected when an alert clinician reported to his local health department that he had identified 10 cases of HAV within a few days, as compared with 1 case of hepatitis A in the entire previous year. Six of these recent cases had reported eating in two separate groups at the same restaurant. A case-control study suggested that all of the customers who became ill had eaten salsa containing raw green onions that had been imported from four farms in Mexico, where hepatitis A is endemic; the FDA subsequently banned imports from these farms. In response to these events, Mexico established a mandatory food safety program.

This process revealed several opportunities for improving the safety of the food supply, much as did the previously discussed investigations of cyclosporiasis outbreaks. Molecular methods for HAV detection hastened tracing the cases back to their source, but a more sensitive surveillance program could reveal an outbreak consisting of more sporadic cases, including those that occur in other countries (Bell, 2005). Preventive measures taken on the farm, such as providing access to adequate sanitary facilities for field workers and using clean water for irrigation and for the rinsing of harvested produce, could also have mitigated this outbreak. Finally, as Bell observed, simply telling the story of the outbreak can increase the public health community's awareness of this and other food safety issues.

FOODBORNE ATTACKS: SCENARIOS AND CONSEQUENCES

Despite the comparative rarity and mildness of previous incidents of intentional food adulteration, little imagination is required to conceive the possibility of a major attack featuring the U.S. food supply. Workshop participants considered accounts of intentional foodborne illness, as well as likely scenarios for food adulteration with both biological and chemical agents at vulnerable points in the U.S. food supply chain. These discussions revealed needs that must be addressed to reduce the potential for such attacks and to mitigate their consequences should they occur.

Incidents of intentional food adulteration reviewed at the workshop included the following:

- The 1984 contamination of an Oregon salad bar with *Salmonella typhimurium* by members of the Rajneesh religious cult, who intended to sway an election by incapacitating voters. A limited "trial run" of their plan sickened more than 700 people (Torok et al., 1997).
- The intentional infection of 12 employees by a coworker who left pastries tainted with *Shigella dysenteriae* in their break room at a large Texas medical center laboratory in 1996 (Kolavic et al., 1997).
- Several incidents in China in which food products were contaminated with rat poison by business competitors (Osterholm, 2005). In 2001, 120 people were sickened after being poisoned by the owners of a noodle factory (Death sentence, 2002a). In 2002, a similar incident took place when a snack store owner spiked a competitor's breakfast foods with rat poison resulting in the deaths of at least 38 people and causing over 300 to become seriously ill (Death sentence, 2002a,b).

The consequences of these and other actual foodborne attacks pale in comparison with the potential human (and/or animal) morbidity, mortality, and socioeconomic consequences that could unfold from an intentional act of adulteration targeting the U.S. food supply chain (Breeze, 2004; Chalk, 2005). A thwarted attempt at such an event, or even a credible hoax, would probably have severe economic repercussions for growers and processors of the affected foods, given previous consumer reaction to perceived threats such as BSE in beef (see subsequent discussion and Chapter 6) or the ripening agent Alar in apples.[2]

[2]Alar (Uniroyal's brand name for the chemical daminozide) was sprayed on apples as a ripening agent to regulate fruit growth and color and to simplify harvest. Registered with the FDA in 1963, Alar was removed from the U.S. market by its manufacturer in 1989 in response to safety concerns. The alarm was raised by media reports of a study by the Natural Resources Defense Council that implicated Alar as a dangerous carcinogen, especially in children. U.S. apple sales and prices plummeted and the EPA moved to ban Alar; Uniroyal pulled its product from the market before the ban could take effect. Years later, the extent to which Alar constituted a public health threat continues to be debated. Some organizations, most notably the industry-funded American Council on Science and Health, contend that the Alar "scare" was unfounded. Others, including the Consumers Union, contend that Alar poses a significant public health risk according to government standards, thus the EPA's actions were appropriate. For a more in-depth discussion of this issue see, Ashton L. 1999 (February 28). Alar scare 10 years past, but food safety debate goes on. *Yakima Times* [online] (excerpts.) Available: http://www.ecologic-ipm.com/APyw22899.html; Environmental Working Group. 1999. Ten years later, myth of 'Alar scare' persists. [Online] Available: http://www.ewg.org/reports/alar/alar.html; and, Wikipedia, accessed March 4, 2006. Daminozide. Available: http://en.wikipedia.org/wiki/Alar.

Food could provide an extremely effective vehicle for delivery of a variety of pathogens, such as anthrax (Osterholm, 2005), as well as for noninfectious, chemical agents including biological toxins (e.g., botulinum toxin) and poisons (e.g., cyanide, dioxin) directly to humans (Khan et al., 2001). To identify the likeliest combinations of foods and adulterants that might be vulnerable, the FDA employs risk management protocols, described by speaker David Acheson and detailed in Chapter 4. Characteristics of high-risk food products include large batch size, short shelf life (which implies rapid turnover), the potential for uniform mixing of a contaminant into the food, and a production process that would permit the agent to be added, undetected, in sufficient quantities for it to be effective (see also Osterholm in Chapter 1). As Acheson and other workshop participants noted, however, no food can be considered risk free, either with regard to intentional or accidental adulteration. The FDA uses these food vulnerability assessments to develop guidance documents and training for state and local regulatory officials and the food industry, to focus the agency's emergency response planning, and to set research priorities.

Many workshop participants expressed concern about a range of potential attackers of the U.S. food supply from al-Qaeda and other foreign nonstate actors, to radical animal rights groups, to homegrown "lone wolf" perpetrators. The transient nature of the food industry workforce is particularly worrisome, according to Osterholm, who noted the ease with which members of terrorist groups could be employed within food-processing companies and obtain "insider knowledge" of the vulnerable "choke points" in the production process.

Botulinum Toxin in Milk: A Possible Bioterrorism Scenario

Three workshop presentations (see Acheson, Leitenberg, and Detlefsen in Chapter 4) addressed a single, highly publicized scenario for foodborne terrorism: the intentional contamination of the U.S. milk supply with botulinum toxin. A May 2005 *New York Times* op-ed essay on this subject by Lawrence Wein (2005) raised heated controversy as to the appropriateness of its publication, as well as the accuracy of its conclusion that milk represents "a uniquely valuable medium for a terrorist" (Leitenberg and Smith, 2005). Six weeks later, the controversy was further fueled by the delayed publication of a peer-reviewed paper (Detlefsen, 2005; Wein and Liu, 2005) in the *Proceedings of the National Academy of Sciences* (Alberts, 2005). Based on a mathematical model of a "cows-to-consumers supply chain," the authors predicted that "if terrorists can obtain enough toxin, and this may well be possible, then rapid distribution and consumption [will] result in several hundred thousand poisoned individuals if detection from early symptoms is not timely."

Discussants Milton Leitenberg and Clay Detlefsen disputed several claims made by Wein and Liu. Leitenberg identified what he considered were numerous inaccuracies and improperly sourced citations in their work; he also questioned the ability of terrorist groups such as al-Qaeda to prepare botulinum toxin according to the "Jihadi manual" mentioned in Wein's op-ed essay, since it requires such technology as a refrigerated cold room, a vacuum refrigerated ultracentrifuge, and a mouse colony. Detlefsen argued that the dairy industry, in partnership with the U.S. government, have taken extensive measures to ensure the security of the milk supply following the terrorist attack of September 11, 2001. These efforts included the determination that higher pasteurization temperatures can be used to denature type A botulinum toxin while retaining milk's familiar flavor and texture. Many milk producers have already adopted this practice, Detlefsen explained, but because it is voluntary, it is not universal.

David Acheson presented the FDA's analysis of the milk production process and recommendations for improving its biosecurity. These include greater awareness of the threat posed by bioterrorism, locks on vulnerable production and storage facilities, thermal destruction of pathogens, and the development of cost-effective tools for the surveillance and mitigation of multiple agents. That Wein and Liu may have overstated a specific threat of foodborne bioterrorism and understated the preparations in place against it does not contradict the argument, made by several workshop participants, that the food supply must be protected without unduly burdening industry or frightening the public.

Food Safety vs. Food Biosecurity

The early detection of foodborne disease, resulting either from accidental contamination (food safety) or from deliberate attack (food biosecurity), demands sensitive surveillance systems for communicable disease at both local and national levels, and it depends on close cooperation and communication among clinicians, laboratories, and public health officials (WHO, 2002c). The particulars of these needs—for the organization of food safety systems, surveillance, reporting, and response to foodborne disease outbreaks—are discussed in greater detail below and in contributions to Chapters 2 and 5–7.

Preventing or mitigating the impact of deliberate food adulteration requires greater attention to such threats on the part of the food industry, according to workshop participants. Industrial food safety standards focus on accidental foodborne disease, a relatively common occurrence with mild to moderate impact on the average affected individual; bioterrorism, by contrast, is a rare, potentially high-impact event. This distinction increases the already daunting challenge of ensuring food safety, of balancing the risk of harm against the cost of protection, and of implementing and paying for cost-effective safeguards.

SURVEILLANCE OF FOODBORNE THREATS TO HEALTH

Two categories of tools and practices are used to detect threats to the food supply: farm-to-table food safety systems and human disease surveillance (Besser,

2005). Although theoretically capable of providing primary prevention, farm-to-table systems—which include food pathogen monitoring, animal disease surveillance, the testing of food during processing and distribution, and the analysis of consumer complaints of adulterated food—can be insensitive because of typically low pathogen loads in contaminated food, according to speaker John Besser (see Chapter 5). The presence of foodborne pathogens, symptoms of foodborne illness, and illness-related behaviors in humans are comparatively sensitive indicators of foodborne outbreaks, but usually take so long to be recognized that they afford only secondary prevention. Several workshop presentations discussing the benefits, limitations, and accomplishments of specific food and disease surveillance tools sparked discussion on obstacles to timely foodborne threat detection and how such challenges might be overcome.

Monitoring Food Safety from Farm to Fork

In framing his description of food surveillance—which focused on microbial threat agents—speaker Robert Buchanan noted its key role in verifying the effectiveness of food safety systems, as well as in preventing foodborne disease. However, he observed, effective food surveillance requires a clear understanding of its strengths and limitations, and the simultaneous use of complementary preventive strategies and public health surveillance methods. The acquisition of food surveillance data occurs through the same multi-step process of sampling and analysis regardless of whether the potential contamination is likely to be intentional or accidental. Thanks to major advances in detection technology over the last decade, several methods can now be used to identify food contaminants in "real time"—a relative term in the food industry, measured by the length of time the monitoring agency has to act upon detecting contamination. For a product that can remain in a warehouse for two weeks after it is tested for safety, "real time" is 13 days; for perishable products such as fruits, vegetables, and milk, "real time" is nearly instantaneous.

Considerably less research has gone into improving sampling methods for food surveillance, which Buchanan characterized as the heart of the surveillance process. An effective sampling plan takes into account the probability of finding a contaminated sample, known as the defect rate. Given the ability of very small numbers of certain microbes to cause foodborne illness, the detection rate for many foods is miniscule. The odds of detecting contamination in these cases can be increased by taking more samples, larger samples, or by focusing on the likeliest trouble spots in the food chain, Buchanan said. Targeted "smart" sampling techniques can be further adapted to provide information, such as baseline contamination rates, that cannot be determined by traditional batch testing methods. In addition to the defect rate, the cost and effectiveness of any food surveillance protocol depends upon the degree of confidence required to ensure safety.

Analyzing Consumer Complaints

Speaker Kimberly Elenberg described a new tool used by the USDA's Food Safety and Inspection Service (FSIS) to rapidly track and analyze consumer complaints regarding adulterated food (see Chapter 5). The analytical component of the Consumer Complaint Monitoring System (CCMS), called Emerging Patterns in Food Complaints (EPFC), employs computational methods to detect patterns in complaints received by CCMS—data that are too voluminous and complex for the human mind to grasp. EPFC examines reports of such "adverse food events" as foreign objects in food and symptoms of illness for mathematical patterns associated with foodborne outbreaks. The system includes decision trees that can identify likely chemical or microbial contaminants from symptom descriptions and onset times, Elenberg explained.

Recent tests demonstrate that EPFC can resolve faint signals amid the flood of noisy data it encounters, permitting it to generate useful alerts based on fewer adverse reports than would be required to obtain a similarly reliable result by other means, including typical syndromic surveillance methods. For example, when presented with historical data, the system immediately identified a foodborne *E. coli* outbreak that had originally taken two weeks of skilled analysis to identify. In the future, Elenberg and colleagues hope to greatly expand the application of their analytical methods, and eventually to enable the real-time integration of data on animal, plant, and human disease.

Public Health Surveillance

As defined by speaker Robert Tauxe, public health surveillance is "the monitoring of health events in humans, linked to action." Information gained from public health surveillance is used to measure the magnitude and burden of foodborne illness, to identify outbreaks, and to evaluate the impact of prevention and control efforts. In the United States, authority to conduct public health surveillance rests with state governments. Surveillance data is derived from a number of different sources including: complaints from citizens to local health departments; formal reporting systems for diseases deemed notifiable; reports from physicians and laboratories to various jurisdictions upon the identification of certain specific diseases, as required by law; microbial strains referred to state public health laboratories for characterization; and reports of outbreaks under investigation. Although voluminous, these data are highly heterogeneous and typically of limited quality.

Since 1996, public health surveillance in the United States has been substantially strengthened through the establishment of standard notifiable disease reporting in all 50 states, as well as the creation of FoodNet, PulseNet, and the electronic food outbreak reporting system known as eFORS (CDC, 2003c; Tauxe, 2005). FoodNet is an active surveillance system that collects data about sporadic cases of foodborne illness, as it is diagnosed (CDC, 2006; see Tauxe in Chapter

3). It is composed of 10 sentinel sites that collectively sample 14 percent of the U.S. population; these sites are operated jointly by state health departments, the FDA, and the USDA under the aegis of the CDC Emerging Infections Program. Information derived from FoodNet is used to estimate the burden of foodborne illness and to monitor epidemiological trends in foodborne disease. FoodNet also serves as a platform for conducting specialized studies of emerging pathogens.

PulseNet, the national molecular subtyping network for bacterial foodborne pathogens, is a digital repository for the genetic fingerprints of several pathogen strains, collected by state and some city public health laboratories and managed by the CDC (CDC, 2005b; see Tauxe in Chapter 3). The analysis and comparison of such fingerprints has greatly improved outbreak detection and investigation, particularly when contaminated foods are widely distributed and the attack rate is low, such as in the previously discussed case of nationally distributed ice cream. A complex multistate outbreak investigation generally follows such a discovery. PulseNet currently monitors five foodborne pathogens—*Escherichia coli* O157:H7, *Salmonella*, *Shigella*, *Listeria*, and *Campylobacter*—and more are expected to be added, as are increasing numbers of molecular subtypes of pathogens found throughout the food chain, in addition to those isolated from people with foodborne disease. Global networks for foodborne disease surveillance typically focus on human pathogens, but some programs monitor animals as well. These include the WHO *Salmonella* surveillance network—Global Salm-Surv (WHO, 2006) and Med-Vet-Net (Med-Vet-Net, 2005), a project of the European Union that examines foodborne infections of both humans and livestock, with a special emphasis on zoonoses (King, 2005). Global Salm-Surv, which now also covers other pathogens including *Campylobacter*, has accumulated data for 565,000 human and 102,000 nonhuman isolates, Jørgen Schlundt noted.

Surveillance of Foodborne Outbreaks

Approximately 1,200 outbreaks of foodborne disease are reported to the CDC each year, each of which, on average, affects 20 to 30 people (Tauxe, 2005). Better surveillance results in more outbreaks being detected, which in turn increases the possibility of preventing future outbreaks, Tauxe explained. Research on foodborne outbreaks leads to targeted prevention strategies for known and emerging pathogens on an ongoing basis. Although most outbreak investigations occur after the fact, they enable public health authorities to discover new combinations of foods and pathogens, identify gaps in the food safety system, and to develop new processes and regulations that improve the safety of the food supply.

This process of continual improvement has been expedited by eFORS, a system by which local or state health departments report foodborne outbreaks to the CDC via a Web-based interface (CDC, 2003c). Diffuse outbreaks continue to challenge surveillance systems, however. An outbreak of foodborne disease that occurs among 250 people within a one-block radius is easily detected, Tauxe observed, but if the same number of people fell ill across the United States, only a highly sophisticated surveillance system could discern the "signal" of such an outbreak from the "background noise" of unrelated, sporadic cases of foodborne illness.

Progress and Roadblocks

FoodNet data reveal that incidences of some foodborne diseases have declined since the network's advent (Tauxe, 2005). Since baselines were established in 1996–1998, cases of *Campylobacter* have dropped by 31 percent, *Listeria* by 40 percent, *E. coli* by 42 percent, and there has been a marginal but statistically significant decrease in *Salmonella* cases. Control of *E. coli* O157:H7 in ground beef has improved, although it is not yet adequate, as is the control of *Campylobacter* in poultry, *Salmonella* in eggs, and *Listeria monocytogenes* in processed meats, Tauxe noted; control remains elusive for multi-drug resistant *Salmonella* in ground beef, a wide array of different pathogens and different problems in produce, and *Vibrio* in raw shellfish.

A variety of constraints that limit the effectiveness of foodborne disease surveillance will not be easily overcome, workshop participants acknowledged. Chief among these is that detection largely depends upon people getting ill; sometimes this occurs after a long period of incubation, further complicating the determination of an outbreak's source. People often delay seeking medical attention, after which considerable time may elapse before a physician or a laboratory can render a diagnosis, and even more time for a public health laboratory to determine its subtype—a necessity for recognizing the "signal" of a diffuse outbreak. Once such an outbreak is suspected, investigators must trace the contaminant to its source. For some foods with many unsourced components, such as ground beef, this task is nearly impossible to perform, Tauxe said.

Improving Foodborne Threat Surveillance

Several opportunities for enhancing foodborne disease surveillance identified by workshop participants included the following:

- Increase the capacity and resources of regulatory agencies for skilled trace-back of food contaminants.
- Decrease the anonymity of foods to make them more readily traceable.
- Provide the resources necessary to bring every state up to the highest current standards of foodborne disease epidemiology, and create a national network capable of real-time surveillance.
- Expand molecular subtyping to include a broader variety of pathogens, fingerprinting pathogens derived from foods and livestock in real time, and linking these subtypes to those in human databases.

- Use faster, automated methods for fingerprinting and the detection of illness clusters (the CDC is currently evaluating several such methods).
- Expand global and regional networks for foodborne disease surveillance, and in particular increase funding for PulseNet, which has already expanded into Canada, Europe, Asia, and Latin America (Besser, 2005; Tauxe, 2005).

Having reflected on the inherent benefits and limitations of the various approaches for detecting and investigating foodborne illness, workshop participants affirmed the need for multiple, integrated surveillance systems. The value of such systems was demonstrated in the 2005 recalls of ice cream, packaged salad, and juice based on PulseNet findings (Besser, 2005). Increasingly sensitive detection methods are blurring the line between outbreaks and sporadic cases of foodborne disease, according to Besser, making real-time surveillance of foodborne illness an achievable goal.

REPORTING FOODBORNE THREATS: THE CASE OF BSE

Among all the resources brought to bear on the control of foodborne illness, time is perhaps the most precious. The rapid reporting of foodborne threats is therefore essential to reducing the burden of foodborne illness, but it also carries inevitable and significant costs to individuals, industry, and national economies. Initial costs such as the value of lost production and expenses associated with the destruction and containment of contaminated and potentially adulterated products (which in some cases translates into acres of crops or herds of livestock) are easily appreciated and often compensated—in which case those costs are often borne by taxpayers.

A variety of indirect costs can also result from outbreaks of foodborne illness, not all of which are incurred by the producer of the affected food. These include the loss of export markets due to restrictions on products associated with disease threats, loss of consumer confidence and market share (which may extend to related products that have never been contaminated), and multiplier effects on businesses and individuals with economic ties to the affected products, from food processors and distributors to business owners and nonfarm workers who serve farming communities (Chalk, 2005; Monke, 2005).

The balance of costs and benefits associated with reporting foodborne threats is clearly illustrated by the recent and ongoing global experience with the neurological disease of BSE. After Canada announced the discovery of BSE in cattle in May 2003, farm-level prices for Canadian beef declined by nearly half. Beef prices in the United States remained very strong until December of that year, when a cow with BSE was discovered within its borders; although U.S. beef prices did not fall as far as Canada's, a trade model developed at Kansas State University estimated the total BSE-associated loss incurred by the U.S. beef industry in 2004 at more than $3.2 billion (Coffey et al., 2005; Hanrahan and Becker, 2005; Monke, 2005).

Although the United States and Canada have clearly incurred substantial costs associated with the reporting of BSE, the benefits of the initial report and ongoing investigation in the United Kingdom were demonstrated nearly a decade later, when the disease was linked with a human variant of Creutzfeldt-Jakob disease (vCJD) (Brown et al., 2001). The establishment of a causal association between BSE and vCJD has led to the establishment of a variety of infection control and surveillance measures, as well as efforts to determine the extent of the vCJD epidemic for the purpose of public health planning. However, it is clear that the disincentives for reporting BSE, discussed below, still greatly outweigh the incentives for doing so. Through a series of presentations, workshop participants explored the biology of BSE and its implications for food safety, international perspectives on BSE surveillance and prevention, and public health lessons learned from this disease, and its consequences.

BSE Biology and Food Safety Implications

A member of the family of diseases known as transmissible spongiform encephalopathies (TSEs, also known as prion diseases), BSE was first identified in 1986 in the United Kingdom and has since been detected in 26 countries (GAO, 2005c). In the early 1980s, speaker Stanley Prusiner proposed that the pathogens that cause two TSEs— Creutzfeldt-Jakob disease (CJD) and scrapie, a disease of sheep—consist entirely of an "infectious" change in the conformation of a protein that he termed the prion (Prusiner, 2004). Researchers have since learned that in addition to scrapie and CJD, prions apparently cause BSE and its human variant, vCJD, as well as chronic wasting disease in deer and elk (see Chapter 6).

Scientists have also discovered that the prion protein is encoded in the genome of every animal studied to date and is expressed, in its normal form, in nerve cells. Prion disease arises when a prion protein in an abnormal, disease-causing conformation induces normal prion proteins to refold (Prusiner, 2004, 2005). Abnormal prion proteins form complexes that resist heat, radiation, and chemicals that would destroy viruses and other pathogens. These complexes build up in nerve cells, causing them to rupture, and producing the characteristic plaques (masses of protein) and vacuoles (microscopic holes) found in the brains of animals with TSEs. Prion diseases may be of spontaneous, infectious, or inherited origin; in the case of BSE, both spontaneous and infectious cases appear to have occurred. Because prion diseases have incubation periods that can exceed 40 years and are invariably fatal, no exposure to prions should be considered acceptable, Prusiner argued (Prusiner, 2005).

In his workshop presentation, Prusiner described the experimental evidence for this model of TSE etiology and efforts to develop rapid, low-cost diagnostic tests for BSE (see Chapter 6). Some recently developed tests are able to detect sufficiently low levels of disease-causing prions in brain tissue to permit the identification of infected but asymptomatic cattle within hours of slaughter. A far better—and as yet unrealized—alternative would detect minute amounts of abnormal prions in the blood and urine of live animals, including humans.

International Perspectives on BSE and vCJD

Speakers Steven Collins, an Australian expert on BSE and vCJD, and Maura Ricketts, a Canadian authority on prion diseases, shared their perspectives on the response to these health threats (see Chapter 6). As a preface to his remarks, Collins described an epidemic of the prion disease kuru in the Eastern Highlands of Papua, New Guinea. The disease, recognized in the 1950s, has since been linked with the practice of ritualistic cannibalism, which was successfully outlawed 50 years ago. Nevertheless, cases are still occasionally diagnosed, suggesting that there may be no finite incubation period for kuru (and perhaps for other TSEs as well). Despite its low transmissibility compared to microbial infections, kuru produced high mortality rates in villages where the disease was endemic. The disease is now thought to be nearly eliminated.

Collins recalled the false reassurance offered in the early years of the BSE epidemic by the lack of documented evidence for the animal-to-human transmission of the related disease, scrapie, which had been recognized for more than a century. Under this mistaken assumption, approximately 200 million infected cattle reached the human food chain during the epizootic (Collins, 2005). In 1996, a researcher at the National CJD Surveillance unit in Edinburgh recognized a case of CJD of an unusual form now known as vCJD; preliminary research soon suggested a link between vCJD and BSE. Based on this experience, Collins said, it should be assumed that all TSEs are capable of breaching species barriers; thus, it is now important to determine whether chronic wasting disease has been transmitted from deer to humans.

To date, 158 cases of vCJD have been diagnosed in the United Kingdom (Collins, 2005). The mean age at onset is 26 years. Two presymptomatic cases may be linked to blood transfusions, raising the possibility that a much larger population than initially thought is at risk of developing vCJD, despite appearances that the epidemic is declining. Australia has conducted surveillance for all human forms of TSEs since 1996, taking a variety of approaches described in detail by Collins in Chapter 6. To date, no probable or definite case of vCJD has been diagnosed in Australia, nor has any endogenous case of BSE or scrapie been found.

In the course of describing the Canadian response to BSE and vCJD, detailed in her contribution to Chapter 6, Ricketts emphasized the social and political forces that shaped the public health response to this threat. Although far from cautious in their individual behaviors, the Canadian public clearly dreaded vCJD and supported the expenditure of $18 billion per year for protection from the disease. Ricketts conjectured that this support was driven in part by public outrage against agricultural and food companies that reaped huge profits selling products that made unsuspecting consumers ill.

Trade-based economies resist the disclosure of threats to public health and the adoption of preventive measures due to their short-term costs, Ricketts observed. Thus government support for disease prevention and surveillance is essential; however, it is often difficult to obtain because the affected country must acknowledge that it has a foodborne disease problem.

Lessons from BSE

Speaker Wil Hueston, of the Center for Animal Health and Food Safety at the University of Minnesota, shared insights gained from 16 years of involvement with BSE and the interface between animal and human health. He distilled this experience into the following seven lessons, summarized here and discussed in detail in Chapter 6:

1. **Detecting a new animal disease is extremely difficult,** for a host of reasons ranging from the fact that animal disease is typically diagnosed and treated on the farm, where sick animals are usually sold, eaten, or buried, to the lack of support for the diagnosis of emerging animal diseases.
2. **Recognizing BSE in a low-incidence country (such as the United States) is difficult,** because most countries use passive surveillance and confuse the absence of evidence for the disease with evidence for its absence. There are huge disincentives for expanding national surveillance, however: it is expensive to do, and it increases the potential for economic losses if BSE is discovered before there is a plan in place to address it.
3. **Most farmers are honest, but disincentives for reporting BSE greatly outweigh incentives.** Possible incentives for reporting BSE, such as treatment or the certification of herds (rather than nations) as BSE-free, do not exist, while controls mandated by the government raise the cost of production in an economy that values cheap food. At the same time, producers that report BSE lose the market for their product and face costs associated with investigation, destruction, and disposal of infected animals.
4. **Testing can become an end unto itself** unless its purpose is clarified; even then, it is not a panacea. It must be backed up with animal and public health measures to reduce the burden of disease.
5. **Effective protective measures focus on reducing the risk of infectious disease, not the presence or absence of disease in a country.** Trade bans do not work because infectious diseases can cross any border.
6. **Opportunity costs.** Every dollar spent on BSE is not available to address other threats to human and animal health. The cost of BSE testing is currently disproportionate to its public health benefit.

7. High health status is a curse because, once attained, the impetus for maintaining a public health infrastructure is lost.

Hueston also presented a series of actions that could be taken to address key issues raised by BSE and that are generally applicable to improving the response to infectious disease. They included the following:

- Surveillance strategies that reflect purpose and scientific validity, as well as the recognition that no single strategy fits all circumstances;
- Incentives for reporting disease, rather than regulatory demands;
- To gain a better understanding of the sociology and psychology of disease reporting and compliance, greater collaboration among biological, medical, and social scientists;
- Replacement of the nationalistic, "zero-risk" paradigm of infectious disease response with global risk management and science-based regulation; and
- Recognizing that all animal health issues are potential public health issues, an emphasis on transdisciplinary approaches to all animal diseases (not just zoonoses).

RESEARCH AND POLICY OPPORTUNITIES

Previously noted workshop presentations and discussions addressed the role of food safety oversight, surveillance, and reporting in protecting the food supply. Additional research and policy opportunities for reducing foodborne threats were raised in subsequent workshop presentations on animal health, food defense, and food safety science. The emphasis on risk assessment in the latter presentation provides a framework for addressing several key challenges to food safety, as well as opportunities for protecting the food supply, identified by workshop participants.

Animal Health at the Crossroads

Following closely on the discussion of BSE and its implications for food safety, Lonnie King's presentation highlighting the recently published NRC report, *Animal Health at the Crossroads* (2005), magnified and reinforced participants' understanding of the critical linkage between animal and human health. The report, summarized in Chapter 7, used case studies of key animal diseases to evaluate existing prevention and detection systems and identify opportunities and barriers to their improvement. Many of the report's findings directly address the reduction of foodborne illness, including the identification of the following needs:

- Greater collaboration and integration between public health and animal health officials and between biomedical and veterinary research communities;

- New technologies and scientific tools to detect, diagnose, and prevent animal diseases and zoonoses;
- Expanding and strengthening the animal health laboratory network;
- Global systems that prevent, detect, and diagnose known and emerging disease threats to animal and public health; and
- The improved and expanded use of predictive, risk-based tools and models to develop strategies to address health threats.

Food Protection and Defense

In contrast to earlier discussion stressing the importance of a unified effort to detect and respond to both accidental and deliberate foodborne threats, speaker Frank Busta focused on research needs and opportunities that, while they might also reduce accidental foodborne illness, are specifically directed toward reducing and mitigating attacks on the food supply. This is the purpose of the National Center for Food Protection and Defense (NCFPD), which Busta directs at the University of Minnesota. The NCFPD pursues this goal through a series of strategies, including the rapid and accurate detection of attacks, the minimization of consequences, and the rapid implementation of recovery measures.

The research needs identified by Busta, detailed in his contribution to Chapter 7, involve tools and technologies necessary to answer key questions prompted by a foodborne attack. Sampling, detection, and tracing technologies can help determine how an attack was staged and what agent was involved. Studies of decontamination and disposal methods can indicate how to protect public health and food workers from the threat agent. Risk communication and economic research can inform optimum approaches to recovery from a foodborne attack. Such information is currently being pursued by many different agencies, and could be collected, coordinated, and shared—rather than duplicated—through the establishment of a multidimensional database, Busta noted.

Food Safety Science

Contending that food safety "is an intellectual concept, not an inherent biological property of a substance," speaker Sanford Miller noted the profound influence of such nonscientific issues as politics, economics, and social values on perceptions of risks to the food supply. The clear identification of foodborne threats and the accurate estimation of the risks they present require a new approach; Miller has collected these functions into a new academic discipline that he calls food safety science. This nascent field integrates nutrition, microbiology, toxicology, molecular biology, genetics, functional biology, and conventional food science and brings these sciences to bear on the problem of ensuring a safe food supply.

Miller, along with several other workshop participants, emphasized the importance of risk assessment to the strategic protection of the food supply. "We all feel comfortable talking about science," he observed, "but the moment comes when science has to be translated into risk and risk has to be translated into public policy. That is when we run into trouble, because we as scientists don't really understand that process and its dynamics." A case in point, one participant noted, is the common pursuit of food safety and security, a goal for which risk assessment provides the intellectual underpinning (Taylor, 2005).

Assessing Needs and Opportunities

The following summary comprises needs and policy opportunities for reducing foodborne threats to health that were most frequently mentioned by workshop participants. In the spirit of the discussion that followed Miller's presentation, the items below can be most appropriately viewed through the lens of risk assessment. That paradigm is the key to appropriately prioritizing needs and anticipating the cost-effectiveness of research and policy opportunities to enhance food safety and biosecurity (protection of the food supply from deliberate adulteration).

1. Prevention:
    a. Create positive incentives for safe food production; encourage industry to recognize and address vulnerabilities, either through regulation or through market forces.
    b. Organize responsibilities for food safety and biosecurity oversight into a single independent government agency (but maintain surveillance separately; see below).
    c. Build capacity to support food safety in developing countries.
    d. Manage risks with the understanding that zero risk cannot be achieved.
    e. Adopt multilevel (domestic) and coordinated (global) approaches to protecting the food supply.

2. Detection:
    a. Improve the cost-effectiveness of surveillance by focusing on the greatest or most likely risks.
    b. Use common agencies, mechanisms, and resources to address accidental and deliberate foodborne illness.
    c. Make all food products more traceable, less anonymous.
    d. Separate surveillance from food safety oversight to permit objective evaluation of protective measures.
    e. Emphasize coordination, communication, and collaboration among local, state, federal, and international food safety authorities.

3. Response:
    a. Create incentives for reporting apparent and actual threats to the food supply.
    b. Coordinate animal and public health responses to foodborne outbreaks.
    c. Use validated risk-based approaches for mitigating foodborne threats.

4. Research:
    a. Investigate the biology and natural history of emerging foodborne pathogens such as *Cyclospora* and prions.
    b. Examine the ecology of foodborne diseases to inform the integration of animal and health surveillance.
    c. Advance techniques for real-time surveillance of foodborne threats to health.
    d. Define the role of water as a source of foodborne illness.

5. Policy opportunities:
    a. Create interdisciplinary animal-public health programs.
    b. Conduct training programs in food safety for public health officials in developing countries, veterinarians, and the animal health community.
    c. Strengthen and integrate laboratory networks that diagnose food-borne and animal diseases.
    d. Enhance communication and collaboration among all geographic levels, all scientific and medical disciplines, and all public and private sectors, toward the common goal of safe food.

REFERENCES

Alberts B. 2005. Modeling attacks on the food supply. *Proceedings of the National Academy of Sciences* 102(28):9737–9738.

Bailar J. 2005 (October 26). *Session V: Who Is Responsible for Ensuring the Wholesomeness of the Food Supply? Domestic and International Perspectives.* Presentation at the Forum on Microbial Threats Workshop Meeting, Foodborne Threats to Health: The Policies and Practices of Surveillance, Prevention, Outbreak Investigations, and International Coordination, Washington, D.C., Institute of Medicine, Forum on Microbial Threats.

Bell B. 2005 (October 25). *Session III: The Food Supply "Threat Spectrum"—Case Studies: Cyclosporiasis in Imported Produce—Hepatitis A from Imported Green Onions.* Presentation at the Forum on Microbial Threats Workshop Meeting, Foodborne Threats to Health: The Policies and Practices of Surveillance, Prevention, Outbreak Investigations, and International Coordination, Washington, D.C., Institute of Medicine, Forum on Microbial Threats.

Besser J. 2005 (October 25). *Session IV: What Are the Tools and Technologies for "Real Time" Surveillance of the Food Supply for Conventional and Unconventional Adulterants?* Presentation at the Forum on Microbial Threats Workshop Meeting, Foodborne Threats to Health: The Policies and Practices of Surveillance, Prevention, Outbreak Investigations, and International Coordination, Washington, D.C., Institute of Medicine, Forum on Microbial Threats.

Branigin W, Allen M, Mintz J. 2004 (December 3). Tommy Thompson resigns from HHS: Bush asks Defense Secretary Rumsfeld to stay. *Washington Post.* [Online]. Available: http://www.washingtonpost.com/wp-dyn/articles/A31377-2004Dec3.html [accessed April 27, 2006].

Breeze R. 2004. Agroterrorism: Betting far more than the farm. *Biosecurity and Bioterrorism: Defense Strategy, Practice, and Science* 2(4):1–14.

Brown P, Will RG, Bradley R, Asher DM, Detwiler L. 2001. Bovine spongiform encephalopathy and variant Creutzfeldt-Jakob disease: Background, evolution, and current concerns. *Emerging Infectious Diseases* 7(1):6–16.

Buzby JC. 2001. Effects of food-safety perceptions on food demand and global trade. In: Regmi A, Ed. *Changing Structure of Global Food Consumption and Trade.* WRS-01-1. Washington, D.C.: Economic Research Service. Pp. 55–66.

CDC (Centers for Disease Control and Prevention). 1986. Aldicarb food poisoning from contaminated melons—California. *Morbidity and Mortality Weekly Report* 35(16):254–258.

CDC. 2003a. Nicotine poisoning after ingestion of contaminated ground beef—Michigan, 2003. *Morbidity and Mortality Weekly Report* 52(18):413–416.

CDC. 2003b. Hepatitis A outbreak associated with green onions at a restaurant—Monaca, Pennsylvania, 2003. *Morbidity and Mortality Weekly Report* 52(47):1155–1157.

CDC. 2003c. *Foodborne Outbreak Response and Surveillance Unit.* [Online]. Available: http://www.cdc.gov/foodborneoutbreaks [accessed May 3, 2006].

CDC. 2005a. *Foodborne Illness. Division of Bacterial and Mycotic Diseases.* [Online]. Available: http://www.cdc.gov/ncidod/dbmd/ diseaseinfo/foodborne infections_g.htm#foodborne disease [accessed April 27, 2006].

CDC. 2005b. *PulseNet Homepage.* [Online]. Available: http://www.cdc.gov/pulsenet/ [accessed May 3, 2006].

CDC. 2006. *FoodNet–Foodborne Diseases Active Surveillance Network Homepage.* [Online]. Available: http://www.cdc.gov/foodnet/ [accessed May 3, 2006].

Chalk P. 2004. *Hitting America's Soft Underbelly: The Potential Threat of Deliberate Biological Attacks Against the U.S. Agricultural and Food Industry.* Santa Monica, CA: RAND Corporation.

Chalk P. 2005. The U.S. agricultural system: A target for al-Qaeda? *Terrorism Monitor* 3(5):4–6.

Coffey B, Mintert J, Fox S, Schroeder T, Valentin L. 2005. *The Economic Impact of BSE on the U.S. Beef Industry: Product Value Losses, Regulatory Costs, and Consumer Reactions.* [Online]. Available: http://www.oznet.ksu.edu/library/agec2/mf2678.pdf [accessed May 4, 2006].

Collins S. 2005 (October 26). *Session VI: What Are the Incentives and Disincentives Associated with Disease/Contamination Reporting? Impacts on Human Health and International Trade—BSE as a "Case Study"?* Presentation at the Forum on Microbial Threats Workshop Meeting, Foodborne Threats to Health: The Policies and Practices of Surveillance, Prevention, Outbreak Investigations, and International Coordination, Washington, D.C., Institute of Medicine, Forum on Microbial Threats.

Cook J. 2005 (June 28). *Session I: Threats to Crops.* Presentation at the Forum on Microbial Threats Working Group Meeting, Food Supply Terrorism as a Biosecurity Issue: Assessing the Problem and the Ethical Considerations of Infectious Disease Research and Surveillance, Washington, D.C., Institute of Medicine, Forum on Microbial Threats.

CSPI (Center for Science in the Public Interest). 2006. *Safe Food International.* [Online]. Available: http://safefoodinternational.org/guidelines_for_consumer_ organizations 20050727.pdf [accessed May 3, 2006].

Death sentence for China poisoning. 2002a (September 30). *BBC News.* [Online]. Available: http://news.bbc.co.uk/2/hi/asia-pacific/2287801.stm [accessed April 26, 2006].

Death sentence over Chinese poisonings. 2002b (September 30). *CNN News.* [Online]. Available: http://edition.cnn.com/2002/WORLD/asiapcf/east/09/30/china.poison/ [accessed May 4, 2006].

DeLauro R. 2005 (May 17). Testimony before the House Government Reform Subcommittee on the Federal Workforce and Agency Organization oversight hearing on "Question: What Is More Scrambled Than an Egg? Answer: The Federal Food Inspection System." [Online]. Available: http://www.hhs.gov/asl/testify/t050517.html [accessed July 6, 2006].

Detlefsen C. 2005. Dairy industry vigilant in addressing food security. *Cheese Market News* 25(22):1.

FDA (Food and Drug Administration). 2002. *The Bioterrorism Act of 2002.* [Online]. Available: http://www.fda.gov/oc/bioterrorism/bioact.html [accessed May 3, 2006].

GAO (Government Accountability Office). 2004. *Federal Food Safety and Security System: Fundamental Restructuring Is Needed to Address Fragmentation and Overlap.* GAO-04-588T. Washington, D.C.: GAO.

GAO. 2005a. *Overseeing the U.S. Food Supply: Steps Should Be Taken to Reduce Overlapping Inspections and Related Activities.* GAO-05-549T. Washington, D.C.: GAO.

GAO. 2005b. *Oversight of Food Safety Activities: Federal Agencies Should Pursue Opportunities to Reduce Overlap and Better Leverage Resources.* GAO-05-213. Washington, D.C.: GAO.

GAO. 2005c. *Mad Cow Disease: FDA's Management of the Feed Ban Has Improved, but Oversight Weaknesses Continue to Limit Program Effectiveness.* GAO-05-101. Washington, D.C.: GAO.

Hanrahan C, Becker GS. 2005 (March 10). *Mad Cow Disease and U.S. Beef Trade.* CRS report RS21709. Washington, D.C.: Library of Congress.

Hedberg CW, MacDonald KL, Osterholm MT. 1994. Changing epidemiology of foodborne disease: A Minnesota perspective. *Clinical Infectious Diseases* 18(5):671–680.

Hennessy TW, Hedberg CW, Slutsker L, White KE, Besser-Wiek JM, Moen ME, Feldman J, Coleman WW, Edmonson LM, MacDonald KL, Osterholm MT. 1996. A national outbreak of *Salmonella enteritidis* infections from ice cream. The Investigation Team. *New England Journal of Medicine* 334(20):1281–1286.

Henry C. 2005 (October 25). *Session I: The Current U.S. Food Supply.* Presentation at the Forum on Microbial Threats Workshop Meeting, Foodborne Threats to Health: The Policies and Practices of Surveillance, Prevention, Outbreak Investigations, and International Coordination, Washington, D.C., Institute of Medicine, Forum on Microbial Threats.

Herwaldt BL. 2000. *Cyclospora cayetanensis:* A review, focusing on the outbreaks of cyclosporiasis in the 1990s. *Clinical Infectious Diseases* 31(4):1040–1057.

Herwaldt BL. 2005 (October 25). *Session III: The Food Supply "Threat Spectrum"—Case Studies: Cyclosporiasis in Imported Produce—Fresh Basil.* Presentation at the Forum on Microbial Threats Workshop Meeting, Foodborne Threats to Health: The Policies and Practices of Surveillance, Prevention, Outbreak Investigations, and International Coordination, Washington, D.C., Institute of Medicine, Forum on Microbial Threats.

INFOSAN (International Food Safety Authorities Network). 2006. *INFOSAN Homepage. World Health Organization.* [Online]. Available: http://www.who.int/foodsafety/fs_management/infosan/en/ [accessed May 3, 2006].

IOM (Institute of Medicine). 2004. *Learning from SARS.* Washington, D.C.: The National Academies Press.

IOM/NRC (National Research Council). 1998. *Ensuring Safe Food from Production to Consumption.* Washington, D.C.: National Academy Press.

Khan AS, Swerdlow DL, Juranek DD. 2001. Precautions against biological and chemical terrorism directed at food and water supplies. *Public Health Reports* 116(1):3–14.

King L. 2005 (October 25). *Session VII: Threat Reduction Research and Policy Opportunities.* Presentation at the Forum on Microbial Threats Workshop Meeting, Foodborne Threats to Health: The Policies and Practices of Surveillance, Prevention, Outbreak Investigations, and International Coordination, Washington, D.C., Institute of Medicine, Forum on Microbial Threats.

Kolavic SA, Kimura A, Simons SL, Slutsker L, Barth S, Haley CE. 1997. An outbreak of *Shigella dysenteriae* type 2 among laboratory workers due to intentional food contamination. *Journal of the American Medical Association* 278(5):396–398.

Leitenberg M, Smith G. 2005 (June 17). "Got toxic milk?": A rejoinder. Federation of American Scientists. Available: http://www.fas.org/sgp/eprint/milk.html [accessed May 3, 2006].

Mead PS, Slutsker L, Dietz V, McCaig LF, Bresee JS, Shapiro C, Griffin PM, Tauxe RV. 1999. Food-related illness and death in the United States. *Emerging Infectious Diseases* 5(5):607–625.

Med-Vet-Net. 2005. *Med-Vet-Net Homepage*. Available: http://www.medvetnet.org/cms/ [accessed May 3, 2006].

Monke J. 2005. *Agroterrorism: Threats and Preparedness*. CRS Report RL32521. Washington, D.C.: The Library of Congress.

NRC. 2002. *Countering Agricultural Bioterrorism*. Washington, D.C.: The National Academies Press.

NRC. 2005. *Animal Health at the Crossroads: Preventing, Detecting, and Diagnosing Animal Diseases*. Washington, D.C.: The National Academies Press.

Osterholm M. 2005 (October 25). *Session II: The Food Supply "Threat Spectrum."* Presentation at the Forum on Microbial Threats Workshop Meeting, Foodborne Threats to Health: The Policies and Practices of Surveillance, Prevention, Outbreak Investigations, and International Coordination, Washington, D.C., Institute of Medicine, Forum on Microbial Threats.

Prusiner S. 2004. Detecting mad cow disease. *Scientific American* 291(1):86–93.

Prusiner S. 2005 (October 25). *Session VI: What Are the Incentives and Disincentives Associated with Disease/Contamination Reporting? Impacts on Human Health and International Trade—BSE as a "Case Study"?* Presentation at the Forum on Microbial Threats Workshop Meeting, Foodborne Threats to Health: The Policies and Practices of Surveillance, Prevention, Outbreak Investigations, and International Coordination, Washington, D.C., Institute of Medicine, Forum on Microbial Threats.

Regmi A, Deepak MS, Seale JL Jr., Berstein, J. 2001. Cross-country analysis of food consumption patterns. In: *Changing Structure of Global Food Consumption and Trade*. Regmi A, Ed. Market and Trade Economics Division, Economic Research Service, U.S. Department of Agriculture, Agriculture and Trade Report. WRS-01-1. Pp. 14–22.

Rosegrant, M, Paisner, MS, and Meijer, S. 2001. Long term prospects for agriculture and the resource base. *Rural Development Strategy Background Paper* No. 1. Washington, D.C.: The World Bank. P. 150.

Schlundt J. 2005 (October 26). *Session V: Who Is Responsible for Ensuring the Wholesomeness of the Food Supply? Domestic and International Perspectives*. Presentation at the Forum on Microbial Threats Workshop Meeting, Foodborne Threats to Health: The Policies and Practices of Surveillance, Prevention, Outbreak Investigations, and International Coordination, Washington, D.C., Institute of Medicine, Forum on Microbial Threats.

Smith-DeWaal C. 2005 (October 26). *Session V: Who Is Responsible for Ensuring the Wholesomeness of the Food Supply? Domestic and International Perspectives*. Comment from a representative of the Center for Science in the Public Interest at the Forum on Microbial Threats Workshop Meeting, Foodborne Threats to Health: The Policies and Practices of Surveillance, Prevention, Outbreak Investigations, and International Coordination, Washington, D.C., Institute of Medicine, Forum on Microbial Threats.

Sobel J. 2005. Food and beverage sabotage. In *Encyclopedia of Bioterrorism Defense*, RF Pilch and RA Zilinskas, Eds. New York: Wiley-Liss, Inc. Pp. 215–220.

Sobel J, Khan AS, Swerdlow DL. 2002. Threat of a biological terrorist attack on the U.S. food supply: The CDC perspective. *Lancet* 359(9309):874–880.

Tauxe R. 2005 (October 25). *Session II: The Food Supply "Threat Spectrum."* Presentation at the Forum on Microbial Threats Workshop Meeting, Foodborne Threats to Health: The Policies and Practices of Surveillance, Prevention, Outbreak Investigations, and International Coordination, Washington, D.C., Institute of Medicine, Forum on Microbial Threats.

Taylor T. 2005 (October 26). *Session VII: Threat Reduction Research and Policy Opportunities*. Comment from a Forum member at the Forum on Microbial Threats Workshop Meeting, Foodborne Threats to Health: The Policies and Practices of Surveillance, Prevention, Outbreak Investigations, and International Coordination, Washington, D.C., Institute of Medicine, Forum on Microbial Threats.

Torok T, Tauxe RV, Wise RP, Livengood JR, Sokolow R, Mauvais S, Birkness KA, Skeels MR, Horan JM, Foster LR. 1997. A large community outbreak of salmonellosis caused by intentional contamination of restaurant salad bars. *Journal of the American Medical Association* 278(5):389–395.

USDA (U.S. Department of Agriculture). 2005a. *National Agriculture Statistics Service: Workforce Plan for FY 2005–2009*. Available: http://www.nass.usda.gov/About_Nass/Strategic_Plan/nassworkforceplanfy2005.pdf [accessed April 26, 2006].

USDA. 2005b. *Global Food Markets: International Consumer and Retail Trends*. Economic Research Service. Available: http://www.ers.usda.gov/briefing/globalfoodmarkets/consumer.htm [accessed May 3, 2006].

USDA. 2006a. *Agricultural Outlook: Key Statistical Indicators*. Economic Research Service Available: http://www.ers.usda.gov/publications/AgOutlook/AOTables/ [accessed April 27, 2006].

USDA. 2006b. *Foreign Agricultural Trade of the United States: Monthly Summary*. Economic Research Service. Available: http://www.ers.usda.gov/Data/FATUS/MonthlySummary.htm [accessed April 27, 2006].

U.S. Senate. 2005. *Safe Food Act of 2005*. 109th Congress. S. 729. Introduced April 6, 2005. Sponsor: Sen. Richard Durbin. Co-sponsor: Sen. Hillary Clinton. Available: http://www.govtrack.us/congress/bill.xpd?bill=s109-729 [accessed May 3, 2006].

Vogt DU. 1998. *Food Safety: Recommendations for Changes in the Organization of Federal Food Safety Responsibilities, 1949–1997*. Congressional Research Service.. Washington, D.C.: Library of Congress.

Vogt DU. 2005. *Food Safety Issues in the 109th Congress*. Congressional Research Service. Washington, D.C.: The Library of Congress.

Wang MJ, Moran GJ. 2004. Update on emerging infections: News from the Centers for Disease Control and Prevention. *Annals of Emergency Medicine* 43(5):660–663.

Wein L. 2005 (May 30). Got toxic milk? *New York Times*, Op-Ed Section.

Wein LM, Liu Y. 2005. Analyzing a bioterror attack on the food supply: The case of botulinum toxin in milk. *Proceedings of the National Academy of Sciences* 102(28):9984–9989.

WHO (World Health Organization). 2002a. *WHO Global Strategy for Food Safety*. Geneva: WHO. Available: http://www.who.int/foodsafety/publications/general/global_strategy/en/ [accessed May 3, 2006].

WHO. 2002b. *Food Safety and Foodborne Illness*. Available: http://www.who.int/mediacentre/factsheets/fs237/en/ [accessed May 3, 2006].

WHO. 2002c. *Terrorist Threats to Food*. Geneva: WHO. Available: http://www.who.int/foodsafety/publications/general/en/terrorist.pdf [accessed May 3, 2006].

WHO. 2006. *Global Salm-Surv (GSS) Homepage*. Available: http://www.who.int/salmsurv/en/ [accessed May 3, 2006].

1

The U.S. Food System

OVERVIEW

Aside from the prospect of terrorism, the U.S. food supply is vulnerable to myriad threats. As Dr. Michael Osterholm observes in the first contribution to this chapter, unintentional foodborne illness kills thousands of people each year in this country and sickens millions more. The vastness and complexity of modern food production provides abundant opportunity for contamination; consider, for example, the intricate path from farm to table taken by processed food products, comprising multiple ingredients from around the world. At the same time, the breadth and swiftness of modern food distribution networks make outbreaks of foodborne illness difficult to detect and all but impossible to contain, as illustrated by the histories of several recent foodborne outbreaks.

Intentionally adulterated food could be delivered to thousands, perhaps millions, of Americans within days. Osterholm notes that such an outright attack on the food supply could cause higher morbidity and mortality, and a far greater economic impact, than is associated with all-too-common outbreaks of accidental foodborne illness. Although most previous acts of foodborne terrorism have involved local attacks staged by lone perpetrators, Osterholm argues that the relative ease by which food could be used to harm societies and economies, as well as individuals, necessitates the development of effective measures to prevent, detect, and respond to potential bioterrorist attacks to the food system. In the course of this process, policy makers will need to assess the risks and benefits of possible safeguards and consider how the costs of safer foods will be borne by the food industry and, ultimately, the public.

The benefits of modern food production and distribution, which balance the aforementioned risks, are considered in the second paper in this chapter. Dr. Craig Henry demonstrates that increasingly globalized and sophisticated food supply chains have afforded cheaper food for much of the world's population. He also discusses consumer and demographic trends that affect the food supply, including growing global demand for products that are not only tasty, convenient, and inexpensive, but safe as well.

THE FOOD SUPPLY AND BIODEFENSE: THE NEXT FRONTIER OF THE FOOD SAFETY AGENDA

Michael T. Osterholm, Ph.D.[1]
University of Minnesota

The interface between the international food supply system and terrorism has the potential to produce a catastrophic impact on both the health of consumers and the availability of and confidence in specific food products.

Former Secretary of Health and Human Services Tommy Thompson observed upon his resignation in 2004, "I, for the life of me, cannot understand why the terrorists have not, you know, attacked our food supply, because it is so easy to do" (Branigin et al., 2004). A few months later, Michael Chertoff, Secretary of Homeland Security, said that he "didn't want to get up in public and say the sky is falling if it is not falling," and stated that he was going to be "realistic and sensible and serious about the kinds of trade-offs that we have to consider when we are making decisions about protecting ourselves." Although superficially contradictory, I would argue that these two remarks are consistent. They reflect the recognition that, four years after September 11, 2001, we cannot guarantee the safety of everyone and everything within our borders. We have to make critical decisions about which critical components of our everyday world to accord priority in protection or in response should an attack occur. I believe that the security of our food supply must be at the top of such a list.

Lester Crawford, a former commissioner of the Food and Drug Administration (FDA), said in 2002, "To conclude that the use of food as an instrument of terror is unlikely would be looking at the world of today through the prism of the past. The terror of these times is based on a different note on a different scale." The occurrence of unintentional foodborne illness already kills thousands of people each year in this country and sickens millions more. However, an inten-

[1]Director, Center for Infectious Disease Research and Policy; Associate Director, Department of Homeland Security National Center for Food Protection and Defense; Professor, University of Minnesota.

tional terrorist attack on the food supply is likely to have very different ramifications in terms of morbidity and mortality, and a far greater economic impact than unintentional foodborne illness.

The Food System

Figure 1-1, which depicts key global trends between 1850 and the present, places our food system in a historical context. The right vertical axis shows the number of days required to circumnavigate the globe; in 1850 it took approximately one year to accomplish an around-the-world trip; by 1950 that same feat could be accomplished in less than 48 hours. Although the time to circumnavigate the world has been essentially the same since 1950, we now move substantially more people and goods around the world today than we did even 30 years ago. The left vertical axis shows the world's population in billions; in the past century the world population has grown from less than 1 billion to more than 6.5 billion people. The commensurate growth in need for protein and carbohydrate has important implications for the origins of food and its patterns of consumption.

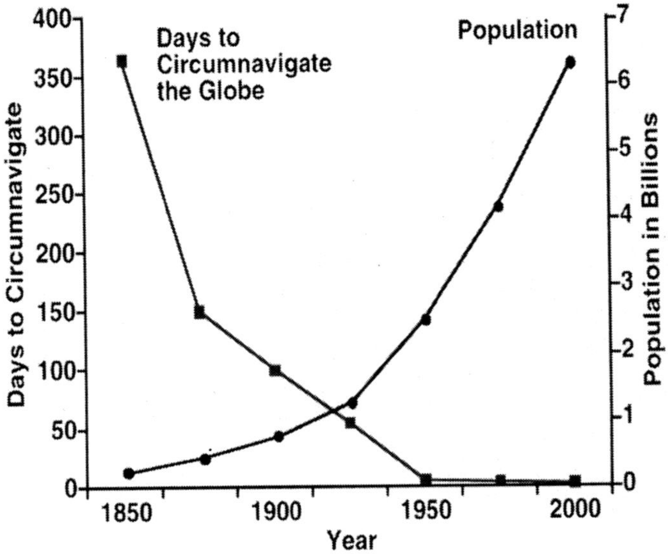

FIGURE 1-1 Speed of global travel in relation to world population.
SOURCE: Murphy and Nathanson (1994). Reprinted with permission from Elsevier.

Today's global food system constitutes the world's most complicated industrial infrastructure. The following framework identifies the major components of the food supply and highlights their vulnerability to intentional harm:

- **Pre-farm inputs** include cattle feed, agricultural chemicals such as fertilizers and pesticides, and water supplied for irrigation.
- **Farming practices** include intensive animal production (zoonoses[2]), the raising of animals and crops in close proximity (fecal contamination of plant products), and corporate farming (products are widely distributed). The recent introduction of foot-and-mouth disease in Great Britain serves as an example of the severe effects upon the food supply that can result from a disease that is limited to livestock.
- **Transportation** is critical to maintaining the U.S. food supply. This was clearly illustrated when, in response to Hurricane Katrina, the Federal Emergency Management Agency (FEMA) requested that private fleet refrigerated trucks locate themselves in several holding areas in the impacted states of Louisiana and Mississippi so they could be used if needed for cold storage of human bodies and food and ice. Although a limited number of independent truckers—the main movers of goods from wholesale to retail grocery stores—answered the call, a major shortage of overland transportation occurred, resulting in an interruption of the food supply when food failed to be delivered from processors to retail locations.
- **Processing** encompasses the preparation of myriad foods in thousands of locations around the globe, any of which represents potential targets for sabotage.
- **Wholesale distribution** occurs with such rapidity and over such great distances that the process resembles an aerosol release. In the case of some products, a terrorist could assume overnight delivery of an adulterant to many thousands, if not millions, of people—a product that would be difficult to detect and remove from market before considerable harm was done.
- **Retail** includes both groceries and prepared food: a huge and complex system of outlets for an equally vast array of foods, provided by a largely low-paid and transient workforce. This is particularly the case in restaurants, which account for nearly half of all U.S. food expenditures. Most foodborne attacks to date have occurred at this level, or thereafter at the point of consumption.

The Global Food Supply

The global nature of the U.S. food supply adds further layers of complication to the farm-to-table framework, thereby magnifying concerns for its safety. The U.S. agricultural sector annually produces more than $1 trillion dollars in eco-

---

[2]Zoonoses is defined as "diseases of non-human animals that may be transmitted to man or may be transmitted from man to non-human animals." (http://cancerweb.ncl.ac.uk/cgi-bin/omd?zoonoses).

nomic activity. Agriculture accounts for 13 percent of the U.S. gross domestic product and employs more than 16 percent of the nation's workforce (USDA, 2005a). In 2004, the nation's agricultural exports, at $62.3 billion, exceeded agricultural imports by $9.6 billion.

The United States is also a major importer of food. Currently, the number of foreign food facilities that have registered with the FDA as required under the Biopreparedness Act of 2002—more than 130,000—outnumbers the number of domestic registrations. Figure 1-2 shows the main regions from which the United States imports significant amounts of several key foods. The supply of these foods may be disrupted by a variety of factors, including variables rarely considered in the United States, such as political instability or the interruption of electrical power. It is also important to note that domestically produced food is no less vulnerable to adulteration than imported products. As Figure 1-3 demonstrates, sanitary standards at some U.S. food production facilities are vastly inferior to others in foreign sites.

The global food supply exemplifies cost containment, with the result that food in the United States and throughout much of the world has become increasingly cheaper. Figure 1-4 shows that while the United States spent an increasing amount of money on food over the past two decades, the percentage of disposable income represented by food expenditures has fallen dramatically over the same period. The expectation of inexpensive food as part of the global just-in-time economy means that there is little resiliency in our food supply, however. Food once stored in warehouses for weeks or months is now shipped overnight, around the world, a situation that makes it difficult to detect a contaminated product and remove it from commerce before it is widely consumed; thus today's food recall typically documents last week's outbreak.

For a terrorist, the number of foods that move from "farm to fork" within days to weeks represents an opportunity. In many instances, an adulterated food could be guaranteed overnight delivery to thousands, if not millions, of Americans.

Previous Outbreaks and Attacks

The single largest outbreak of salmonellosis documented in the United States to date stands as an example of the potential of a foodborne illness to occur among many thousands of consumers before it is detected. In 1994, ice cream mix produced in a Minnesota plant was shipped before final freezing and packaging as a pasteurized product in trucks that had previously carried raw egg mix without being adequately cleaned. There were more than 200,000 cases of illness among those who ate the ice cream (Hennessy et al., 1996).

As is typical in foodborne outbreaks, humans serve as the bioassay for contamination. Routine enteric disease surveillance conducted by the Minnesota Department of Health identified an increased occurrence of cases of *Salmonella*

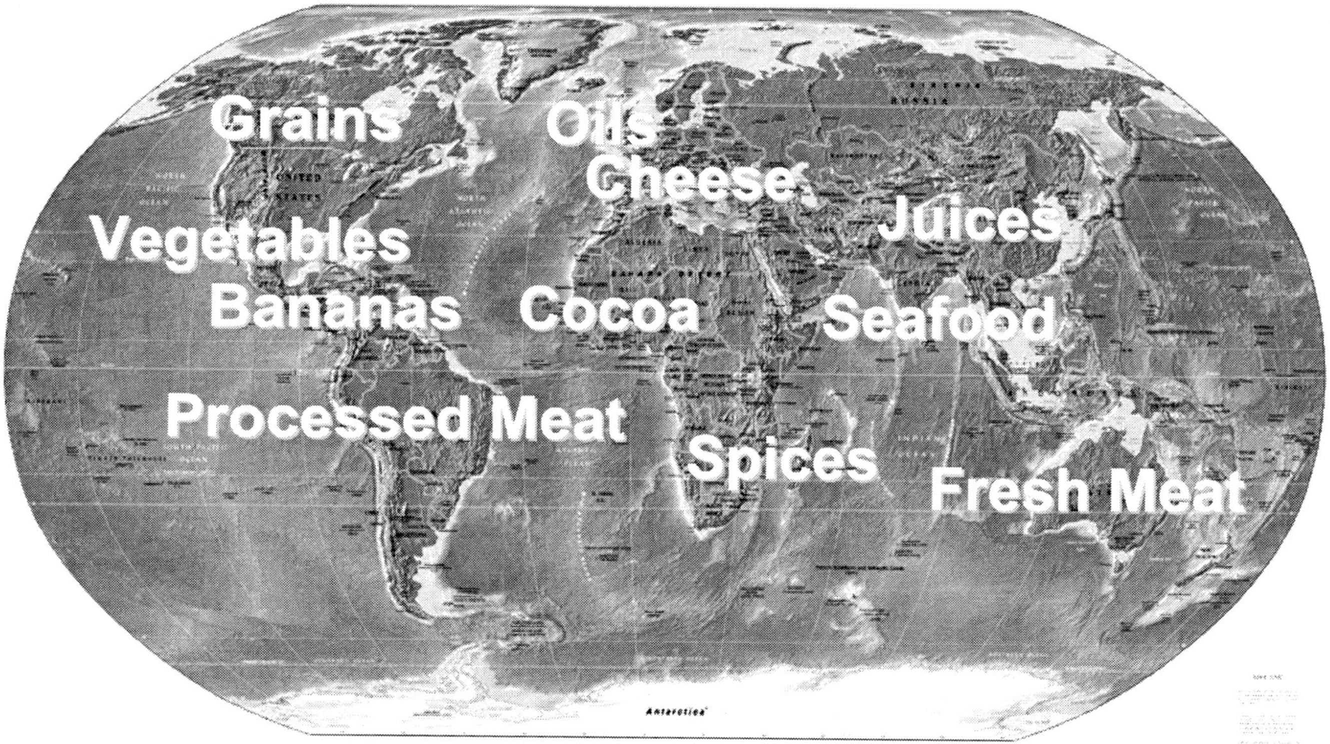

FIGURE 1-2 The problem: Global food systems.
SOURCE: Osterholm (2005).

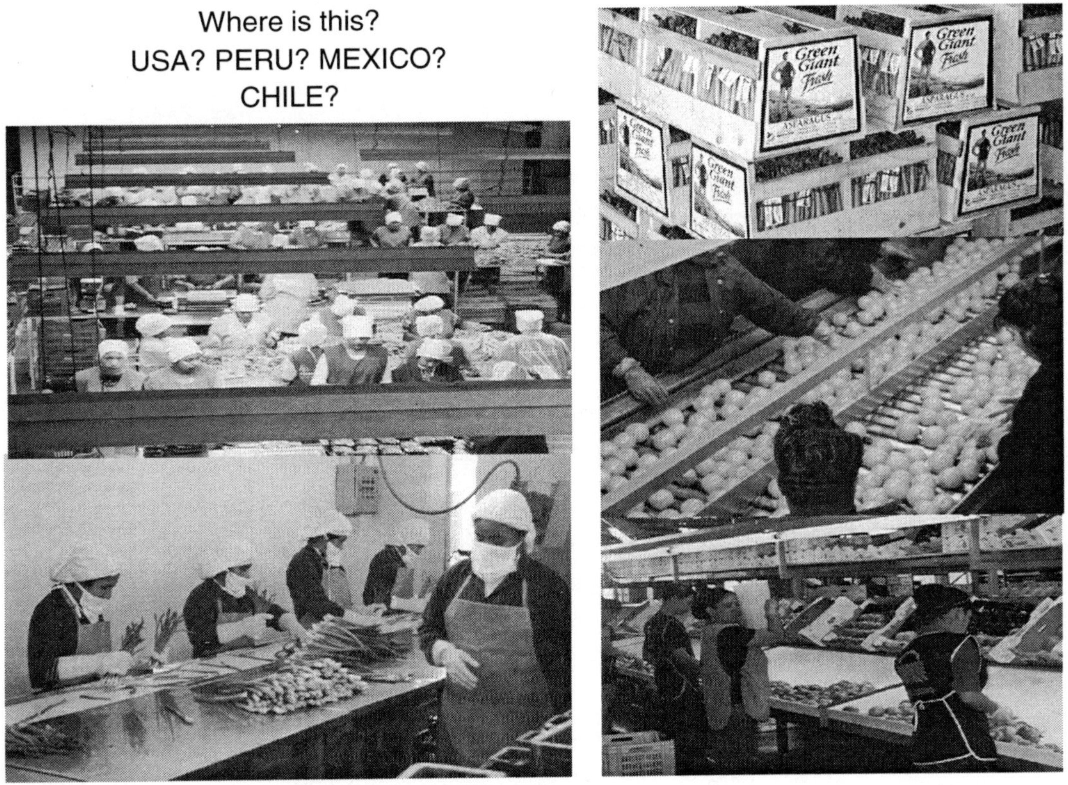
Where is this?
USA? PERU? MEXICO?
CHILE?
Green Giant Fresh

FIGURE 1-3 Identifying the source of food in a global system is challenging.
SOURCE: Sholl (2005).

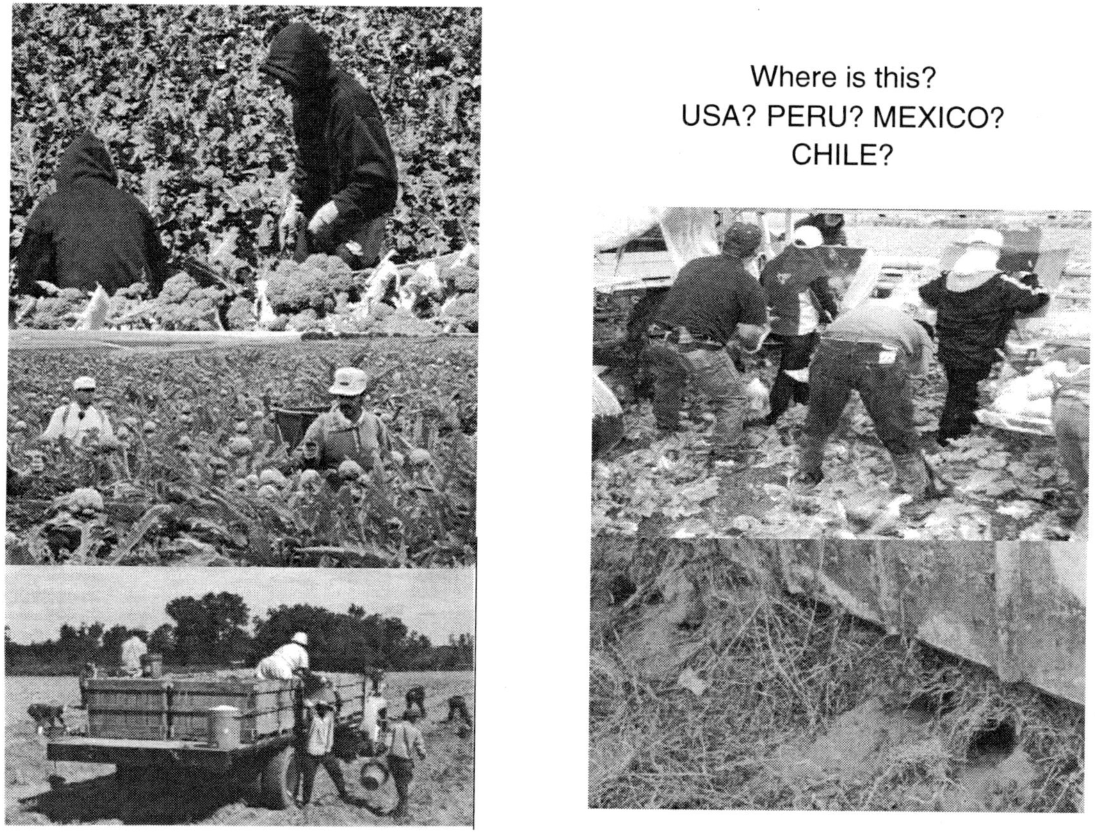

FIGURE 1-3 Continued.

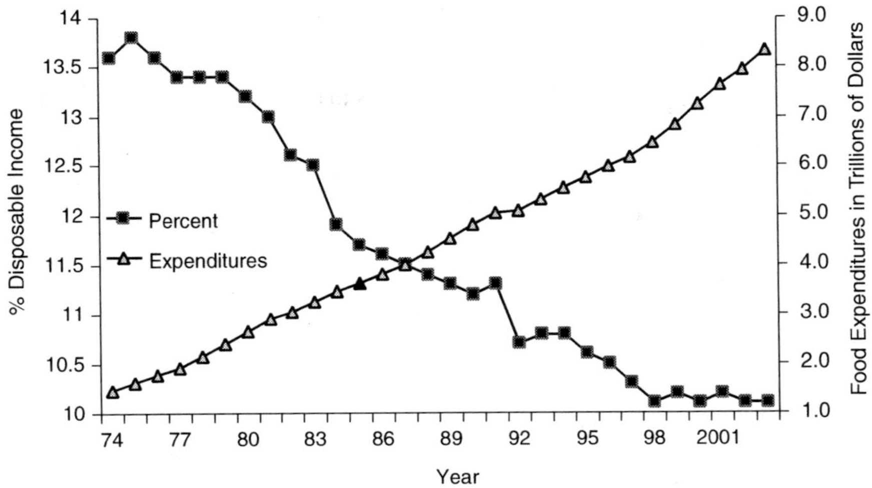

FIGURE 1-4 Food expenditures as a share of disposable personal income, United States, 1974–2003.
SOURCE: Adapted from USDA (2004).

serotype *enteritidis* infection. An epidemiologic investigation led to the identification of *Salmonella* serotype *enteritidis* contamination in selected lots of ice cream. Epidemiologic data provided the only indication that ice cream was the vehicle, as the bacterium was found in less than two percent of samples tested. Nevertheless, despite the low attack rate, a large number of people were sickened because of the large volume of contaminated ice cream. An intentional attack would probably feature higher concentrations of such an agent, with predictably devastating consequences.

To date intentional foodborne attacks have not produced a major catastrophe. Instead, they have been largely localized events, staged by individuals. For example, a postgraduate student in parasitology scattered his roommate's food with the roundworm *Ascaris suum*; four persons became seriously ill, and two suffered respiratory failure (Phills et al., 1972). Although *Ascaris* is not an agent of particular concern, this example reminds us that many individuals have access to infectious and noninfectious adulterants that could easily be added to many foods.

A well-known incident occurred in Oregon, in 1984, when members of the Rajneesh religious cult contaminated a salad bar with *Salmonella*, causing 751 illnesses (Torok et al., 1997). This attack was actually a limited "trial run" of a plan to sway an election by incapacitating voters.

In 1996, a disgruntled Texas lab worker intentionally contaminated pastries with *Shigella dysenteriae* and left them for her coworkers to eat. Twelve people became infected (Kolavic et al., 1997); the culprit was ultimately sentenced to 20 years in prison (Ex-lab worker, 1998).

As the following examples illustrate, chemical contamination of the food supply may pose an even much greater risk than many biologic agents:

- In Holland and Germany, in 1978, a dozen children were hospitalized after citrus fruit from Israel was intentionally contaminated with mercury (Khan et al., 2001).
- In China, in 2001, 120 people became ill after specific food products were laced with rat poison by makers of competing products (Death sentence, 2002a). In 2002, a similar rat poisoning incident killed at least 38 people and made more than 300 seriously ill (Death sentence, 2002a, 2002b).
- In Michigan, the contamination of 200 pounds of ground beef with insecticide containing nicotine by a disgruntled employee in a supermarket sickened 111 people, including 40 children (CDC, 2003).

Foodborne Attack Scenarios

Terrorists could achieve mass human casualties by adding a class A bioterrorism agent such as botulinum toxin during the processing or transportation of a variety of vulnerable foods. This is not an artificial scenario, given the previously described account of milk adulteration. It is of grave concern to analysts who have researched its possibility and projected consequences, some of whom feel that such attack scenarios should not be publicly discussed.

Economic disruption is a likely outcome of any foodborne attack, and it could be achieved without directly harming humans by spreading pathogens specific to livestock (e.g., foot-and-mouth disease) or crops (e.g., soybean rust). Such diseases could have critical implications for the food supply system. Economic consequences would also likely result from mass anxiety, which could be generated with a credible hoax that targeted popular food products or a popular restaurant. Previous incidents have shown that consumers react intensely to the mere suggestion that a food has been or will be contaminated and may extrapolate an isolated incident of contamination to a nationwide scale.

An ideal food or beverage vehicle for a foodborne terrorism attack would have the following characteristics:

- It would be produced in such a way that a perpetrator would have the ability to adulterate it beyond control steps that would eliminate or disable the potential agent. Although food processes such as heat treatment are designed to deactivate pathogens, most do not specifically target chemical contaminants.
- It would be a large volume of a widely distributed product, allowing the agent to be disseminated to the largest possible population.

- It would be able to preserve the agent's potency until it is consumed.
- It would be a product that is rapidly distributed and consumed, thus unlikely to be detected until considerable damage is done.
- The product would be consumed disproportionately by high-risk populations (e.g., children or the elderly).

In addition to *Clostridium botulinum* (botulism) and its toxin, biological agents for such attacks could include *Bacillus anthraces* (anthrax) and other enteric bacterial species. Gastrointestinal anthrax represents a relatively effective foodborne weapon; while not as deadly as its aerosol counterpart, it can result in significant morbidity, mortality, and economic disruption. Although only 22 cases of anthrax occurred in this country in 2001, those cases resulted in a dramatic impact on the U.S. postal system; even a few cases of food-related anthrax in a single food commodity would do the same, if not more. At the same time, common enteric bacterial species, such as *Salmonella*, could produce mass illness, as demonstrated by the previous example of the Rajneesh cult attack Such an outbreak may not be recognized as an attack, and therefore fail to cause panic and fear.

Chemical adulterants pose an even greater risk to the food supply than many biologic agents. A vast number of potentially deadly chemicals could be introduced into a number of widely distributed foods, to devastating effect.

Food Biosecurity

In recent years in the United States, food biosecurity has traditionally been defined as the development of effective measures to prevent, detect, and respond to potential bioterrorist attacks to the food system. However, it is important to recognize a more essential, global definition of food biosecurity: the availability of sufficient food. While the United States attempts to protect its food supply from bioterrorism, we must also bear in mind that security for much of the world is compromised by the lack of an adequate food supply.

The World Health Organization (WHO) in a 2002 document entitled *Terrorist Threats to Food* (WHO, 2002) concluded that the early detection of disease resulting from covert food terrorism requires sensitive surveillance systems for communicable disease at the local and national levels, with close cooperation and communication among clinicians, laboratories, and public health officials. These conclusions apply to food safety in general, not just protection against deliberate attacks, reinforcing the need for a comprehensive system for foodborne disease surveillance.

Detecting and responding to an act of foodborne terrorism will depend on the type of agent, the efficiency of the attack, and the geographic distribution of cases. If an attack produces a few unusual, distinctive cases, it is more likely to be detected than one that sickens many people with a common foodborne illness. A large number of acute cases of foodborne illness, clustered by time and location, will trigger an immediate response. However, it may take weeks to recognize an epidemic of foodborne disease: from the time the contaminated food is eaten until symptoms appear; from the time a person seeks medical attention until the results of a stool sample can be interpreted; from the time public health officials receive laboratory results until case interviews can be conducted.

Improving systems for food defense requires us to decide how we determine what constitutes acceptable risk, as well as what measures best serve the public good. Today, the U.S. food industry emphasizes food safety, which is not the same thing as food biosecurity. For example, a standard tool for identifying potential sources of foodborne illness, called Hazard Analysis and Critical Control Point (HACCP) (FDA, 2006), focuses on exposures that are reasonably likely to occur, regardless of impact. Bioterrorism, while an extremely rare event, would be expected to have a severe impact.

Should food producers be required, or merely encouraged, to invest resources in protecting their products against the risk of terrorism? Are food defense systems public goods that warrant public support? They are unlikely to yield measurable benefits to a company. Representatives from the food industry have stated that they would prefer legislative requirements for such safeguards, so that every company bears the same burden as its competitors. Under such conditions, food defense would be treated as a cost of doing business. No such regulation has yet been formally proposed, nor has the level of "tolerable risk" been defined, except to note that risk cannot be entirely eliminated. However, it is clear that an effective response to the threat of foodborne terrorism requires collaboration and greater efficiency among the federal agencies responsible for food safety and for transportation, as well as among state and local health departments.

Despite all we know about the potential for various agents to cause foodborne illness, we do not know the identity of tomorrow's terrorist today. He or she could be a member of an animal liberation group who is working in a food-processing plant, waiting for an opportunity to act. An unbalanced individual with expertise in microbiology could be planning to stage a small-scale attack with an infectious agent just to see what happens. An international terrorist organization could be readying an attack. That is why Paul Wilkinson, from the Centre for the Study of Terrorism and Political Violence, said more than a decade ago, "Fighting terrorism is like being a goalkeeper. You can make a hundred brilliant saves, but the only shot that people remember is the one that gets past you" (Wilkinson, 1992).

THE U.S. FOOD SUPPLY—HOW CHANGING DEMOGRAPHICS AND CONSUMER DEMAND POSE NEW CHALLENGES FOR FOOD SAFETY

Craig W. Henry, Ph.D.[3, 4]
Food Products Association

Summary

When purchasing food, U.S. consumers consider a variety of product attributes, including taste, convenience, cost, and safety. Increasingly, this is true around the world, as consumers seek to purchase high-quality, safe foods.

Regardless of income, families in countries around the world are spending less on food as a percentage of total expenditures, as they benefit from the lower cost of food production and increased competition in the retail marketplace. However, the fact remains that lower-income families, on average, spend approximately 2.5 times more on food as a percent of total expenditures than do higher-income families. Conversely, higher-income families spend more on meat and seafood products than do lower-income families.

Process attributes related to the manner in which a food is grown, raised, processed, and marketed are becoming increasingly important to consumers globally. For example, there is a growing demand for "organically" grown food products, particularly in the United States and Europe.

The food purchased and consumed in the United States increasingly is imported. From 2000 to 2004, food imports into the United States increased substantially, with meat, fresh fruit, and vegetables leading in sales growth.

Demographic changes in the United States are reflected by the marketplace. For example, the number of single-parent households in the United States continues to grow. By 2030, it is anticipated that only 17 percent of U.S. households will be single-earner married couples, with almost 30 percent of households headed by unmarried individuals. With more households where both parents work and more single-parent households in the future, less time will be available for meal preparation.

Clear, concise, and accurate information must be communicated among the United States and countries around the world to help ensure compliance with regulatory requirements. Additionally, stakeholders must coordinate the approach to addressing threats such as mad cow disease and avian influenza. Only through

[3]Senior vice president of Scientific and Regulatory Affairs.

[4]The Food Products Association (FPA) is the largest trade association serving the food and beverage industry in the United States and worldwide. FPA's laboratory centers, scientists, and professional staff provide technical and regulatory assistance to member companies and represent the food industry on scientific and public policy issues involving food safety, food security, nutrition, consumer affairs, and international trade.

a collaborative effort and the proper allocation of resources can the United States and other countries meet the challenge of ensuring a safe, abundant, and nutritious world food supply.

Global Consumption Trends

Gathering accurate and up-to-date statistics on global food consumption trends is challenging. However, using statistics from a number of sources—in particular, information compiled and published by the Food Marketing Institute (FMI)—allows us to examine some emerging trends regarding global food consumption (Tables 1-1 through 1-3).

It is clear that some "health-oriented" foods—such as soy-based drinks and yogurt beverages—have enjoyed substantial growth during this period. Demographics certainly play an important role in food expenditures. The U.S. Department of Agriculture (USDA) report for March 2005 provided excellent insight into global buying habits. First, we see the predominant income groups in a variety of countries (Table 1-2). Following the breakdown of income groups, we see the food expenditure patterns among the selected countries (Table 1-3).

Although food expenditures have declined for all income groups, the decline is more pronounced for the low-income group. Tables 1-4 through 1-9 provide more insight into the type of foods being purchased by the various levels of income (see Annex 1-1).

If we look at the trends as far as a summary of this is concerned, between 1997 and 2003 there is a clear decline of 2.5 percent of income spent on the major food groups. However, the question remains, why are the costs of food expenditures declining? More efficient production, leading to lower food prices, and/or increased competition in the retail food marketplace likely have had an impact. Certainly, the global food industry has done an excellent job of enhancing efficiencies related to farming practices and food production.

TABLE 1-1 Food Categories with the Fastest Growing Global Sales and Growth Rate Between 2003 and 2004

Categories with Fastest Growing Sales	Growth Rate 2003–2004 (%)
Soy-based drinks	31
Drinkable yogurts	19
Eggs	14
Cereal, muesli, fruit bars	10
Sports energy drinks	10
All others	6–9

SOURCE: Nielson (2004).

TABLE 1-2 Food Expenditure Patterns Among Selected Countries

High	Upper Middle	Lower Middle	Low Income
Japan	Mexico	Colombia	Ukraine
United States	Czech Republic	Russia	Indonesia
United Kingdom	Hungary	Romania	India
Germany	Chile	Bulgaria	Vietnam
France	Brazil	Morocco	
Singapore	South Africa	Philippines	
South Korea	Turkey	China	

SOURCE: USDA (2005b).

Data indicates that growing wealth in countries around the world is creating a growing demand for food attributes beyond taste and cost. Worldwide, we see growth in consumer demand for foods with various attributes, such as the increased demand for soy-based drinks. Convenience and safety are another two key attributes that are having a growing effect on consumer buying habits.

According to the FMI's *Grocery Shopper Trends for 2005*, single men and women without children, account for 25 percent of the 81.9 million working households in the United States. Since 1940, single-parent families have doubled and now account for 16 percent of the households in the United States. The issue is: who is buying and who is preparing meals in our domestic economy? Married couples with and without children account for 37 percent of U.S. households. By 2030 it is expected that 17 percent of households with married couples will have a single earner. Forty-five percent will be dual-earner married couples, and 30 percent will be unmarried individuals. Single-parent households will exceed 18 percent (FMI, 2005).

In the United States, female "bread winners" are far more common today than in the past. Twenty percent of U.S. households currently are supported by a single female earner. This equates to close to 3.6 million or 8 percent of all the total current working households. This results in fewer adults at home with a primary focus on family care and meal preparation. In turn, this creates a change in how meals are prepared and, subsequently, creates time constraints for meal

TABLE 1-3 Food Expenditure Patterns Among Selected Countries, Food Share of Total Expenditures

	1997 (%)	2003 (%)
High-income average	11.7	11.1
Upper-middle income average	22.2	19.5
Lower-middle income average	35.4	32.0
Low-income average	41.7	38.3

SOURCE: USDA (2005b).

preparations. Let's consider how meals are actually sourced and prepared within the home. Surprisingly only 1.5 evening meals per week are consumed away from home. Thirty-nine percent of the shoppers, on a weekly average, eat out less than once per week. On the weekly average, 15 percent of single mothers eat at fast food restaurants at least three times a week. Let us look at the various sources of food for the U.S. household (Table 1-10).

Ninety-two percent of households eat home-cooked meals one or more times a week; 79 percent eat home-cooked meals at least three times a week. This indicates that a significant percentage of the time, people are preparing their meals at home. An equal number, 22 percent, eat at least one meal a week at either a fast-food or full-service restaurant. And nearly a quarter of U.S. households eat at least one "ethnic" meal at home or at a restaurant each week; Chinese and Mexican cuisine have become part of the mainstream America diet. *Grocery Shopper Trends for 2005* also indicates that income, age, region, residence, and ethnicity affect food buying decisions.

The NPD Group recently released findings from its *20th Annual Report on Eating Patterns in America* (NPD Group, 2006). It is interesting to see what has changed over the past 20 years. Today, 53 percent of consumers say they try to avoid snacking as opposed to 71 percent in 1985. The annual number of main meals skipped per person rose from 102 in 1985 to 114 in 2005. Meals cooked in microwave ovens doubled from 10 percent in 1985 to 20 percent today. To me, this is surprising, in that I would have expected it would have been a much higher increase than just a doubling.

Clearly, saving time is important for most consumers. What has the food industry done to respond to consumer demand for more convenient but still good-tasting foods? Joy Zacharia, associate editor of *Cooking Light* magazine, says consumers are taking advantage of prewashed salads, precut and washed vegetables, pork tenderloins and boneless, skinless chicken breast and thighs.

Consumers in developed countries around the world increasingly look for convenient, high-quality foods that are safe. There is also a growing market for foods perceived to support healthy lifestyles. The food industry continues to develop and market new products to meet evolving consumer demands.

TABLE 1-10 Grocery Shopper Trends for 2005

	1 or More Times/Week (%)	At Least 3 Times/Week (%)
Eat home-cooked meals at home	92	79
Eat out at fast-food establishments	22	5
Dine out at full-service restaurants	22	4
Purchase items at gourmet coffee shops	7	3
Eat ethnic meals at home or out	24	6

SOURCE: FMI (2005).

TABLE 1-11 Trends in Proportion of Shoppers Who Purchased Organic Food Within the Past Six Months

Number of Organic Foods Purchased	2000 (%)	2003 (%)	2004 (%)
None	47	50	48
One or two categories	24	24	26
Three or four categories	16	15	14
Five or more categories	13	11	12
Total	100	100	100

SOURCE: FMI et al. (2004).

Demand for Organic Foods

In recent years, there has been conflicting conclusions regarding the trends in organic food consumption. The Organic Trade Association (OTA) states that the organic industry grew by 20 percent and attained $10.8 billion in sales in 2003 (OTA, 2003). However, according to FMI et al. (2004) organic food sales have remained steady (Table 1-11).

The organic market survey of 2005 indicates 37 percent of U.S. shoppers expressed an interest in buying organic fruits and vegetables, 24 percent are interested in or have bought organic cereals and breads, and 23 percent either purchased or would purchase organic packaged foods. Interestingly, 18 percent of consumers surveyed indicated they would be interested in purchasing organic meats, but this product line has grown by only 5 percent since 2000. Apparently, the organic demand for meats is driven by availability. Shoppers indicate that, if there was a greater availability of organic meats, they would take advantage of it. Going forward, we are likely to see steadily increasing demand for organic food and other foods with attributes related to health or a healthy lifestyle.

Global Demographics

Research by the American Enterprise Institute (AEI) indicates that, to sustain the current global population, every woman must bear 2.1 children (Eberstadt, 2004). Nearly half of the developed world has birth rates below that figure. In the United States, population growth is being fueled by immigration and by a higher birth rate for minorities.

Another factor to take into consideration regarding global demographics is the male-to-female ratio. Today more boys than girls are being born. The populations of most nations have an average of 105 boys for every 100 girls born. This imbalance is particularly pronounced in nations such as China (with 121 boys born for every 100 girls) and India (with 126 boys born for every 100 girls).

AEI research also indicates that HIV and AIDS are definitely affecting mortality rates in a number of countries, which has the potential to affect global food demand in the future.

What about the U.S. workforce and the ratio of workers to retirees? In 1950, the United States had 16 workers for every retiree. In 2005, that number is down to three workers for every retiree, which poses enormous challenges for continued funding of the Social Security system and its benefits to retired workers. This issue is even more pronounced in other countries. For example, in Italy it is projected that there will be 0.7 active workers for each retiree by 2030. This indicates there is a very serious economic problem on the horizon.

According to the USDA Economic Research Service, in the last three decades we have seen a tremendous growth in food sales worldwide. In the processed food area, sales are now $3.2 trillion, or about three-fourths of the total world food sales. However, we have not seen significant overall growth in global trade during the same time period. For most countries, the vast majority of processed food consumed is produced within that country.

This is not true for the United States. Between 2000 and 2004, U.S. food imports significantly increased by 29 percent, according to the USDA Foreign Agriculture Service, with meat, fresh vegetables, and fruits leading this growth. Without question, U.S. consumers have become accustomed to having year-round access to fresh produce. We must pay very close attention to the production and the quality of such products as they come through our system.

Food Safety

Food is handled at multiple points throughout the food chain, from farm to fork. This is a factor on an international basis that must be addressed to meet customer and regulatory requirements. Look at most seafood products as an example. It is typical to have oceangoing vessels with full processing and even packaging capability. The product is handled in one particular area on the vessel and then shipped for further processing, potentially in two or more countries, before the finished product actually reaches the retail market. This creates a challenge that needs to be considered as far as food safety and quality are concerned.

Imported food products meet consumer demand for varied foods—including fresh fruits and vegetables year-round. Ensuring the safety of imported foods is an absolute priority for the U.S. food industry. When it comes to imported foods, vigilance, verification, and validation of sound food safety systems and practices is a necessary part of doing business.

Verifying that food safety systems in countries around the world are equivalent to those in the United States is an important aspect of ensuring that the foods sold in the United States are safe, be they imported or domestically produced. This can be a challenge. For example, in 2004 U.S. meat inspectors reported that meat facilities in France do not meet USDA food safety sanitation standards, and therefore banned the sale of processed meats from France in the United States. In 2005, Brazil voluntarily suspended meat exports to the United States for similar reasons.

Proper allocation of resources to enhance food safety is paramount. All stakeholders need to work together in addressing the challenges that lie before the United States and the global community. Mad cow disease and the potential emergence of pandemic avian flu are just two examples of those challenges. Only if we apply the appropriate collaborative effort, and certainly the proper allocation of resources, are we going to make progress in addressing the key food safety challenges facing the United States and the global community.

ANNEX 1-1

TABLE 1-4 Food Expenditure Patterns Among Selected Countries, Bread and Cereals

	1997 (%)	2003 (%)
High-income average	16.5	15.9
Upper-middle income average	21.9	21.1
Lower-middle income average	17.7	18.0
Low-income average	26.1	25.6

SOURCE: USDA (2005b).

TABLE 1-5 Food Expenditure Patterns Among Selected Countries, Meat and Seafood

	1997 (%)	2003 (%)
High-income average	35.2	34.3
Upper-middle income average	27.3	28.9
Lower-middle income average	31.4	29.8
Low-income average	19.4	20.3

SOURCE: USDA (2005b).

TABLE 1-6 Food Expenditure Patterns Among Selected Countries, Dairy and Eggs

	1997 (%)	2003 (%)
High-income average	11.5	11.3
Upper-middle income average	15.5	14.9
Lower-middle income average	12.0	11.3
Low-income average	12.8	11.9

SOURCE: USDA (2005b).

TABLE 1-7 Food Expenditure Patterns Among Selected Countries, Oils and Fats

	1997 (%)	2003 (%)
High-income average	2.8	2.8
Upper-middle income average	5.2	4.8
Lower-middle income average	5.6	5.7
Low-income average	6.4	5.3

SOURCE: USDA (2005b).

TABLE 1-8 Food Expenditure Patterns Among Selected Countries, Fruits and Vegetables

	1997 (%)	2003 (%)
High-income average	18.6	18.8
Upper-middle income average	19.0	19.1
Lower-middle income average	18.0	17.6
Low-income average	24.6	24.1

SOURCE: USDA (2005b).

TABLE 1-9 Food Expenditure Patterns Among Selected Countries, Sugar and Confectionary

	1997 (%)	2003 (%)
High-income average	7.5	7.6
Upper-middle income average	6.6	6.4
Lower-middle income average	5.0	5.1
Low-income average	4.5	5.9

SOURCE: USDA (2005b).

REFERENCES

ACNielsen. 2004. *What's Hot Around the Globe: Insights on Growth in Food and Beverages 2004.* [Online]. Available: http://www2.anielsen.com/reports/documents/2004_whatshot_food-bev.pdf [accessed April 14, 2006].

Branigin W, Allen M, Mintz J. 2004 (December 3). Tommy Thompson resigns from HHS: Bush asks Defense Secretary Rumsfeld to Stay. *The Washington Post.* [Online]. Available: http://www.washingtonpost.com/wp-dyn/articles/A31377-2004Dec3.html [accessed August 2, 2006].

CDC (Centers for Disease Control and Prevention). 2003. Nicotine poisoning after ingestion of contaminated ground beef—Michigan, 2003. *Morbidity and Mortality Weekly Report* 52(18): 413–416.

Chertoff M. 2005 (March 17). Homeland security chief to shift from "sky is falling" approach. *New York Times*. P. A21.

Crawford LM. 2002 (September 6). *A Conversation on Food Safety and Global Security. Secretary's Open Forum, Department of State, Washington, D.C.* [Online]. Available: http://www.fda.gov/oc/speeches/2002/state0906.html [accessed June 28, 2006].

Death sentence for China poisoning. 2002a (September 30). *BBC News*. [Online]. Available: http://news.bbc.co.uk/2/hi/asia-pacific/2287801.stm [accessed April 26, 2006].

Death sentence over Chinese poisonings. 2002b (September 30). *CNN News*. [Online]. Available: http://edition.cnn.com/2002/WORLD/asiapcf/east/09/30/china.poison/ [accessed May 4, 2006].

Eberstadt N. 2004 (August 20). *Four Surprises in Global Demography*. Washington, D.C.: AEI. [Online]. Available: http://www.aei.org/publications/pubID.21076,filter.all/pub_detail.asp [accessed June 28, 2006].

Ex-lab worker tainted food. 1998 (September 12). *Houston Chronicle*. P. A48.

FDA (Food and Drug Administration). 2006. *Hazard Analysis and Critical Control Point*. Available: http://www.cfsan.fda.gov/~lrd/haccp.html [accessed May 5, 2006].

FMI (Food Marketing Institute). 2005. *Grocery Shopper Trends for 2005*. [Online]. Available: http://www. fmi.org/ [accessed April 14, 2006].

FMI, Prevention Magazine, and Rodale, Inc. 2004. The organic market. Ch. 4 In: *Shopping for Health: Making Sense of Nutrition News and Health Claims*. Washington, D.C.: The Food Marketing Institute. Pp. 55–62.

Hennessy TW, Hedberg CW, Slutsker L, White KE, Besser-Wiek JM, Moen ME, Feldman J, Coleman WW, Edmonson LM, MacDonald KL, Osterholm MT. 1996. A national outbreak of Salmonella enteritidis infections from ice cream. The Investigation Team. *New England Journal of Medicine* 334(20):1281–1286.

Khan AS, Swerdlow DL, Juranek DD. 2001. Precautions against biological and chemical terrorism directed at food and water supplies. *Public Health Reports* 116(1):3–14.

Kolavic SA, Kimura A, Simons SL, Slutsker L, Barth S, Haley CE. 1997. An outbreak of Shigella dysenteriae type 2 among laboratory workers due to intentional food contamination. *Journal of the American Medical Association* 278(5):396–398.

Murphy FA, Nathanson N. 1994. The emergence of new virus diseases: An overview. *Seminars in Virology* 5(2):87–102.

NPD Group. 2006. *NPD Group Homepage*. [Online]. Available: http://www.npdfoodworld.com/foodServlet? nextpage=pr_body.html&content_id=2228 [accessed April 14, 2006].

Osterholm MT. 2005. (October 25). *Session I: The Current U.S. Food Supply*. Presentation at the Forum on Microbial Threats Workshop Meeting, Foodborne Threats to Health: The Policies and Practices of Surveillance, Prevention, Outbreak Investigations, and International Coordination, Washington, D.C., Institute of Medicine, Forum on Microbial Threats.

OTA (Organic Trade Association). 2003. *Organic Trade Association Homepage*. [Online]. Available: http://www.ota.com/index.html [accessed April 14, 2006].

Phills JA, Harrold AJ, Whiteman GV, Perelmutter L. 1972. Pulmonary infiltrates, asthma and eosinophilia due to Ascaris suum infestation in man. *New England Journal of Medicine* 286(18): 965–970.

Sholl J. 2005 (June 28). *Session III: Vulnerabilities of the Ready to Eat Food Supply*. Pictures taken by Jeff Sholl and presented at the Forum on Microbial Threats Working Group Meeting, Food Supply Terrorism as Biosecurity Issue—Assessing the Problem and the Ethical Considerations of Infectious Disease Research and Surveillance (slide 31), Washington, D.C., Institute of Medicine, Forum on Microbial Threats.

Torok TJ, Tauxe RV, Wise RP, Livengood JR, Sokolow R, Mauvais S, Birkness KA, Skeels MR, Horan JM, Foster LR. 1997. A large community outbreak of salmonellosis caused by intentional contamination of restaurant salad bars. *Journal of the American Medical Association* 278(5): 389–395.

USDA (U.S. Department of Agriculture). 2004. *Food CPI, Prices and Expenditures: Food Expenditures by Families and Individuals as a Share of Disposable Personal Income*. Economic Research Service. [Online]. Available: http://www.ers.usda.gov/Briefing/CPIFoodAndExpenditures/data/table7.htm [accessed July 25, 2006].

USDA. 2005a. *National Agriculture Statistics Service: Workforce Plan for FY 2005–2009*. [Online]. Available: http://www.nass.usda.gov/About_Nass/Strategic_Plan/nassworkforceplanfy2005.pdf [accessed April 26, 2006].

USDA. 2005b. *Global Food Markets: International Consumer and Retail Trends*. [Online]. Available: http://www.ers.usda.gov/Briefing/ globalfoodmarkets/consumer.htm [accessed April 14, 2006].

WHO (World Health Organization). 2002. *Terrorist Threats to Food: Guidelines for Establishing and Strengthening Prevention and Response Systems*. [Online]. Available: http://www.who.int/foodsafety/publications/fs_management/terrorism/en/ [accessed April 28, 2006].

Wilkinson P. 1992 (September 1). British Scholar, author on terrorism. *The Daily Telegraph*. [Online]. Available: http://www.bartleby.com/66/25/64725.html [accessed May 5, 2006].

2

Food Safety Oversight

OVERVIEW

In the United States, the oversight of food safety at the national level presently involves at least 12 agencies,[1] of which 4 predominate: the U.S. Department of Agriculture (USDA), the Food and Drug Administration (FDA), the Environmental Protection Agency (EPA), and the National Marine Fisheries Service. Many of the more than 70 agreements intended to coordinate food safety activities among federal agencies are not fully implemented or enforced, resulting in considerable waste, confusion, and inefficiency. Therefore, it is not surprising that over the past six decades more than 20 proposals have advocated a reorganization of the federal food safety system. Prominent among these calls for reform was a 1998 report of the Institute of Medicine (IOM) and National Research Council (NRC), entitled *Ensuring Safe Food from Production to Consumption* that recommended the integration of food safety oversight into a single, independent agency (IOM/NRC, 1998). In the first paper in this chapter, Dr. John Bailar, chairman of the study committee, discusses the committee's findings and considers why little progress has been made toward implementing the report's recommendations in the seven years since its publication.

---

[1]The major federal agencies involved include: the Agricultural Marketing Service, the Animal and Plant Health Inspection Service, the Agricultural Research Service, the Cooperative State Research, Education and Extension Service, the Economic Research Service, the Food Safety and Inspection Service, and the Grain Inspection, Packers, and Stockyards Administration of the United States Department of Agriculture; the Centers for Disease Control and Prevention, the Food and Drug Administration, and the National Institutes of Health of the Department of Health and Human Services; the National Marine Fisheries Service of the Department of Commerce; and the Environmental Protection Agency.

The subsequent contribution by Dr. Jørgen Schlundt, director of the food safety program of the World Health Organization (WHO), offers a global perspective on the burden of foodborne illness and progress toward the development of international systems to respond to foodborne outbreaks. WHO has assumed a central role in global food safety through its organization of Global Salm-Surv, a network linking *Salmonella* surveillance efforts in 141 countries, and the International Food Safety Authorities Network (INFOSAN), which disseminates information related to food safety. Pending forthcoming revisions to the international health regulations due to take effect in 2007, WHO will serve as the hub of a global system for reporting public health emergencies including foodborne illness.

Although each country needs to defend its food supply from deliberate contamination, Schlundt maintains that these efforts should be undertaken as part of a comprehensive food safety agenda that extends to the international level. The WHO Global Strategy for Food Safety takes a largely preventive approach, combining surveillance, communication among all stakeholders, and rapid response to foodborne outbreaks. Rather than rely on food testing to intercept contaminated products, the inherent inefficiency of which Schlundt demonstrates, WHO seeks to build capacity for safe food production and outbreak detection and alert, particularly in developing countries in recognition of their increasing contribution to global food trade.

THE U.S. FOOD SAFETY SYSTEM

John Bailar, M.D., Ph.D.[2]
Professor Emeritus, University of Chicago

The focus of my remarks to the Forum on Microbial Threats was the 1998 report entitled *Ensuring Safe Food from Production to Consumption* (IOM/NRC, 1998). That report was issued by a committee assembled jointly by the Institute of Medicine and the National Research Council, which I chaired, and which included at least three participants in this workshop: Lonnie King, Sanford Miller, and Michael Osterholm. My brief presentation, summarized below, described the long-recognized need for a complete overhaul of the U.S. food safety system, including the integration of widely scattered responsibilities for food safety oversight into a single, independent federal agency.

How the System Falls Short

The problems that must be addressed by the U.S. food safety system were discussed in detail in several workshop presentations (see Summary and Assess-

[2]Scholar in Residence, The National Academies.

ment, as well as Osterholm in Chapter 1, Tauxe in Chapter 3). Briefly, they include the tens of millions of cases, the thousands of deaths, and the billions of dollars lost every year because of foodborne illness, as well as the possibility of deliberate harm to our food system. To address these challenges, we have a food safety system that involves at least 12 different agencies (of which four have major responsibilities) that conduct monitoring, surveillance, inspection, enforcement, outbreak management, research, and education. These agencies work under a total of 35 food safety-related statutes and more than 50 interagency agreements and working groups; they report to a total of 28 House and Senate committees. A variety of federal-state programs, international treaties and agreements, and voluntary programs are also involved in ensuring food safety.

Clearly, there is an absence of focused leadership in food safety oversight. The federal agencies that share responsibility for food safety are poorly integrated, as are federal, state, and local food safety agencies. Moreover, each federal agency with food safety responsibilities has other missions that are generally regarded as more important. This situation has numerous and serious repercussions: surveillance of known, existing problems is inadequate; food safety standards are inconsistent, uneven, and archaic; resources available for food safety are lacking; consumers have limited knowledge about food safety; and there is poor adherence to even the minimum food safety standards currently in place.

The lack of integration and clear leadership among federal agencies responsible for food safety is demonstrated in Table 2-1, which lists the various offices and agencies involved in ensuring the safety of various food categories and contaminants through monitoring and surveillance, risk assessment, research, inspection and enforcement, and education. None of the four major elements of food safety—type of hazard, food category, nature of activity, or program responsibility—lines up with any of the others. Is anyone surprised that foodborne illness remains so common? Overlap occurs for every specific function listed in the table (e.g., four offices and three different agencies are responsible for risk assessment in seafood). Inconsistencies appear in each column; for example, in several cases, agencies responsible for monitoring and surveillance for a given commodity are not responsible for risk assessment, and some of these agencies in turn differ from those involved in research, inspection, enforcement, and education. Looking across the rows in Table 2-1, the group of agencies sharing responsibility for a function in one commodity (e.g., inspection of fruits and vegetables) does not match the agencies responsible for the same function in another commodity (e.g., inspection of seafood).

Reorganizing the U.S. Food Safety System

Prominent among the recommendations made in *Ensuring Safe Food from Production to Consumption* seven years ago is the following statement:

TABLE 2-1 Overlap in Federal Food Safety Oversight

Selected Food Products							Food Contaminants	
Fruits and Vegetables	Dairy Products	Eggs & Egg Products	Meat & Poultry	Seafood	Grain, Rice & Related Commodities	Imported Foods	Animal Drugs & Feeds	Pesticide Residues
CDC; CFSAN/FDA	CDC; CFSAN & CVM/FDA	CDC; CFSAN/FDA; AMS/USDA	CDC; CFSAN/FDA; USDA: FSIS, ERS	CDC; CFSAN/FDA; NMFS/NOAA	CDC; CFSAN/FDA	CDC, CFSAN & ORA/FDA; FSIS/USDA	CDC; CVM/FDA; FSIS/USDA; APHIS	CDC; FSIS/USDA; CFSAN/FDA
CFSAN/FDA; ARS/USDA	CFSAN; CVM/FDA; ARS/USDA	ARS & FSIS/USDA; ORACBA; CFSAN/FDA	USDA: ARS, CSREES, FSIS, ERS, ORACBA; CFSAN/FDA	CFSAN/FDA; NMFS/NOAA; ARS/USDA	ARS/USDA; CFSAN/FDA	Same as domestic food products	CVM/FDA; ARS/USDA/ APHIS	OPPTS/EPA; USDA: AMS, ARS, ERS, NASS
CFSAN, NCTR/FDA; ARS, CSREES/ USDA	CFSAN; CVM/FDA, CSREES & ARS/USDA	CFSAN/FDA; ARS/USDA CSREES	USDA: ARS, CSREES	CVM & CFSAN/FDA; NMFS/NOAA; CSREES & ARS/USDA	ARS, CSREES/ USDA; CFSAN/FDA	Same as domestic food products	CFSAN & CVM/FDA; ARS & CSREES/ USDA	ORD/EPA; CSREES & ARS/USDA; CFSAN/FDA
CFSAN & ORA/FDA	CFSAN, ORA, & CVM/FDA	FSIS/USDA; FDA: CVM, CFSAN & ORA	FSIS/USDA; CFSAN & CVM/FDA	ORA & CFSAN/FDA; NMFS/NOAA	GIPSA/USDA; ORA & CFSAN/FDA	FSIS/USDA; CFSAN & ORA/FDA	ORA & CVM/FDA; FSIS/USDA; APHIS	USDA:FSIS, AMS/ FDA: CFSAN, CVM, & ORA; OECA/EPA
CFSAN/FDA; CSREES, ARS/USDA	CFSAN/FDA; CSREES, ARS/USDA	CFSAN/FDA; FSIS & CSREES, ARS/USDA	USDA: FSIS, CSREES, ARS, ERS, ORACBA; CFSAN/FDA	CFSAN/FDA; CSREES, ARS/USDA; NMFS/NOAA	CSREES, ARS/USDA; CFSAN/FDA	CSREES, ARS/FDA; CFSAN/FDA	CSREES, ARS/USDA; CVM/FDA	CFSAN/FDA; FSIS & CSREES, ARS/ USDA

NOTE: Acronym list is provided in Appendix B.

SOURCE: IOM/NRC (1998).

> Congress should establish, by statute, a unified and central framework for managing food safety programs, one that is headed by a single official and which has the responsibility and control of resources for all federal food safety activities, including outbreak management, standard-setting, inspection, monitoring, surveillance, risk assessment, enforcement, research, and education (IOM/NRC, 1998).

This committee was not the first body to call for such reform. At that time, we knew of nearly 20 commissions, committees, and studies dating back to 1949 that had made similar recommendations (Vogt, 1998); more recently, the Government Accountability Office (GAO) has taken up this issue (GAO, 2004, 2005a,b). However, I would like to emphasize one of the important points that came out of our report: the need to have an independent agency, one that will not be influenced by competing priorities within agencies where the work of ensuring food safety is currently carried out.

I will conclude with a personal observation as to why, despite the many calls for reorganization, our food safety system remains fragmented and inadequate. I believe that the following three reasons lie at the heart of this problem:

1. Bureaucratic inertia—It will take time, effort, and money to implement the major reorganization that has been recommended.
2. Turf battles—Federal agencies and congressional committees that currently oversee various aspects of food safety do not want to give up funds, personnel positions, authorities, and responsibilities.
3. Industrial inertia—Regulated industries have adapted to the present system and its constraints. Companies do not welcome change, even when it is in the public interest.

Although none of these obstacles constitutes an acceptable excuse for postponing needed reform, they clearly must be overcome in order to create the unified, independent federal program that is needed to truly ensure the safety of the U.S. food supply.

FOOD SAFETY THREATS—INTERNATIONAL COORDINATION

Jørgen Schlundt, Ph.D.[3]
World Health Organization

Summary

Food safety relates to both human health and economic development. Countries all over the world are affected by a range of diseases related to food, in effect

[3]Director, Department of Food Safety, Zoonoses and Foodborne Diseases.

causing a very significant disease burden that seems to have been on the rise in both developed and developing countries over the most recent decades. Outbreaks of foodborne diseases most often originate in natural or accidental contamination events, but the potential for intentional contamination of the food chain is present, as documented by previously recorded—although relatively minor—such outbreaks. The developments towards a more global food market underlines that it is in the best interest of all countries to strengthen the international capacity for foodborne outbreak alert and response. Such capacity is built most efficiently through unified systems dealing with all forms of outbreak—intentional as well as unintentional. The role of the WHO is to provide advice on strengthening national systems to prevent and respond to foodborne outbreaks, including intentional contamination events. The WHO is in a unique position to coordinate existing international systems for public health disease surveillance and emergency response. The revised WHO International Health Regulations provides the legal platform for all countries to declare public health emergencies of international concern. The WHO INFOSAN offers a system for alert action and response to public health emergencies involving food, related to both intentional and unintentional contamination events.

Existing Foodborne Disease Burden

Food safety is an important public health problem that relates to both human health and economic development (WHO, 2002a). Countries all over the world are affected by a range of diseases related to food, in effect causing a very significant disease burden that seems to be increasing both in developed and developing countries.

Food safety problems can cause a number of different diseases, from relatively mild cases of food poisoning to deadly infections and cancer. Diarrheal diseases—almost all caused by food- or waterborne microbial pathogens—are leading causes of illness and death in less developed countries, killing an estimated 1.8 million people annually at the global level (WHO, 2005). Even in developed countries it is estimated that up to one-third of the population is affected by microbiological foodborne disease each year (Mead et al., 1999). The majority of the pathogens causing this significant disease burden are now considered to be zoonotic pathogens. The occurrence of some of these zoonotic pathogens seems to have increased significantly over recent years.

Although a significant fraction of diarrhea is caused by food, this still only constitutes part of the total foodborne disease burden. Other parts of the burden relate to a number of important, and often more chronic, diseases caused by not only microorganisms but also chemical contaminants in our food. The disease burden related to chemical contaminants and chemical constituents in our food is very difficult to estimate, but it is likely that this part of the total burden could be as big as the microbiological burden.

The reporting of foodborne disease is typically based on the number of laboratory confirmed cases, only representing a fraction of the real cases. The factor between reported and real cases is called the underreporting factor. Few thorough epidemiological estimations of the national underreporting factor have been made, but there are significant variations in the factor presented. One example of such variation is that for salmonellosis the factors can vary from 3.2 fold from a study in the United Kingdom (Wheeler et al., 1999) to 38 fold from a study in the United States (Mead et al., 1999). It is not easily evaluated whether differences in the underreporting factor between countries is a reflection of real differences in the performance of health systems or a reflection of differences in methodology used to estimate the factor.

Although some national foodborne disease surveillance systems mainly collect information on the number of outbreaks and the number of cases involved in the outbreaks, for most foodborne diseases the majority of cases are sporadic. Surveillance systems must include measures to estimate also the sporadic part of the foodborne disease burden. New, active surveillance systems are likely in the future to blur the difference between what has traditionally been referred to as outbreaks and sporadic cases. The possibility of comparing types of pathogens (e.g., pulsed-field gel electrophoresis typing) isolated from human cases in a broad national system enables the linking of cases, previously considered single or sporadic in nature, and present them as part of an outbreak spread over a larger geographical area (Gerner-Smidt et al., 2005). It is thus likely that our understanding of the relative importance of outbreaks and sporadic cases will change in the near future.

As a result of the increased global trade in food it is also likely that outbreaks covering larger areas and affecting several countries will be recognized in larger numbers in the future. Surveillance of foodborne diseases provides information for action. The use of laboratory data in surveillance enables the identification of pathogens and the potential sources of infection. In the future, integrated surveillance including human data as well as animal- and food-monitoring data can also provide the basis for preventive action along the entire food chain. In 2000, WHO initiated the Global Salm-Surv, which provides targeted efforts to national typing laboratories, and the sharing and analysis of such results has recently lead to the recognition of trade and foreign travel as factors related to the international emergence of certain *Salmonella* serotypes as well as to multicountry outbreaks of *Salmonella* (WHO, 2006).

The Global Salm-Surv network builds laboratory and epidemiological capacity for integrated laboratory-based foodborne disease surveillance. The network presently has almost 900 members from 141 countries. The Global Salm-Surv maintains a database that in its first five-year period (2000–2004) recorded 565,042 isolates from humans and 102,113 nonhuman isolates (mainly from food).

As an integral part of foodborne disease surveillance there is a need to enable precise and timely information sharing between countries of outbreak-related data. At the global level such systems do not yet exist, but WHO efforts related to the new International Health Regulations and the newly formed INFOSAN should be seen in this light. These initiatives will be described further in Chapter 4.

Deliberate Contamination of Food: Recent Concern—Old Problem

The "deliberate contamination of food" is sometimes used synonymously with food terrorism or food bioterrorism. Food terrorism is defined as an act or threat of deliberate contamination of food for human consumption with chemical, biological, or radionuclear agents for the purpose of causing injury or death to civilian populations and/or disrupting social, economic, or political stability. Threats from terrorists, criminals, and other antisocial groups who target the safety of the food supply are already a reality. During the past two decades, WHO member states have expressed concern about the possibility that chemical and biological agents and radionuclear materials might deliberately be used to harm civilian populations. In May 2002, the 55th World Health Assembly (WHA) adopted a resolution that expressed serious concern about threats against civilian populations by deliberate use of biological, chemical, or radionuclear agents (WHO, 2002b). It noted that such agents can be disseminated via food, and the WHA requested the Director General to provide tools and support to member states, particularly developing countries, in strengthening their national systems.

In the past food supplies have often been contaminated deliberately, historically during military campaigns and, more recently, to terrorize or otherwise intimidate civilian populations (Khan et al., 2001). Deliberate contamination of food by chemical, biological, or radionuclear agents can occur at any vulnerable point along the food chain, from farm to table, depending on both the food and the agent. For example, in 1984, members of a religious cult contaminated salad bars in the United States with *Salmonella typhimurium*, causing 751 cases of salmonellosis. The attack appeared to be a trial run for a more extensive attack intended to disrupt local elections. The cult was also in possession of strains of *Salmonella typhi*, the causative organism of typhoid fever, a severe invasive illness (Torok et al., 1997).

The impact on human health of the future deliberate contamination of food can be estimated by extrapolation from the many documented examples of unintentional outbreaks of foodborne disease. The largest, best-documented incidents include an outbreak of *S. typhimurium* infection in 1985, affecting 170,000 people, caused by contamination of pasteurized milk from a dairy plant in the United States (Ryan et al., 1987). An outbreak of hepatitis A associated with consumption of clams in Shanghai, China, in 1991 affected nearly 300,000 people and may be the largest foodborne disease incident in history (Halliday et al., 1991). In 1994, an outbreak of *S. enteritidis* infection from contaminated pasteurized liquid ice cream that was transported as a premix in tanker trucks caused illness in 224,000 people in 41 states in the United States (Hennesy et al., 1996). In 1996, about 8,000 children in Japan became ill, including some deaths, with *Escherichia coli* O157:H7 infection from contaminated radish sprouts served in school lunches (Mermin and Griffin, 1999).

Episodes of foodborne illness caused by chemicals have also been reported in the published literature. The chemicals that can contaminate food include pesticides, mycotoxins, heavy metals, and other acutely toxic chemicals. In perhaps one of the most deadly incidents, over 800 people died and about 20,000 were injured, many permanently, by a chemical agent present in cooking oil sold in Spain in 1981 (WHO, 1983). In 1985, 1,373 people in the United States reported becoming ill after eating watermelon grown in soil treated with aldicarb (Green et al., 1987).

There are also many examples of outbreaks resulting from imported foods. In 1989, staphylococcal food poisoning in the United States was associated with eating mushrooms that had been canned in China (Levine et al., 1996). Outbreaks of cyclosporiasis in the United States in 1996 and 1997 were linked to consumption of Guatemalan raspberries (Herwaldt and Ackers, 1997). In the early 1990s epidemiological investigations of an increased human incidence of *Salmonella berta* in England and Wales was traced to chicken imported from Denmark (Threlfall et al., 1992).

In general, contamination of food may also have enormous economic implications. In an effort to damage Israel's economy in 1978, some citrus fruit exported to several European countries was contaminated with mercury, leading to significant trade disruption. In 1998, a company in the United States recalled 14 million kilograms of frankfurters and luncheon meats potentially contaminated with *Listeria*, resulting in a total cost of approximately US$50–70 million (CDC, 1999). An outbreak of *E. coli* O157:H7 infection in the United States in 1997 resulted in the recall of 11 million kilograms of ground beef (CDC, 1997). The crisis in Belgium in which dioxin-contaminated meat and dairy products were recalled around the world demonstrates not only the extensive costs to individual countries, but also the extent of disruption of global trade that can be caused by this type of incident (WHO, 2004a). From October 1996 to November 2002, 139 cases of variant Creutzfeldt-Jakob Disease have been reported globally, mainly in the United Kingdom, and most likely linked to exposure through food to the causative "agent" of bovine spongiform encephalopathy (BSE) in cattle (WHO, 2002c). Consequent consumer concern about consumption of meat has had a significant long-term impact on meat production in many countries.

In less developed countries, the economic consequences of major food contamination events could—in addition to human suffering and costs—also affect development and exacerbate poverty as well as food availability. Likewise the loss of export earnings can be very substantial both as a result of substantiated as well as unsubstantiated import restrictions. The lost revenues from food (especially fish) exports as a result of the 1991 cholera epidemic in Peru has been estimated to be US$700 million (Motarjemi, 1993). In a less well documented case, fish import restrictions in the European Union were upheld for a significant period of time following the publication of reports of cholera in East Africa, resulting in significant economic losses.

Prevention and Response Systems

All countries must have basic systems to prevent or deter deliberate contamination of their food supplies and, if attacked, to respond rapidly to minimize the health, economic, and other effects of such contamination.

However, counterterrorism should be seen as only one aspect of a broader, comprehensive food safety program in national and global contexts. WHO and a number of member states have addressed this issue with strategies to reduce the increasing burden of foodborne illness. The WHO Global Strategy for Food Safety, endorsed in January 2002 by the WHO executive board, comprises a preventive approach to food safety, with increased surveillance and more rapid response to outbreaks of foodborne illness. This approach could substantially expand the abilities of member states to protect the safety of their food supplies against natural and accidental threats and provides a framework for addressing terrorist threats to food.

Food production systems have become longer and more complicated over the latest decades. These changes in the way food is produced, processed, distributed, and sold have occurred at the same time as rapidly expanding international trade, the emergence of new transboundary food scares, greater international travel, and changing consumer preferences—all serving to draw new attention to the importance and challenge of ensuring food safety at the international level.

The recognition of the source and potential intention behind an outbreak or contamination event will in many cases only be possible at a very late stage. Although deliberate contamination presents a special set of issues, the same detection and response systems need to tackle outbreaks or contamination events whether the event is intentional or unintentional. Sensible precautions, coupled with strong surveillance and response capacity, constitute the most efficient and effective way of countering all such emergencies, including deliberate contamination of food.

For both developed and developing countries, guidance is needed to strengthen surveillance, preparedness, and response systems to meet the threat of any food safety emergency. Unfortunately, the tragic events in the United States on September 11, 2001, have focused a new angle to the debate of food safety: the issue of bioterrorism or other forms of intentional contamination of food. Agricultural production systems and food-processing facilities are potentially at risk. Efforts towards prevention should be integrated in existing systems, for example critical points for control should be defined within existing Hazard Analysis and Critical Control Point (HACCP) systems. Likewise existing surveillance and monitoring systems for foodborne disease and food contamination should be expanded to include the threats related to potential intentional contamination. This integrated approach would result in activities supporting the general food safety efforts instead of detracting from them.

Strengthening of such integrated systems and programs will both increase a country's capacity to reduce the increasing burden of foodborne illness and help to address the threat of intentional food contamination. It is important to reiterate that any intentional contamination event would probably always initially be considered as a natural or unintentional event, and that such events must therefore be managed on the food side through one, coherent system with relevant links to other authorities (police, intelligence services, etc.) in case of suspicious events.

Prevention, although never completely effective, is the first line of defense. The key to preventing food terrorism is establishment and enhancement of existing food safety management programs and implementation of reasonable security measures—not the setting up of new separate systems potentially detracting from existing efforts and scarce resources.

Prevention is best achieved through a cooperative effort between government and industry, given that the primary means for minimizing food risks lie with the food industry. Policy advice should be aimed at strengthening existing emergency alert and response systems by improving links with all the relevant agencies and with the food industry. This multistakeholder approach will strengthen disease outbreak surveillance, investigation capacity, preparedness planning, effective communication, and response (WHO, 2002d).

There is a growing realization that existing systems for food animal production in many countries do not correspond to the prevalent food control systems that are often centered around efforts at the slaughter house. The importance of small-holder production systems and animal markets has been clearly outlined, especially in an Asian context and in relation to recent outbreaks of highly pathogenic H5N1 avian influenza. A recent WHO report underlines the need for WHO and countries to improve current regulatory frameworks related to the marketing of live birds and other animals for food, including guidance applicable in developing countries (WHO, 2004b). Again the links between countries through increased food trade should be recognized, as should the need for timely international information sharing and coordinated response.

A growing share of the food consumed in industrialized countries today comes from developing and transition countries, and this trend is likely to intensify in the future. Clearly, it is in the best interest of us all to strengthen the capacity of the public and private sector in developing countries to produce food that meets international safety and quality standards. Consumers and importers in industrialized countries stand to benefit from increased access to an affordable, diverse, and safe supply of food products. Developing countries will benefit from access to new markets and greater foreign exchange earnings through trade.

International Preparedness

Contrary to popular beliefs the effect of food control systems based on testing is not very efficient. The reason for this relates to the fact that for many food types the prevalence of pathogens potentially causing disease can be very low. *Salmonella* in eggs causes a very large proportion of the human salmonellosis cases in most countries. Nevertheless, the prevalence of *Salmonella*-positive eggs is often 1:1,000 or even down to 1:10,000. In effect, you would therefore have to test a very large number of eggs to have any chance to find positive eggs, and the effect of removing such (few) eggs from the market is negligible. Even for foods with higher prevalence of pathogens, control based on testing is inefficient, and the main positive effect of such systems lies in a potential for (economic) punishment leading to changes in the production systems. For example, it is likely that the classification of enterohemorrhagic *Escherichia coli* as an adulterant in the United States and the resulting economic disasters for certain producers found to be in violation could have resulted in changes in the production systems leading to the avoidance of some of the previous problems. However, in many of these cases it is difficult to measure objectively the effect of such strategies as these problems are often affected by many different factors at the same time.

Since test-and-eliminate strategies are often not very efficient, it follows that prevention of outbreaks solely based on border control in most cases will not provide the level of protection sought after. New—and more efficient—food safety systems try to focus on preventative efforts as close to the source as possible, such as in industrial production settings through the introduction of HACCP systems. Because many food contamination events have international implications and because a significant fraction of food for consumption in many countries are imported, it follows that the most efficient way for any country to prevent intentional or unintentional foodborne outbreaks is to strengthen food safety in the country of origin and to ensure efficient international systems for outbreak alert and necessary response. A result of the global food market is that we now have a joint interest in building capacity to prevent and detect foodborne outbreaks in all countries through relevant international mechanisms.

In general, the need for international exchange of experience and scientific information in the food safety area is evident. The recent 2nd Global Forum for Food Safety Regulators in Bangkok, Thailand, is an example of such exchange of experience with a view of building efficient food safety capacity in all countries (FAO/WHO, 2004). Based on the outcome of this meeting the newly established INFOSAN, hosted by WHO, will continue a real-time interaction between the food safety authorities of the world (WHO, 2004c).

INFOSAN is intended to be an information network for the dissemination of important information about global food safety issues. INFOSAN members (of which each country can have several) receive information notes on current issues of interest for food safety authorities. Recent examples of information note subjects include avian influenza, *Enterobacter sakazakii* in powdered infant formula, acrylamide in food, antimicrobial-resistant *Salmonella*, and evaluation of genetically modified food. The INFOSAN focal points are expected to disseminate INFOSAN information to interested parties and stakeholders in their country, as appropriate. INFOSAN focal points may be located in several ministries, such as ministries of health, commerce, agriculture, and trade (see Figure 2-1).

A new emergency arm of the INFOSAN network (INFOSAN Emergency) will enable timely sharing of information and coordinated response in the case of major international foodborne outbreaks or food contamination events (WHO, 2004c). INFOSAN Emergency contact points are expected to function as two-way action points for emergency information. They should alert relevant food safety authorities within their country to foodborne disease outbreaks or food contamination events of international public health significance as reported to them by INFOSAN Emergency. And they should convey to the network information of national outbreaks or contamination events with a potential to become international events. Only one INFOSAN Emergency contact point has been requested per country in order to facilitate rapid and reliable communication with governments in cases where timeliness is critical. Potential future incidents involving deliberate contamination with international implications would likely be communicated through INFOSAN Emergency.

Relevant past examples of international food-related events that could have benefited from an international system for information sharing include the Chernobyl accident in the former Soviet Union (1986), the BSE outbreak and ban

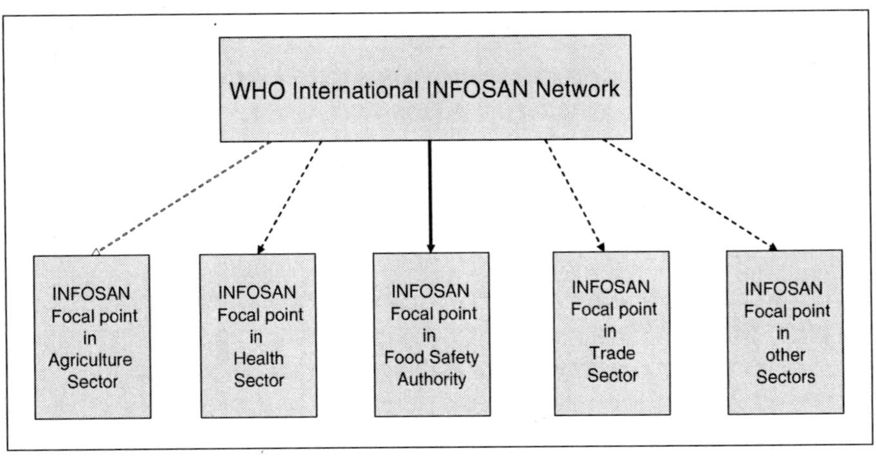

FIGURE 2-1 The WHO International Food Safety Authorities Network (INFOSAN): Set-up of focal points for information sharing.
SOURCE: INFOSAN (2005).

on feeding materials in the United Kingdom (1996), and the dioxin contamination of animal-derived food in Belgium (1997).

Since its inception in October 2004, INFOSAN Emergency has been involved in 11 verification events and sent out 3 notifications alerting from 5 to 32 countries on issues of potential international importance. These issues include powdered infant formula contaminated with *Salmonella*, orange juice contaminated with *Salmonella*, and pork contaminated with *Streptococcus*.

Clear, rapid, reliable, and authoritative information on food emergencies is the essential basis not only for prevention and response measures but also maintaining consumer confidence in the food supply. INFOSAN Emergency will be activated only during major international incidents involving the imminent risk of serious injury or death to consumers. INFOSAN Emergency contact points will be expected to accept some notification and response responsibility and to facilitate the communication of urgent messages during food safety emergencies. Figure 2-2 presents an example of how this may be structured in a country. Because of the potential sensitivity of the information exchanged, communication on this network would be considered confidential.

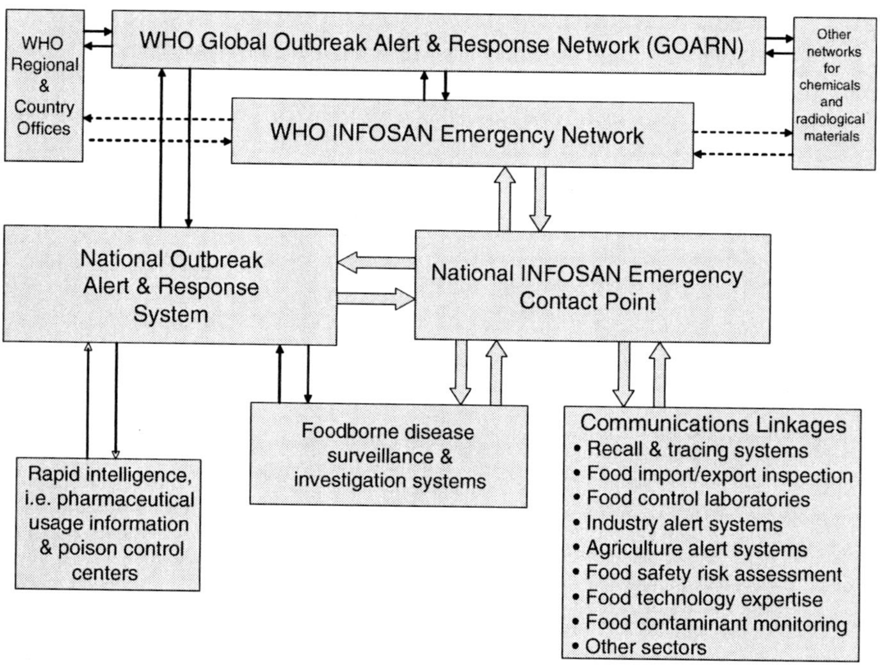

FIGURE 2-2 The WHO International Food Safety Authorities Network (INFOSAN): Potential communication lines for national INFOSAN Emergency Contact Points.
SOURCE: INFOSAN (2005).

INFOSAN Emergency will be closely linked to the alert-and-response activities of WHO and will be—to the extent necessary—functioning in support of the new international health regulations (WHO, 2004d). These regulations stipulate the international rules for sharing information on certain infectious diseases. The existing rules have up until now only covered yellow fever, cholera, and plague, enabling (and demanding) international exchange of information of outbreaks of such diseases. Responding to a realization that many internationally important disease incidents involve other responsible agents, including new agents such as the SARS virus, the need for a revision of international health rules was formulated in the WHA several years ago. The new rules propose the extension of the WHO coordinated public health emergency system to include all public health emergencies of international concern, which has been defined to also include foodborne emergencies or emergencies involving zoonotic diseases. Because of the legal framework of the regulations, there is no need for national ratification, and they will enter into force for all 192 WHO member states in June 2007.[4] All WHO member states will be obliged to declare public health emergencies of international concern to the WHO.

WHO's international systems to minimize impact on public health of international incidents, including the international health rules, INFOSAN, and other networks related to chemical and radiological incidents basically exist to do the following:

- Rapidly detect any international incident;
- Respond in a timely fashion to international emergencies; and
- Decide and inform on the termination of emergency situations.

The systems therefore require:

- Capacity for efficient information gathering and rapid communication;
- Capacity to verify and make decisions;
- Procedures to respond and capacity to assist; and
- Basic platforms of national preparedness with international links.

REFERENCES

CDC (Centers for Disease Control and Prevention). 1997. *Escherichia coli* O157:H7 infections associated with eating a nationally distributed commercial brand of frozen ground beef patties and hamburgers: Colorado, 1997. *Morbidity and Mortality Weekly Report* 46(33):777–778.

CDC. 1999. Update: Multi-state outbreak of listeriosis—United States, 1998–1999. *Morbidity and Mortality Weekly Report* 47(51/52):1117–1118.

---

[4]In May 2006, the WHA in a resolution agreed to: "Call upon Member States to comply immediately, on a voluntary basis, with provisions of the International Health Regulations (2005) considered relevant to the risk posed by avian influenza and pandemic influenza."

FAO/WHO (Food and Agriculture Association and the World Health Organization). 2004. *Second FAO/WHO Global Forum of Food Safety Regulators—A Forum Dedicated to Sharing Experiences in Management of Food Safety.* [Online]. Available: http://www.foodsafetyforum.org/global2/index_en.asp [accessed April 10, 2006].

GAO (Government Accountability Office). 2004. *Federal Food Safety and Security System: Fundamental Restructuring is Needed to Address Fragmentation and Overlap.* GAO-04-588T. Washington, D.C.: GAO.

GAO. 2005a. *Overseeing the U.S. Food Supply: Steps Should be Taken to Reduce Overlapping Inspections and Related Activities.* GAO-05-549T. Washington, D.C.: GAO.

GAO. 2005b. *Oversight of Food Safety Activities: Federal Agencies Should Pursue Opportunities to Reduce Overlap and Better Leverage Resources.* GAO-05-213. Washington, D.C.: GAO.

Gerner-Smidt P, Kincaid J, Kubota K, Hise K, Hunter SB, Fair MA, Norton D, Woo-Ming A, Kurzynski T, Sotir MJ, Head M, Holt K, Swaminathan B. 2005. Molecular surveillance of shiga toxigenic *Escherichia coli* O157 by PulseNet USA. *Journal of Food Protection* 68(9):1926–1931.

Green MA, Heumann MA, Wehr HM, Foster LR, Williams LP Jr, Polder JA, Morgan CL, Wagner SL, Wanke LA, Witt JM. 1987. An outbreak of watermelon-borne pesticide toxicity. *American Journal of Public Health* 77(11):1431–1434.

Halliday ML, Kang LY, Zhou TK, Hu MD, Pan QC, Fu TY, Huang YS, Hu SL. 1991. An epidemic of hepatitis A attributable to the ingestion of raw clams in Shanghai, China. *Journal of Infectious Diseases* 164(5):852–859.

Hennesy TW, Hedberg CW, Slutsker L, White KE, Besser-Wiek JM, Moen ME, Feldman J, Coleman WW, Edmonson LM, MacDonald KL, Osterholm MT. 1996. National outbreak of *Salmonella enteritidis* infections from ice cream. *New England Journal of Medicine* 334(20):1281–1286.

Herwaldt BL, Ackers ML. 1997. An outbreak in 1996 of cyclosporiasis associated with imported raspberries. Cyclospora Working Group. *New England Journal of Medicine* 336(22):1548–1556.

INFOSAN (International Food Safety Authorities Network). 2005. *International Food Safety Authorities Network.* [Online]. Available: http://www.who.int/foodsafety/fs_management/infosan_0705_en.pdf [accessed April 20, 2006].

IOM/NRC (Institute of Medicine/National Research Council). 1998. *Ensuring Safe Food from Production to Consumption.* Washington, D.C.: National Academy Press.

Khan AS, Swerdlow DL, Juranek DD. 2001. Precautions against biological and chemical terrorism directed at food and water supplies. *Public Health Reports* 116(1):3–14.

Levine WC, Bennet RW, Choi Y, Henning KJ, Rager JR, Hendricks KA, Hopkins DP, Gunn RA, Griffin PM. 1996. Staphylococcal food poisoning caused by imported canned mushrooms. *Journal of Infectious Diseases* 173(5):1263–1267.

Mead PS, Slutsker L, Dietz V, McCaig LF, Bresee JS, Shapiro C, Griffin PM, Tauxe RV. 1999. Food-related illness and death in the United States. *Emerging Infectious Diseases* 5(5):607–625.

Mermin JH, Griffin PM. 1999. Public health in crisis: Outbreaks of *Escherichia coli* O157:H7 in Japan. *American Journal of Epidemiology* 150(8):797–803.

Motarjemi Y. 1993. Health and development aspects of food safety. *Archiv für Lebensmittelhygiene* 44(2):35–41.

Ryan CA, Nickels MK, Hargrett-Bean NT, Potter ME, Endo T, Mayer L, Langkop CW, Gibson C, McDonald RC, Kenney RT, Puhr ND, McDonnell PJ, Martin RJ, Cohen ML, Blake PA. 1987. Massive outbreak of antimicrobial-resistant salmonellosis traced to pasteurized milk. *Journal of the American Medical Association* 258(22):3269–3274.

Threlfall EJ, Hall ML, Ward LR, Rowe B. 1992. Plasmid profiles demonstrate that an upsurge in *Salmonella berta* in humans in England and Wales is associated with imported poultry meat. *European Journal of Epidemiology* 8(1):27–33.

Torok T, Tauxe RV, Wise RP, Livengood JR, Sokolow R, Mauvais S, Birkness KA, Skeels MR, Horan JM, Foster LR. 1997. A large community outbreak of *Salmonella* caused by intentional contamination of restaurant salad bars. *Journal of the American Medical Association* 278(5): 389–395.

Vogt DU. 1998. *Food Safety: Recommendations for Changes in the Organization of Federal Food Safety Responsibilities, 1949–1997.* CRS Report 93-955. Washington, D.C.: Library of Congress.

Wheeler JG, Sehti D, Cowden JM, Wall PG, Rodrigues LC, Tompkins DS, Hudson MJ, Roderirick PJ. 1999. Study of infectious intestinal disease in England: Rates in the community, presenting to general practice, and reported to national surveillance. The Infectious Intestinal Disease Study Executive. *British Medical Journal* 318(7190):1046–1050.

WHO (World Health Organization). 1983. *Toxic Oil Syndrome: Mass Food Poisoning in Pain.* Report of a WHO meeting, Madrid, Spain, May 21–25, 1983. Copenhagen: WHO Regional Office for Europe.

WHO. 2002a. *WHO Global Strategy for Food Safety: Safer Food for Better Health. Food Safety Issues Series.* [Online]. Available: http://www.who/int/foodsafety/publications/general/global_strategy/en/ [accessed April 10, 2006].

WHO. 2002b. *World Health Assembly Resolution (WHA55.16): Global Public Health Response to Natural Occurrence, Accidental Release or Deliberate Use of Biological and Chemical Agents or Radionuclear Material That Affect Health.* [Online]. Available: http://www.who.int/gb/ebwha/pdf_files/WHA55/ewha5516.pdf [accessed April 10, 2006].

WHO. 2002c. *Fact Sheet No. 180 on variant Creutzfeldt-Jakob Disease* (Rev. November 2002). Geneva: WHO.

WHO. 2002d. *Terrorist Threats to Food: Guidance for Establishing and Strengthening Prevention and Response Systems, Food Safety Issues Series.* Geneva: WHO.

WHO. 2004a. *Sixth Futures Forum on Crisis Communication.* Report of a WHO meeting, Reykjavik, Iceland, May 10–11, 2004. Copenhagen: WHO Regional Office for Europe.

WHO. 2004b. Food safety. In: *The Work of WHO in the Western Pacific Region, Report of the Regional Director, 1 July 2003–30 June 2004.* Manila, Philippines: WHO. Pp. 80–83.

WHO. 2004c. *INFOSAN: International Food Safety Authorities Network.* [Online]. Available: http://www.who/int/foodsafety/fs_management/infosan/en/ [accessed April 10, 2006].

WHO. 2004d. *IHR: International Health Regulations.* [Online]. Available: http://www.who.int/csr/ihr/en/ [accessed April 10, 2006].

WHO. 2005. *World Health Report 2005. Annexes by Country.* [Online]. Available: http://www.who.int/whr/2005/en/ [accessed April 10, 2006].

WHO. 2006. *WHO Global Salm-Surv Progress Report (2000–2005): Building Capacity for Laboratory-Based Foodborne Disease Surveillance and Outbreak Detection and Response.* Geneva: WHO.

3

Investigating Foodborne Threats

OVERVIEW

Foodborne illness is estimated to affect more than 76 million people in the United States each year, resulting in 325,000 hospitalizations and 5,200 deaths, but its true incidence is unknown (Mead et al., 1999). Because foodborne disease is difficult to diagnose, the vast majority of these illnesses and more than half of such deaths are attributed to "unknown agents" (Mead et al., 1999). The annual cost of medical expenses and productivity losses associated with the five most prevalent, diagnosable foodborne illnesses is nearly $7 billion (Vogt, 2005).

Many people with symptoms of foodborne illness do not seek medical attention, further contributing to underdiagnosis. These circumstances, in addition to the rapid distribution of food on both a national and global scale, make it nearly impossible to detect even a large foodborne outbreak in time to limit its impact; see, for example, the description of the 1994 *Salmonella* outbreak in ice cream, described by Osterholm in Chapter 1. Most often, outbreak investigations occur after the fact. However, as the papers in this chapter illustrate, findings from outbreak investigations enable public health authorities to identify new foodborne pathogens, trace their entry into the food chain, and thereby reveal opportunities to improve food safety.

The first contribution to this chapter, by Robert Tauxe of the Centers for Disease Control and Prevention (CDC), provides an overview of the foodborne threat spectrum and the practices of public health surveillance by which these microbes, and the burden of disease they cause, have become known. Tauxe explores several recent advancements in this field, including the development of information networks for foodborne disease surveillance (see also Besser in Chapter 5) and enhanced outbreak investigations, and their probable link to recent reductions in cases of several major foodborne diseases.

Despite these improvements, the processes of outbreak detection and investigation remain highly challenging, as illustrated in the case studies that make up the remainder of this chapter. The first two papers, by Barbara Herwaldt of the CDC and Roberta Hammond and Dean Bodager of the Florida Department of Health, describe their experiences investigating a relatively new foodborne threat: the coccidian parasite *Cyclospora cayetanensis*. Little was known about the organism when, in the mid-1990s, large, multistate outbreaks of gastroenteritis were recognized. Herwaldt and public health colleagues eventually traced these outbreaks to raspberries from Guatemala, where *Cyclospora* infection is endemic. Several other types of fresh produce have also been identified as vehicles for cyclosporiasis outbreaks. Herwaldt analyzes the challenges presented by foodborne outbreaks (in general, as well as the specific difficulties associated with *C. cayetanensis*) and draws important lessons for the future of public health.

In the subsequent paper, Hammond and Bodager describe the complexities of a recent *C. cayetanensis* investigation. Triggered by an early 2005 report from a private lab of an unusually large number of infections, the investigation ultimately involved county health departments throughout Florida, three different state agencies that regulate food in Florida, and two federal agencies: the CDC and the Food and Drug Administration (FDA). The investigators determined that imported basil provided the vehicle for the parasite; like raspberries, basil is a "stealth" ingredient that many people do not recognize or (because such foods are often served as garnishes) easily forget. Such accounts illustrate the importance of examining seemingly unrelated cases of apparent foodborne illnesses as indicators of outbreaks and pursuing them to their sources through timely and thorough investigation.

The pathogen discussed in the chapter's final contribution, the hepatitis A virus (HAV), is far better characterized than *Cyclospora*, yet its investigators are faced with a similar array of challenges. This paper, by workshop speaker Beth Bell and Anthony Fiore of the CDC, describes a series of hepatitis A outbreaks in late 2003 that included the largest such outbreak reported in the United States. It involved over 600 patrons of a single Pennsylvania restaurant, and ultimately led the FDA to ban imports from the Mexican farms that grew the tainted green onions that caused the outbreak. Investigators were aided by molecular methods for HAV detection (comparable methods do not exist for *Cyclospora*), but Bell and Fiore note several characteristics of routine hepatitis A surveillance and of the infection itself that continue to hinder its detection and control. The authors conclude that foodborne HAV infection (and those of other enteric pathogens) may be best prevented on the farm by reducing the contamination of produce with fecal material.

Taken as a whole, the papers in this chapter demonstrate both the crucial importance and the daunting difficulty of conducting foodborne outbreak investigations. The success of such investigations depends to a large extent on public and private laboratories that must have adequate resources if they are to quickly and accurately detect threats to our food supply. Indeed, Tauxe observes that future advancements in the detection and investigation of foodborne illness are less likely to be achieved through technical innovation than through the strengthening of public health infrastructure.

THE BURDEN OF ILLNESS ASSOCIATED WITH FOODBORNE THREATS TO HEALTH, AND THE CHALLENGE OF PREVENTION

Robert V. Tauxe, M.D., M.P.H.[1]
Centers for Disease Control and Prevention[2]

Few human endeavors are more complex than the constant, daily, and varied effort to produce and prepare the foods we eat. The many cultural traditions and changing tastes introduce new foods and food-making processes to growing populations around the world. As a result, the foodborne diseases that follow the contamination of the food supply with any of a large number of microbes and toxins present similarly evolving challenges. A new foodborne disease may emerge when a previously unknown pathogen appears in a reservoir related to the food supply or when transmission through a new foodborne pathway is documented for a known pathogen. When a new foodborne disease appears, there is a natural history to the challenge, starting with first detection and description; the development of means to diagnose and treat the new infection; investigations into the sources, reservoirs, and transmission pathways; and finally prevention stratagems that improve to the point that the disease no longer presents an important problem. Each of the many known foodborne diseases is somewhere on this progression, and more are likely to be appreciated in the future. The spectrum of foodborne diseases is a dynamic range of threats.

An array of bacterial, viral, and parasitic pathogens that cause foodborne infections are currently recognized as public health problems in the United States. Among these, an important number have only been recognized as foodborne pathogens in the last three decades (Table 3-1). Some were first detected as pathogens in recent times and may represent the evolution of new combinations of virulence properties. For example, *E. coli* O157:H7, not detected at all before the 1970s and first recognized as a cause of human illness in 1982, became a major foodborne disease with a recognized bovine reservoir on several continents by the 1990s (Griffin and Tauxe, 1991). This pathogen evolved from precursors with

---

[1]Captain, U.S. Public Health Service; Chief of Foodborne and Diarrheal Diseases Branch, Division of Bacterial and Mycotic Diseases, National Center for Infectious Diseases.

[2]The findings and conclusions in this manuscript have not been formally disseminated by CDC and should not be construed to represent any agency determination or policy.

TABLE 3-1 Foodborne Pathogens in the United States

Bacteria	Viruses
Bacillus cereus	*Norovirus**
Brucella	*Rotavirus**
*Campylobacter**	*Astrovirus**
Clostridium botulinum	Hepatitis A
*Clostridium perfringens**	
*Enterobacter sakazakii**	**Parasites**
E. coli O157:H7*	*Anisakis*
E. coli non-O157 STEC*	*Cryptosporidium**
E. coli other diarrheogenic*	*Cyclospora**
Mycobacterium bovis	*Giardia lamblia**
Salmonella Typhi	*Toxoplasma**
Salmonella nontyphoidal	*Trichinella*
Shigella	
Staphylococcus aureus	**Prions**
Streptococcus	Bovine encephalopathy agent*
Vibrio cholerae, toxigenic (O1 and O139)*	
*Vibrio vulnificus**	
*Vibrio parahaemolyticus**	
*Yersinia enterocolitica**	

NOTE: Pathogens characterized as foodborne within the last 30 years are indicated with an asterisk.

SOURCE: Tauxe (2005); Adapted from Tauxe (2002).

far less pathogenic potential as the result of several phage-induced mutations (Wick et al., 2005). Though the timing of these modifications remains unproven, several have noted that mobilization of phages and of other transferable genetic elements could be linked to exposure to antimicrobial agents (Zhang et al., 2000; LeFebvre et al., 2005) and therefore perhaps linked to relatively recent changes in agriculture. Another recent example is the emergence of an entirely new toxigenic serotype of *Vibrio cholerae* with epidemic potential. This serotype, O139, first appeared in 1992 in India, and spread rapidly through much of South and Southeast Asia where it was transmitted through water and food (Hoge et al., 1996). This serotype appears to have evolved as the result of a horizontal transfer of the genes that produce the O-antigen, possibly from another *Vibrio*, into several strains of the dominant strain of epidemic toxigenic *V. cholerae* O1 (Faruque et al., 2003).

Other pathogens were recognized as human pathogens well before they were linked to foodborne transmission. For example, *Listeria monocytogenes*, first described as a cause of severe invasive infections in humans in the 1930s, was first linked to foodborne transmission in 1981 in an outbreak associated with cole slaw (Schlech et al., 1983), and more recently it was documented to be primarily foodborne (Slutsker et al., 2000). *Campylobacter jejuni*, described as a cause of invasive infection in immunocompromised hosts in the 1950s, was shown in 1977 to be a common enteric pathogen in normal hosts; the importance of foodborne transmission was established by 1980 (Blaser et al., 1983). The more recent observations of the parasite *Cyclospora cayetanensis* show how a pathogen that was geographically restricted to remote and third-world locations may leap to the forefront as a new food safety challenge, as summarized elsewhere in this report. This means that the new and emerging foodborne pathogens observed elsewhere in the world are of substantial interest and may offer a view into our future. The recent reports of outbreaks of *Yersinia pseudotuberculosis* associated with lettuce in Finland and of hepatitis E infection associated with swine in Japan are worthy of our attention (Nuorti et al., 2004; Yazaki et al., 2003).

Still others represent the recrudescence of foodborne challenges long brought under control, as changing tastes and patterns of trade reintroduce pathogens to the public that we last saw as a significant problem many decades ago. Souvenir seafood brought back in suitcases led to foodborne cholera in New Jersey in the 1990s (Finelli et al., 1992). The recent appearance of bovine tuberculosis in New York City may be a result of the rapid shipment of homemade cheeses from Latin America, made traditionally with unpasteurized milk (CDC, 2005a). The specter of an intentional attack on the population through the food supply has added other pathogens—new and old—to the list of potential threats (Sobel et al., 2002).

We can anticipate new challenges to continue to emerge. A robust and flexible public health surveillance system is an important part of how we will detect, characterize, and ultimately prevent these new challenges.

Public Health Surveillance

Public health surveillance is conducted to define the magnitude and burden of a disease that needs public health action, to identify and investigate outbreaks so that control measures can be rapidly implemented and issues in need of further research swiftly identified, and to measure the impact of control and prevention efforts. The public health surveillance of infections that are likely to be foodborne now includes a substantial list of pathogens whose diagnosis is to be reported to public health authorities, and a new set of national networks for characterizing the pathogens and the illnesses they cause. The recent improvements in surveillance have been summarized in detail in a recent Institute of Medicine (IOM) publication (IOM/NRC, 2003). The following is a brief sketch of some of the improvements.

The primary authority for surveillance rests with the state health departments, which gather information from cities and counties and operate most of the public health laboratories. State and local notifiable diseases laws request or require clinicians and laboratories to report specific infections and to refer isolates of some pathogens to the public health laboratory for further characterization. These laws also typically require the reporting of unusual clusters or outbreaks of disease. In addition, many jurisdictions maintain complaint lines, to which concerned citizens may directly report illnesses or observations they think may need public health attention. Some food testing occurs in the course of routine inspections and as part of process monitoring within food production. This testing may also provide some information about the status of the food supply, though its purpose is usually the ongoing verification of process control, not safety testing of each lot.

Since 1996, the public health surveillance system for foodborne diseases has been strengthened in several ways. Several diseases were added to the standard notifiable disease reporting system, including non-O157 Shiga toxin-producing *E. coli*, hemolytic uremic syndrome, *Cyclospora cayetanensis*, and *Listeria monocytogenes*. The routine public health serotyping of *Salmonella* and *Shigella* was strengthened by the production and distribution of new antisera and training in their use; now new DNA sequence-based methods are being developed for more rapid identification of the serotype of *Salmonella* (McQuiston et al., 2004). Public health monitoring of antimicrobial resistance in several enteric bacterial pathogens has been implemented in parallel with monitoring of resistance in the same pathogens isolated from animals and foods, leading to the identification of such hazards as fluoroquinolone-resistant *Campylobacter jejuni* and multi-drug resistant strains of *Salmonella enteriticas* serotype Typhimurium and *Salmonella enteriticas* serotype Newport (Holmes and Chiller, 2004).

The reporting of outbreaks of foodborne diseases from local and state health departments has been improved by standardized and rapid reporting via the Internet and the Electronic Foodborne Outbreak Reporting System (CDC, 2005d). Enhanced surveillance, including a new collection form and improved close-out procedures doubled the number of foodborne outbreaks reported to more than 1,200 outbreaks each year (Figure 3-1). Now the Electronic Foodborne Outbreak Reporting System has changed an old and slow paper-based system into a more rapid reporting that makes it likely that a cluster of similar outbreaks occurring in several parts of the country at once will be detected and flagged, and also increasing the utility of the surveillance data to track trends in specific foodborne outbreak categories.

PulseNet, CDC's national network for subtyping foodborne bacterial pathogens, has been implemented in all 50 states and a growing number of large city health departments, as well as in the laboratories of the food regulatory agencies at the U.S. Department of Agriculture (USDA) and the FDA (Gerner-Smidt et al., 2006). This network relies on the submission of isolates of *E. coli* O157:H7, *Listeria monocytogenes*, *Salmonella*, and other bacterial pathogens from clinical laboratories to the public health laboratory, where the DNA "fingerprint" is determined using pulsed-field gel electrophoresis. Automated comparison of the digitized DNA pattern with the growing state and national database can swiftly identify strains (and therefore cases) that might be related, detecting clusters spread across multistate jurisdictions that might otherwise have been missed completely. In the 1960s, *Salmonella* serotyping transformed surveillance for that organism by increasing the signal-to-noise ratio and making it possible to pick

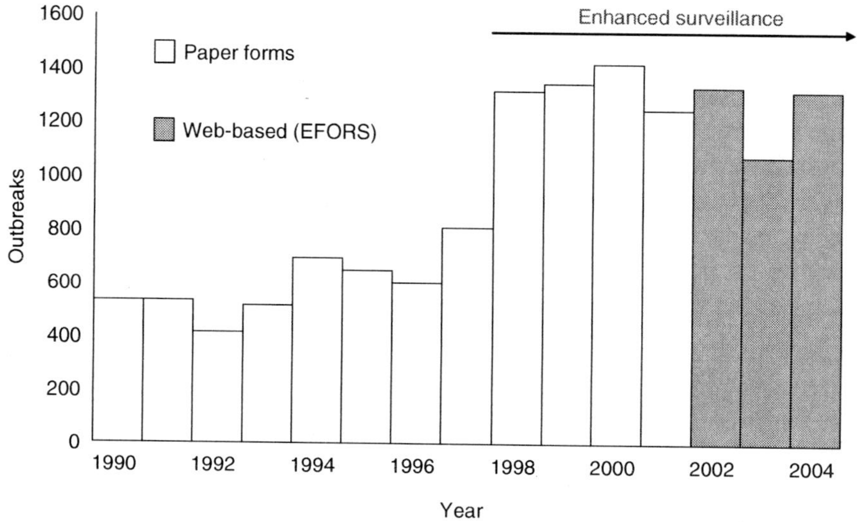

FIGURE 3-1 Reported outbreaks of foodborne diseases, 1990–2004, United States.
SOURCE: Adapted from CDC (2006b).

out outbreaks of one serotype from the background noise of all salmonellosis (CDC, 1965). Now PulseNet provides an additional specificity, with a generally applicable tool for identifying clusters of infections that are likely to be related, even within a single closely-related serotype such as *E. coli* O157:H7, or within individual *Salmonella* serotypes. PulseNet test protocols have now been developed for seven bacterial foodborne pathogens, as well as for *Yersinia pestis* and *F. tularensis*.

PulseNet protocols have now been adopted in Canada, Japan, Australia and other countries and are the heart of international networks for surveillance in Europe, Asia and the Pacific, and Latin America (Swaminathan et al., 2006). This will enhance our own prevention capacity. For example, in 2004, public health laboratories in Japan detected a small cluster of *E. coli* O157:H7 infections in Okinawa that they linked to consuming ground beef from the commissary at a U.S. military base there, and an indistinguishable *E. coli* was detected in ground beef in Japan, which came from the United States (CDC, 2005b). The notification by Japan led to recall of 90,000 pounds of ground beef shipped to the military and other institutions in the United States. The same strain was also identified in two persons in the United States who did eat beef the origin of which was not traceable, and who would not otherwise have been linked.

In the future, routine usage of multilocus variable number tandem repeat assays or other sequence based-methods in state health department laboratories will further refine the speed and precision of the network. However, the promise of real-time results is more dependent on resources, rather than technology, including the vital participation of the private clinical laboratory sector to refer strains rapidly to the public health laboratory and on the laboratory support within the state health department to run the tests swiftly.

Another major advance in foodborne surveillance has been FoodNet, the active sentinel site surveillance system for foodborne illness (Allos et al., 2004). While PulseNet enhances the ability of all states to detect clusters and investigate outbreaks, FoodNet is focused on developing standard and detailed surveillance data on sporadic (nonoutbreak-associated cases) in 10 sites around the country, now representing 14 percent of the U.S. population. Though sporadic cases are far more common than those that are associated with outbreaks, they receive far less attention in general. Active surveillance means that the health department regularly contacts the clinical laboratories to collect reports of what has been diagnosed, rather than relying on the laboratories to report them. In addition FoodNet conducts specialized surveys of the clinical laboratories, of the general population, and of other groups to obtain measures of the frequency of gastroenteritis in general, of specific diagnostic tests, and other measures important to interpreting surveillance data. Data from FoodNet have been critical to refining the overall estimates of the burden of foodborne disease and to tracking trends in specific infections over time. For example, between 1996 and 2004, FoodNet documented a 42 percent decline in diagnosed *E. coli* O157 infections, decreasing to 0.9 per 100,000 in the year 2004; a 40 percent decline in *Listeria* infections; and a 31 percent decline in *Campylobacter* infections (CDC, 2005c). With case-control and other studies, FoodNet also defines the association between infections and specific foods, contributing to the attribution of the burden of specific infections to foods. Increasingly, FoodNet serves as a platform for developing and evaluating improved public health surveillance and investigative and prevention strategies.

Estimating the Burden of Foodborne Diseases

The health burden of an infection includes the morbidity it causes, the hospitalization and other medical care that results, and the mortality, among other measures. Estimating this burden for a given pathogen means going beyond the reported cases. To contribute a reported case, the person must become ill, must seek medical care, the physician must ask for a laboratory test, the patient must provide a specimen for diagnostic study, the specimen must yield evidence of the pathogen, and the case must be reported. Slippage at each point means that the diagnosed cases are likely to represent only a small fraction of the cases that actually occur. Other measures of severe infection, such as hospital discharge summary records and cause of death as reported on death certificates, may be used to estimate the total number of hospitalizations and deaths due to acute enteric disease, but these measures significantly underreport specific infections, as laboratory diagnoses may often not be reflected in the discharge or death certificate coding. In 1999, we published a report estimating the actual acute health burden of foodborne disease in the United States (Mead et al., 1999).

These estimates were assembled from a variety of data collected by FoodNet and other sources. FoodNet population surveys measure the number of cases of acute gastroenteritis that actually occur and the proportion of these that seek care and are cultured (Herikstad et al., 2002). The FoodNet clinical laboratory surveys measure the likelihood that a specimen will be routinely tested for say, *Salmonella* or *Campylobacter* or *E. coli* O157 (Voetsch et al., 2004a). This information can then be used to amplify the number of cases that are diagnosed and reported; in this way FoodNet estimated that there are actually 38 cases of salmonellosis for every one that is diagnosed and reported (Voetsch et al., 2004b). FoodNet data also provide the number of diagnosed salmonellosis cases that lead to hospitalization and the number that lead to death. Doubling that number to account for cases that were not cultured provides a conservative estimate of the total number of hospitalizations and deaths. Using similar data and assumptions, the incidence of other infections under surveillance by FoodNet can also be estimated, and by use of a uniform set of assumptions and expert opinion it is possible to estimate the overall burden of known enteric infections at some 39 million infections per year (Mead et al., 1999).

The next step was to estimate the proportion of these infections that are transmitted through food, rather than through water, direct contact with ill children, or other pathways. The estimated proportion of infections that are transmitted through foods varied by pathogen, and in sum was 38 percent. Thus, of 39 million enteric infections estimated to be caused by the known enteric pathogens, 16 million were attributed to food. A curious observation is that the estimate of acute enteric illness developed pathogen by pathogen (annual incidence of 39 million cases) is substantially less than the total amount of acute gastroenteritis in the population estimated by population survey (annual incidence of 211 million cases) (Mead et al., 1999). This "diagnostic gap" suggests that there are more pathogens yet to be discovered (Tauxe, 2002). The fraction of these other cases not accounted for by known pathogens that might be attributed to food is not directly measurable. The authors of the 1999 estimate chose 38 percent, the summary statistic for the known pathogens, as the best point estimate of what it might be for the other acute illnesses not accounted for by known pathogens. The final estimate, 76 million illnesses, 323,000 hospitalizations, and 5,000 deaths, refers to the year 1997. This comprehensive estimate is now being revised in a similar stepwise approach, starting with the measurement of the overall burden of acute gastroenteritis and with more refined and pathogen-specific approaches to the estimates of unreported illness.

There are other ways of measuring the burden of unreported illness. In the United Kingdom, the Intestinal Infectious Diseases study empanelled a group of citizens who recorded their symptoms prospectively and provided stool specimens for even mild cases of diarrheal illness (Wheeler et al., 1999). The Dutch SENSOR study followed a similar strategy, working with a group of sentinel general practitioners and their patients (de Wit et al., 2001). Both European approaches depended on the national healthcare system itself to provide a population-based framework, and both were sufficiently expensive that they have not been repeated. There are also measures of burden other than simple counts of cases, hospitalizations, and deaths. For example, the health-related costs for the principal bacterial foodborne pathogens (*Salmonella*, *Campylobacter*, *E. coli* O157, other Shiga-toxin-producing *E. coli*, and *Listeria monocytogenes*) have been estimated to be $6.9 billion (ERS, 2000). The cost to society associated with the estimated number of deaths that were not attributed to known etiologies could be as high as $17 billion, underlining the need for further refinement of this sector of the estimate (Frenzen, 2004). Inclusion of the postinfectious sequelae in the estimate can also greatly increase the economic burden. A detailed model developed for *Campylobacter* in the Netherlands included the burden of postinfectious arthritides and Guillain-Barre syndrome and measured the burden in disability-adjusted life years; this estimate indicated that a greater burden was due to the sequelae, rather than the acute illness (Havelaar et al., 2005). The industry costs of disrupted trade and development that can be occasioned by foodborne illness can be enormous, though they usually do not appear on the public health ledger. The costs of antimicrobial resistance associated with foodborne exposures have also not been estimated, but they might include the cost of illness caused by resistant foodborne pathogens and the costs related to the spread of transmissible resistance genes that are present in commensal organisms in the food supply, from which they may transfer to human pathogens.

Prevention of Emerging Foodborne Threats: The Importance of the Outbreak Investigation

The prevention of foodborne diseases in general is a complex effort, involving many different actors along the chain of production from the farm to food service. There are many different pathogens involved, almost none of which are vaccine preventable in the final consumer. Educating consumers, food handlers, and producers about their role in preventing foodborne disease is important, but not sufficient. Contamination of food can occur at many points from farm to table. Often the key to prevention is to understand those mechanisms of contamination well enough to prevent them, before the food reaches the final consumer. Investigation of contamination events, and especially investigation of outbreaks, is critical to understanding the mechanisms of contamination. Prevention often means reengineering food processes and policies for safety, usually with a focus on a specific food and/or pathogen.

The foodborne outbreak investigation is thus a major driver for enhancing overall food safety. When an outbreak is detected, the first priority is to learn enough to prevent further cases from occurring in the current outbreak. However, it is also an opportunity to learn something new, and to open research agendas with impact far beyond the one outbreak. Many foodborne pathogens were first identified in the course of an outbreak investigation. A new combination of pathogen and food may be revealed that needs further study by food scientists, animal and plant pathologists, as well as medical researchers. Just as the National Transportation Safety Board investigates a plane crash thoroughly after the fact to learn how to prevent similar ones, careful investigation even after an outbreak is over can define gaps in the system, stimulate further specific research, and indicate the needs for new processes or regulations. New combinations of specific pathogens and foods identified by outbreak investigations have been critical to guiding research and prevention (see Table 3-2).

As the surveillance systems that we use in the United States have been enhanced in the last 10 years, we have observed a change in the number and nature of outbreaks detected. This is a paradox of surveillance: making surveillance better often reveals more of the problem, so that the actual public health burden appears worse. For example, as noted above, the number of foodborne outbreaks reported through the Electronic Foodborne Outbreak Reporting System doubled following relatively simple improvements in process and participation. PulseNet has caused a more substantial change in the nature of the outbreaks detected. By increasing the signal-to-noise ratio for specific pathogen subtypes, PulseNet makes it far more likely that geographically diffuse outbreaks will be detected. Those diffuse outbreaks are particularly instructive.

PulseNet has had a profound impact on the kind of outbreaks that have been detected because the nature of the outbreaks detected depends critically on the methods used to detect them. If outbreaks only come to the attention of public health when concerned citizens, physicians, or healthcare facilities report them, then only large and locally apparent outbreaks are likely to be detected. These

TABLE 3-2 Some New Pathogen-Food Combinations Characterized During Outbreak Investigations in the United States

Pathogen	Food
E. coli O157	Beef, apple cider, and sprouts
Salmonella serotype Enteritidis	Eggs, broilers, and almonds
Salmonella Poona	Cantaloupe
Multidrug resistant *Salmonella* Newport	Ground beef and raw milk cheese
Salmonella Javiana, Newport, and Braenderup	Tomatoes
Listeria monocytogenes	Sliced luncheon turkey, hot dogs, and Mexican queso fresco
Cyclospora	Raspberries and basil
Norovirus	Raw oysters, salads, and sliced luncheon meats
Hepatitis A	Strawberries and green onions

classic point source outbreaks often affect a single group of people in a single town or city, following a single meal, with a substantial attack rate. Investigating this outbreak proceeds with local authority, and the food-handling problems that are identified are often local in scope. Although important, these investigations may have greatest impact at the local level.

The use of molecular subtyping to compare strains across many jurisdictions has revealed an entirely different kind of outbreak in which a dispersed group of persons who do not know each other are affected at the same time with the same infecting organism in many different locations. In this scenario, no local listening post may perceive more than a few cases, and the local increase is often not apparent against the background of cases. Although each individual case may appear to be sporadic, the outbreak may in fact be very large but dispersed. Investigating these dispersed scenario outbreaks requires the coordinated efforts of many health authorities acting in concert and pooling the information. Though difficult to detect and to investigate, the findings of these outbreaks can be of particular importance. The dispersion may well reflect a contamination event high in the food's chain of production, not just a problem in the final kitchen. Identifying that event can instruct the industry and regulatory authorities about a flaw in the system that was previously unappreciated. Correcting it can lead to lasting and generalized protection across the country.

This means that improved detection and investigation can serve to probe the safety of the food production system at several levels. These investigations, providing information about gaps in the food safety system, drive the cycle of prevention faster and reduce the overall number of infections. The results of enhanced prevention can be seen in the recent declines in the incidence of infections with *Listeria monocytogenes* and *E. coli* O157, the two pathogens tracked most intensively by PulseNet. Following the institution of PulseNet surveillance for *Listeria monocytogenes*, there was an important increase in the number of outbreaks detected (Figure 3-2). Many of these were related to processed meats, focusing prevention efforts on that sector; incidence declined to an all time low of 2.7 per million in 2004, a drop of 40 percent since the baseline period 1996–1998 (CDC, 2005c). The incidence of *E. coli* O157 infections began to decrease sharply after 2002, as the repeated investigations of pulsed-field gel electrophoresis clusters focused attention on more specific controls at the level of ground beef. By 2004, the incidence of *E. coli* O157 infections as measured in FoodNet had dropped 42 percent since the baseline period of 1996–1998, and was 0.9 per 100,0000, below the goals set by Healthy People 2010. It is doubtful that such progress would have been made without PulseNet.

The most recent outbreak surveillance information published for *E. coli* O157:H7 also illustrates how improved surveillance can first produce a sharp increase in reported outbreaks, followed by a drop as better prevention strategies take effect (Figure 3-3) (Rangel et al., 2005). In the 1980s, *E. coli* O157 outbreaks of infection were rare, perhaps because the pathogen itself was less com-

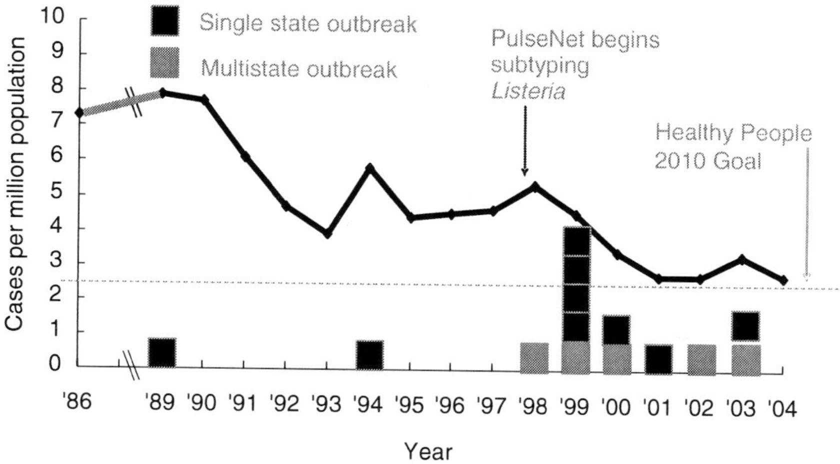

FIGURE 3-2 Reported incidence of *Listeria monocytogenes* infections and reported outbreaks of listeriosis, United States, 1986–2004.
SOURCES: Adapted from Tappero et al. (1995); CDC (2006a,b).

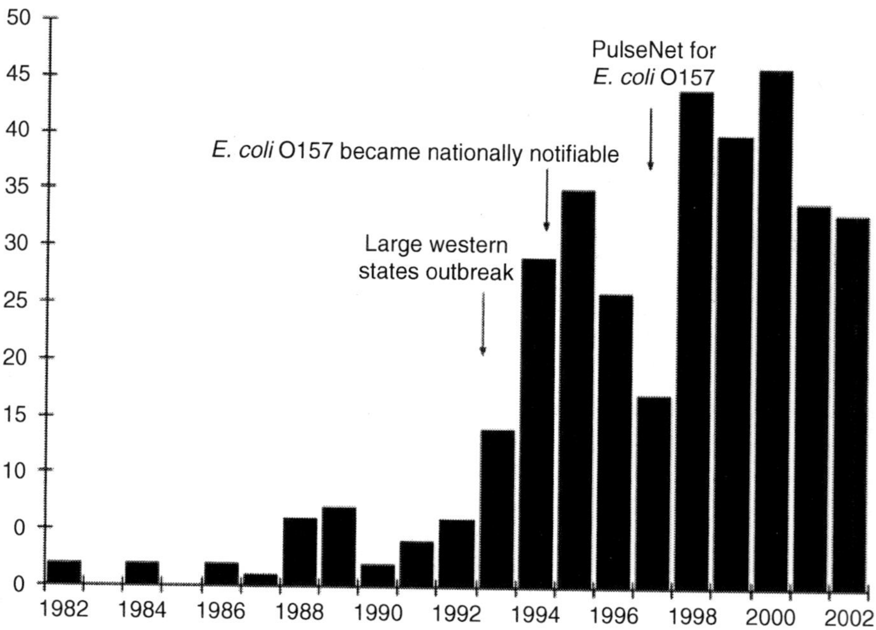

FIGURE 3-3 Reported outbreaks of *E. coli* O157 infections, United States, 1982–2002.
SOURCE: Rangel et al. (2005).

mon, but also because it was not likely to be diagnosed or reported. Washington, the first state to make it a notifiable condition, did so in 1988. After the large Western states outbreak of 1993, centered in Washington, many other states made it notifiable, and it became nationally notifiable in 1994. At the same time, an education effort targeting clinical laboratories promoted simple laboratory screening for the pathogen. It is not surprising that the number of reported outbreaks jumped to more than 30 in 1994, and then began to decline, as many in the fast-food industry and homes changed burger cooking procedures to avoid undercooking. In 1996–1997, in the first FoodNet case-control study of sporadic *E. coli* O157:H7 infections, eating burgers at a fast-food restaurant was no longer associated with illness, though it had been in earlier studies (Kassenborg et al., 2004). Following the launch of PulseNet, the number of reported outbreaks more than doubled again in 1998, and since then has generally trended downwards as other prevention measures have been enacted. As noted above, the biggest decrease may have happened after 2002, after new procedures to reduce the contamination of ground beef were implemented, though the impact of those on *E. coli* O157:H7 outbreaks has not yet been summarized in print.

Constraints and Limitations on Using Outbreaks to Drive Control and Prevention

Detecting and investigating foodborne outbreaks triggers public health intervention, but as a prevention system, this has built in delays. Most obviously, it is not activated until after people are exposed, become ill, and the outbreak is detected. Often the outbreak is actually over by the time it is detected, making the outbreak investigation itself a blunt instrument for achieving control over single brief exposures to contamination. There are biology-dependent delays, like the incubation period between the moment of exposure and the onset of symptoms, which can vary from less than a day for some pathogens to several weeks for others. Delays in diagnosis may depend on when the typical patient feels sufficiently ill to consult a physician and on how long the laboratory tests take to yield a diagnosis. Signal delay depends on the time it takes to accumulate enough cases in one database to be detectable as a distinct cluster and may be longer if cases are more dispersed. There are also the resource-dependent delays that depend critically on support that surveillance gets in the private and public sectors. Clinical laboratories may batch isolates for shipment to the public health laboratory to cut shipping costs, adding delays. The speed of testing strains in public health laboratories also depends on the available resources. Interviewing cases and tracing implicated foods back to their sources depends on the availability of trained and supported investigative staff, for whom this is part of their core work duties, not a distraction from the "real" work they must accomplish.

Many state and local health departments lack sufficient capacity to effectively investigate outbreaks. For example, in a recently published survey of state health departments, 88 percent reported there were barriers to more active case finding, and 30 percent reported that they lacked adequate epidemiological staff to conduct investigations. Outbreaks go uninvestigated for a number of reasons, the most common of which are delayed notification (83 percent of those respondents) and lack of staff (67 percent). Many state public health laboratories are also understaffed and under supported, making real-time testing of submitted strains difficult and leaving them with little surge capacity for emergencies (APHL, 2003).

Pooling Resources

The fundamental ability to detect and investigate outbreaks is critical to the response to any new threat, be it intentional or natural in origin. In the only two intentional foodborne attacks involving bacterial infectious agents in recent experience in the United States, local and state health departments detected and responded to outbreaks as a matter of course; it was not recognized at the outset that the events were intentional in origin (Torok et al., 1997; Kolavic et al., 1997). Some states have recognized that robust public health surveillance is a fundamental part of protecting the public health against both natural and intentional events, and the infusion of new resources to strengthen the response to bioterror threats has improved surveillance and response capacity in general. However, in many others, bioterror response resources have lured staff and attention away from the traditional activities of public health, leaving those systems weaker than before. Yet actual foodborne bioterror events remain remarkably rare. During the last 25 years, two have been documented, while during this same time, applying the recent Electronic Foodborne Outbreak Reporting System number of 1,200 foodborne outbreaks a year, there were an estimated 30,000 nonintentional foodborne outbreaks. Like firefighters in a firehouse restricted to arson fires, the dedicated squad will have to practice its skills in drills and table top exercises, while their less well-equipped and perhaps less well-paid colleagues put out all the fires, which must occur before the fire can be determined to be arson or not.

Enhancing Foodborne Outbreak Investigations

Despite the many constraints, the response to foodborne outbreak investigations can be improved substantially. Expanding routine subtyping to a greater number of isolates and different pathogens may help drive prevention faster and more broadly. Faster and more automated subtyping methods, including sequenced-based methods for both bacteria and viruses, need to be deployed as the cost and complexity of sequencing equipment decreases. Cluster detection can be speeded by providing the resources for swift transport and real-time testing rather than batch processing. Routine case interviews can be made more swift and standardized, and they can be integrated with control interviews to make investigation rapid. Improving the record keeping necessary for accurate tracing of foods to their sources, and increasing the skilled capacity in the state and national regulatory agencies to perform such investigations would speed that critical phase of investigations. Fingerprinting the pathogens isolated from foods and food animals in real time and linking those data with the human isolate database would make it possible to rapidly generate hypotheses about potential sources. Expanding the capacity for surveillance in other countries around the world and expanding regional and global surveillance networks to detect and investigate outbreaks can enhance the detection of foodborne threats at home and abroad (Tauxe and Hughes, 1996).

Conclusion

Enhancing foodborne surveillance, outbreak detection and response means better public health. Outbreaks will continue to occur, and people will continue to get ill, but with effective response, these unfortunate events can drive prevention. FoodNet is providing better data to measure trends and burden of illness and to determine sources of sporadic infections. PulseNet, the new network for molecular subtyping, is blurring the line between obvious outbreaks and apparently sporadic cases, and it is probing more deeply into the safety of the entire food system. Investigating and learning from the outbreaks is critical to achieving continuous improvement in food safety. As the public health system is likely to be the first responders in the event of an intentional attack, as well as for the far more frequent unintentional outbreaks, having a more robust and effective response is better for the public protection in either event.

THE ONGOING SAGA OF U.S. OUTBREAKS OF CYCLOSPORIASIS ASSOCIATED WITH IMPORTED FRESH PRODUCE: WHAT *CYCLOSPORA CAYETANENSIS* HAS TAUGHT US AND WHAT WE HAVE YET TO LEARN

Barbara L. Herwaldt, M.D., M.P.H.[3]
Centers for Disease Control and Prevention[4]

. . . For disease will peer up over the hedge
of health, with only its eyes showing . . .
For there will be computers
For there will be hard data and they will be hard
to understand

[3]Medical Epidemiologist in the Division of Parasitic Diseases.

[4]The findings and conclusions in this manuscript have not been formally disseminated by the CDC and should not be construed to represent any agency determination or policy.

For the trivial will trap you and the important escape you
For the Committee will be unable to resolve the question
For there will be the arts
    and some will call them
    soft data
    whereas in fact they are the hard data
    by which our lives are lived . . .

—John Stone (Stone, 2004)

Prologue: An Ongoing Tale of Two Settings, Viewed from Multiple Perspectives

Cyclospora cayetanensis infection is endemic in many resource-poor and middle-income countries (Bern et al., 1999, 2000; Herwaldt, 2000; Lopez et al., 2003; Ortega et al., 1993). The United States, a resource-rich consumer country, has unwittingly imported this foreign, enigmatic parasite along with fresh produce that has been linked to outbreaks of cyclosporiasis. From the U.S. perspective, the unforeseen emergence of this microscopic pathogen has evolved into an ongoing tale of large foodborne outbreaks, which have entailed crossing jurisdictional borders and working with foreign governments, produce growers, and trade organizations (CDC, 1998, 2004; Herwaldt, 2000; Herwaldt et al., 1997, 1999; Ho et al., 2002; Lopez et al., 2001).

The parasite *C. cayetanensis*, which was christened in 1994 (Ortega et al., 1994), and the precedent-setting series of outbreaks of cyclosporiasis continue to be sources of fascination, frustration, challenges, and learning opportunities for the persons, agencies, industries, and governments they have directly or indirectly affected. The parasite and various aspects of the outbreaks (e.g., coordination of multisite investigations, interactions with foreign sources of implicated produce, regulatory responses when the mode of contamination is unknown, impacts on international trade) have been and continue to be subjects of case studies (Calvin, 2003; Jackson, 2006; Powell, 1998), including a U.S. Senate hearing in 1998 entitled *The Safety of Food Imports: From the Farm to the Table: A Case Study of Tainted Imported Fruit* (U.S. Senate, 1998) and this case study, which was presented in part at the IOM's October 2005 workshop on food safety.[5]

This case study—in which the parasite and the U.S. outbreaks are viewed with a wide-angle lens that includes public health, societal, and historical contexts—focuses on food for thought (e.g., perspectives, principles, and issues for the public health community to ponder) rather than detailed commentary about foodborne threats to health or comprehensive review of the outbreaks of cyclo-

[5]Forum on Microbial Threats. 2005 (October 25–26). "Foodborne Threats to Health: The Practice and Policies of Surveillance, Prevention, Outbreak Investigations, and International Coordination," Washington, D.C.

sporiasis. In the text of the article, selected details about the parasite and the outbreaks are included for illustrative purposes, such as to underscore lessons learned, relearned, or yet to be learned and to highlight common themes (e.g., challenges intrinsic to emerging pathogens). Supplemental details and perspective are provided in figures (Figure 3-4, Figure 3-5) and tables (Tables 3-3 through 3-6, which may be found at the end of this article in Annexes 3-1 through 3-4). Table 3-4 and Table 3-5 represent attempts to list and dissect the elements of foodborne outbreaks and investigations to demonstrate what various ingredients add to the mix (e.g., the challenges, opportunities, and approaches if the etiologic agent is an enigmatic parasite).[6]

Investigating the initial outbreaks in the 1990s would have been even more difficult than it was if *Cyclospora* and cyclosporiasis had emerged in the United States as complete unknowns. The fact that they did not reflects the contributions and astute observations of relatively few persons with expertise in parasitology and tropical medicine, in diverse places such as Papua New Guinea, Peru, and Nepal (Ashford, 1979; Hoge et al., 1995; Ortega et al., 1993, 1994). Their efforts culminated in fundamental scientific and medical advances, described in articles published seemingly just in the nick of time. Through studies in Peru, the confusion about the identity of the organism was resolved: it is not a species of blue-green algae (cyanobacteria); it is a coccidian parasite, the first and only species in the *Cyclospora* genus known to infect humans (Ortega et al., 1993, 1994). In a placebo-controlled clinical trial in Nepal, the antimicrobial combination of trimethoprim-sulfamethoxazole was demonstrated to be highly effective treatment of cyclosporiasis (Hoge et al., 1995), the first and only such therapy to have been documented (Table 3-3, Annex 3-1).

Unfortunately, the parasitologists were not prophets: the experts were as surprised as the novices by the unpredicted U.S. emergence of *C. cayetanensis* and by the unprecedented association between a parasite and large, common-source foodborne outbreaks. Although other enteric parasites are known to be transmissible by contaminated food, nothing remotely comparable to the widespread, recurrent outbreaks of cyclosporiasis has been documented in the United States for any other parasite. The first of the series of major eruptions of *C. cayetanensis* on the international scene occurred in the spring of 1996, after premonitory rumblings earlier in the decade (Herwaldt, 2000; Huang et al., 1995; Koumans et al.,

---

[6]Table 3-4 and Table 3-5, which are complementary, have the same column headings—i.e., outbreaks/investigations in general, the etiologic agent *C. cayetanensis*, fresh produce vehicles, and foreign sources. In Table 3-4, which focuses on the characteristics of outbreaks/investigations, the row headings distinguish outbreaks/investigations in general and outbreaks with various characteristics (i.e., large, multisite, concurrent, recurrent, seasonal, and associated with high attack rates). In Table 3-5, which focuses on the goals of outbreak investigations, the row headings distinguish the processes of identifying food vehicles, their sources, sites/modes of contamination, and control measures. Additional perspectives about the scientific and communication challenges highlighted in Table 3-4 and Table 3-5 are provided in Table 3-3 and Table 3-6, respectively.

1998). The eruption in 1996 took the form of a large (>1,000 reported cases[7]), multinational outbreak of cyclosporiasis in two countries, the United States and Canada, that was linked to a third country, Guatemala, where the epidemiologically implicated raspberries were grown (Herwaldt et al., 1997).

The modus operandi of this pathogen in the United States as the etiologic agent of outbreaks has not changed during the subsequent decade, although the repertoire of food vehicles and sources has expanded beyond raspberries from Guatemala to include assorted types of fresh produce from several middle-income countries (Table 3-4, Annex 3-2; Table 3-5, Annex 3-3). The saga of outbreaks appears to have evolved into an interminable tome, with no end in sight. Its inscrutable chief character, *C. cayetanensis*, a unicellular (protozoan) parasite, continues to wreck havoc, surprise, outsmart, baffle, and bewilder us (Table 3-3, Annex 3-1). As discussed in this article, *Cyclospora* epitomizes the challenges intrinsic to addressing obscure pathogens that appear, seemingly out of nowhere, including how and why the challenges translate into difficulties investigating and preventing outbreaks and communicating among health professionals, the general public, and the produce industry. The scientific unknowns and political overtones are among the factors that have complicated efforts to communicate and collaborate (see Tables 3-4 through 3-6, Annexes 3-2 through 3-4).

Cyclospora, the U.S. outbreaks of cyclosporiasis, and their aftermaths have affected physical, economic, and communal health in exporter and importer nations (Calvin, 2003; Herwaldt, 2000; Jackson, 2006; Powell, 1998) (Table 3-6, Annex 3-4). The need to invest resources to investigate the outbreaks has resulted in increased recognition of and interest in this parasite and its effects on the persons, products, and places where *Cyclospora* infection is endemic. The extent to which the heightened awareness will stimulate long-term investments in multidisciplinary, multilingual research activities; the research will solve remaining mysteries about this elusive pathogen, its quirky human hosts, and their micro- and macrohabitats; and the increased knowledge will be translated into wisdom, vision, and sustainable, effective, transnational prevention and control measures remains to be seen and recorded. The potential for additional scientific advances to have positive ripple effects that extend beyond *Cyclospora* and cyclosporiasis is high.

---

[7]Although the true magnitude of the outbreak in North America in 1996 is unknown, 1,465 cases of cyclosporiasis were reported (including 1,270 [87 percent] in the United States, in 20 states and the District of Columbia), which dwarfed the total number of cases previously documented worldwide (Herwaldt et al., 1997). In the raspberry-associated outbreak in 1997, the case count was 1,012 (including 981 [97 percent] in the United States, in 17 states and the District of Columbia) (Herwaldt et al., 1999). The total number of reported cases in the series of outbreaks in North America from 1995–2005 exceeds 4,000. The admonition to remember that cases occur in real persons bears repeating (Baron, 1985). As expressed by a physician to the medical students she mentors: "... you have not finished your work until you have taken care of the patient, not just the problem" (Treadway, 2006).

Challenges in Addressing Public Health Issues in General and Foodborne Outbreaks of Cyclosporiasis in Particular

Addressing public health issues, even ostensibly straightforward matters, can be difficult in part because of competing demands for scarce resources. The challenges are compounded for chronic issues such as foodborne cyclosporiasis that are associated with confounding complexities and unknowns. Figure 3-4 and the text in this section of the article represent attempts, replete with mixed metaphors, to place the challenges in perspective by depicting and describing the elements of a support structure for a public health bridge between disease and prevention and control. The goal (i.e., to bridge the chasm between disease and prevention and control), the base on which the support structure for the bridge is built (i.e., the public health infrastructure), and the societal and historical contexts for public health activities are not unique to cyclosporiasis.

Building and maintaining a structurally sound, science-grounded bridge are challenging (i.e., are uphill struggles, as depicted by the angle of the bridge). The instability and vulnerability of the base (soil) are major impediments. The infra-

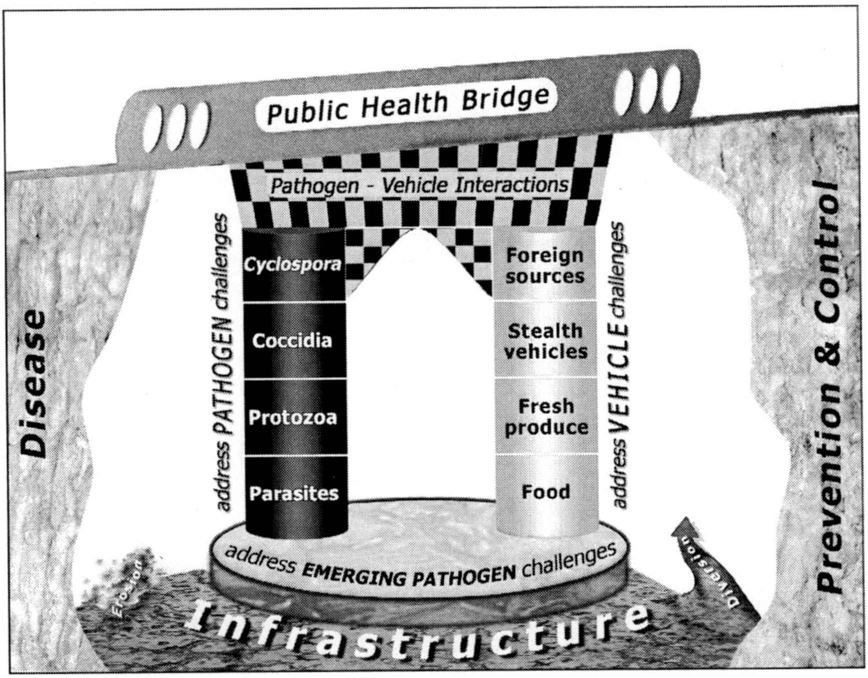

FIGURE 3-4 Generic and *Cyclospora*-specific challenges in bridging the chasm between disease and prevention and control.
SOURCE: B. Herwaldt and D. Juranek, CDC, Division of Parasitic Diseases, April 2006 (see Acknowledgments).

structure is portrayed as underground (unseen), overburdened, stretched, atrophied, eroded, and diverted. The impoverished infrastructure includes the residual resources of all types, at all tiers (e.g., local, state, federal) of the public health system. Core infrastructure constraints can be appreciated through the lens of an analogy, in which the public health system is viewed as an internal combustion engine, subject to the laws of thermodynamics (see footnote for details).[8] Revitalizing the infrastructure will require commitment, concerted effort, and coordination from and among all tiers of the public health system, as well as great wisdom and vision, archetypical eroded, diverted elements.

Addressing foodborne cyclosporiasis entails adding more loads to the overburdened infrastructure in the form of the support elements for the public health bridge between disease and prevention and control. The elements are depicted as:

- a foundation stone, which symbolizes the importance of addressing fundamental constraints intrinsic to emerging pathogens; and
- pathogen and vehicle pillars (support columns), which symbolize the needs to address the superimposed challenges specific to the type of pathogen (the unique peculiarities of the coccidian parasite *C. cayetanensis* [Table 3-3, Annex 3-1]) and the types of food vehicles (not just fresh produce, but imported produce served in inconspicuous ways, such as garnishes [Table 3-4, Annex 3-2; Table 3-5, Annex 3-3]).

A multidimensional, complex web of interactions is depicted by the checkerboard pattern under the bridge. Although the concept of pathogen-vehicle interactions is highlighted, additional types of interactions (synergisms, antagonisms, collaborations, feedback loops) among the elements of the support structure for the bridge, the infrastructure, and society at large are germane (Table 3-4, Annex 3-2; Table 3-5, Annex 3-3). The fact that the parasite *C. cayetanensis* is emerging while parasitologists are becoming an endangered species is an ironic example of a negative pathogen-infrastructure interaction.

The public health infrastructure is further stretched and strained if the challenges associated with emerging pathogens must be addressed in the context of emergencies (the extraordinary demands associated with large, multisite outbreaks [Table 3-4])—i.e., if a base of scientific knowledge about the pathogen

[8]Within the public health system (engine), resources (internal energy) are constantly being consumed (e.g., scarce financial and personnel resources are becoming scarcer), regardless of whether the system is idling or moving an agenda and whether the direction of the movement is forward or backward. Although resources can be converted from one type or state to another (e.g., from dollars to devices and from federal to state programs), as well as redistributed, recycled, and diverted, they cannot be created *de novo*; acquisition of new resources requires infusions from, or collaborations with, other systems. The positive spin on the need for outside input is that it provides opportunities for invaluable perspective and reality checks.

and databases for outbreaks must be created concurrently and on the fly. If the infrastructure withstands the cumulative burden of many converging stresses, outbreak investigations, in concert with basic and applied research activities, provide opportunities to solve mysteries through scientific advances and to identify and reinforce weak elements in the public health system (Buchanan, 1997; Hall, 1997; Tauxe, 1997) (see Table 3-4, Annex 3-2; Table 3-5, Annex 3-3). The yin of outbreaks can be partially converted into yang, by translating challenges into opportunities into advancements in science and the public good.

Challenges in Addressing Emerging Pathogens, Parasites, and *Cyclospora cayetanensis*

Emerging Pathogens

The challenges intrinsic to emerging pathogens—particularly to newly described orphan microbes without close relations—include many constraints, all of which did or still apply, to varying degrees, to *C. cayetanensis*, the quintessential emerging pathogen (Table 3-3, Annex 3-1). The constraints include:

- *lack of* fundamental knowledge about the biology of the organism (e.g., life cycle) and therefore the epidemiology of infection (e.g., modes of transmission), which translate into difficulties predicting the behavior of the organism (e.g., responses to environmental stimuli), determining the pertinent questions to include in epidemiologic surveys, and evaluating the plausibility of competing hypotheses in outbreak investigations (Tables 3-4 through 3-6, Annexes 3-2 through 3-4);
- *lack of* competence and expertise among specialists (e.g., parasitologists), let alone *lack of* general knowledge and familiarity among other health professionals and lay persons (i.e., the little known by supposed experts is not widely known or readily accessible);
- *lack of* tools (e.g., analytic methods, techniques to propagate viable organisms, decontamination strategies); and
- *lack of* research materials (e.g., ample quantities/isolates of the organism).

The handicaps can be restated and classified in such categories as ignorance ("don't have a clue but wish I knew"), uncertainty ("not sure and might be wrong"), unpredictability ("wouldn't even hazard a guess"), unfamiliarity ("don't ask me"), and unavailability ("urgently need but don't have"), further modified by the likelihood the formidable obstacles can be overcome in the foreseeable future.

Parasites, Including Cyclospora cayetanensis

Many of these constraints apply to parasites, even to those not considered emerging pathogens per se. For example, as a broad generalization, health professionals and lay persons are less knowledgeable about and familiar with parasites than bacteria. Addressing foodborne enteric parasites—particularly protozoa, which include the coccidia *C. cayetanensis* and *Cryptosporidium* species[9] (Table 3-3, Annex 3-1)—requires a paradigm shift. Although the statement that protozoa are not bacteria is a truism, the ramifications of the fact that protozoa do not behave like bacteria (e.g., do not multiply outside the host, in the environment, or in food) have been difficult to communicate.

The scientific and communication challenges posed by foodborne outbreaks of cyclosporiasis have been exacerbated by the different characteristics and behaviors of the major enteric coccidia (Table 3-3, Annex 3-1). An example of a fundamental biologic difference with epidemiologic ramifications is that *Cryptosporidium* oocysts (the environmental stage of coccidia) in freshly excreted stool are infective, whereas *Cyclospora* oocysts are not; they must mature (sporulate) outside the host to become infective, which is thought to require days to weeks under favorable environmental conditions (Table 3-3, Annex 3-1; Figure 3-5). The identified differences between *Cyclospora* and *Cryptosporidium* species in the realms of what is known about them underscore the potential risks of extrapolating from the knowns about *Cryptosporidium* species to fill gaps in knowledge about *Cyclospora*. The persistence of many enigmas about *C. cayetanensis* reflects the elusive search for pertinent model systems, the paucity of *Cyclospora* oocysts available for research purposes, and the pathogen's short recorded history, as recounted below.

Challenges Entailed in Discovering and Classifying *Cyclospora cayetanensis* (1977–1994)

Reverberating Themes

Portions of the chronicle of the (re)discovery and (re)classification of the pathogen christened *C. cayetanensis* in 1994 are retold and dissected here to underscore recurring themes in the ongoing saga of cyclosporiasis, including common themes for emerging pathogens. Examples of such themes include the importance of:

- distinctions between signals and noise and the difficulties encountered in detecting and identifying previously undescribed, nondescript, rare signals (e.g.,

[9]In this article, the terminology "*Cryptosporidium* species" refers to *C. hominis/parvum*.

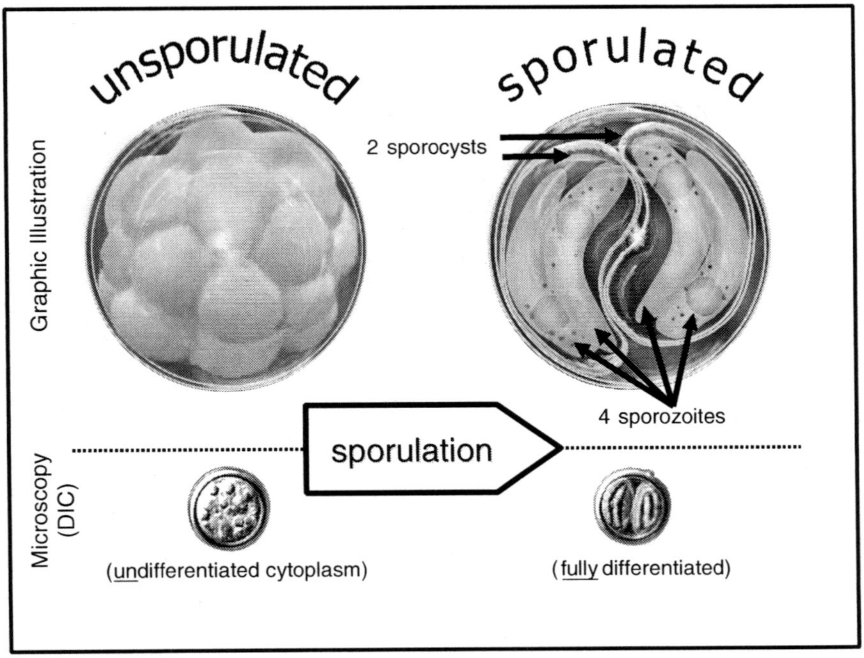

FIGURE 3-5 Sporulation of *Cyclospora cayetanensis* oocysts. Unsporulated and sporulated *C. cayetanensis* oocysts are shown in graphic illustrations (top) and photographs (bottom), as viewed by differential interference contrast (DIC) microscopy, a specialized type of microscopy that markedly accentuates morphologic features (Herwaldt, 2000). Persons infected with *Cyclospora* shed immature, unsporulated oocysts (8–10 μm in diameter), which are thought to require days to weeks in favorable environmental conditions to sporulate and become infective (Ortega et al., 1993) (Table 3-3, Annex 3-1).
SOURCE: B. Herwaldt and D. Juranek, CDC, Division of Parasitic Diseases, April 2006 (see Acknowledgments).

pathogens, outbreaks, contaminated produce) in complex mixtures of noise (e.g., stool specimens, surveillance data, salads);

- careful observations by trained, experienced persons (e.g., clinicians, laboratorians, epidemiologists), who, at a minimum, realize they are seeing something that is or might be unusual and know where to turn for help and confirmation (Table 3-3, Annex 3-1; Table 3-4, Annex 3-2);
- basic skills (e.g., looking, seeing, watching, waiting, counting, thinking, writing, reading);
- basic materials (e.g., stool specimens for diagnostic purposes and oocysts for research purposes [Table 3-3, Annex 3-1]); and
- basic tools (e.g., microscopes for detecting oocysts and telephones for expeditious reporting of cases and potential outbreaks of cyclosporiasis).

Distinguishing Signals and Noise: Detecting Parasites Amidst the Sea of Specks in Stool Specimens

Detection and identification of protozoa, even those already known to be pathogens, by light-microscopic examination of stool specimens, is labor intensive and challenging. When viewed by light microscopy, stool specimens appear to be seas of specks; environmental samples have even more specks, lures, and pathogen imposters. Determining which of the specks are or might be parasites is difficult, especially if methods for highlighting or tagging the pertinent specks are unavailable (Table 3-3, Annex 3-1). *Cyclospora* oocysts (8–10 µm in diameter) can easily be missed; the oocysts in freshly excreted stool (i.e., those seen by clinical microbiologists) are unsporulated, with undifferentiated, nondescript cytoplasm and typically are shed at low levels (Table 3-3, Annex 3-1; Figure 3-5) (Herwaldt, 2000).

The Ashford and Ortega Chapters

In retrospect,[10] the first three described cases of *C. cayetanensis* infection were detected in 1977 and 1978, by Ashford, a British parasitologist working in Papua New Guinea (Ashford, 1979). If someone without Ashford's extraordinary eye for detail and parasitologic expertise had looked through the oculars of the microscope during "routine stool examination" of the patients' specimens, the presence and importance of the odd, "scanty" structures in the specimens almost assuredly would have been missed or dismissed. Ashford's discovery is all the more remarkable because techniques that facilitate detection and identification of this organism were not yet available (Table 3-3, Annex 3-1).

Explicitly listing the steps (ingredients) entailed in Ashford's discovery is illustrative.

- He took the time to examine the stool specimens (i.e., he had to "look" to be able to "see").
- He found/saw the "scanty" structures (unsporulated oocysts) in the sea of specks (i.e., he detected the "signal" despite the "noise").
- He took note of them and realized that they were microbes, not debris (i.e., he both "saw" and "perceived").
- He recognized that they were unusual ("distinct") (i.e., he had sufficient experience to distinguish "usual/typical" from "unusual/atypical").
- He recognized that they had features suggestive of coccidian oocysts (i.e., he had sufficient knowledge to begin to categorize the structures).

---

[10]Some aspects of the *Cyclospora* chronicle are clear only if viewed through the retrospectoscope, which underscores the importance of reevaluating conclusions (e.g., from ongoing and prior outbreak investigations [Table 3-4]), as additional data and insights become available.

- He monitored the structures to see whether they would sporulate (i.e., he knew how to test the hypothesis that they were coccidian oocysts and had sufficient interest to do so).
- He did not yield to the temptation to discard the specimens before sporulation finally was demonstrable (at 8 days in 1 case and 11 in another).
- He recognized his limitations: he could not discern, with confidence, the number of sporozoites (i.e., two) in each of the two sporocysts in a sporulated oocyst and realized that his tally (i.e., four) might be (and was) incorrect.
- He understood the ramifications of his limitations: he could not place the organism in a genus or christen it because precise counts of the numbers of sporozoites and sporocysts, not best guesses, are required for taxonomic classification of coccidia by traditional morphologic criteria.[11]
- But he also recognized the importance of publishing his observations, with conservative conclusions, which he did in 1979, in the *Annals of Tropical Medicine and Parasitology*, in an article entitled "Occurrence of an undescribed coccidian in man in Papua New Guinea" (Ashford, 1979).

Ashford's report (signal) about the anonymous organism he noticed was virtually unnoticed (undetected) for over a decade,[12] as, presumably, the organism had been for much longer. The Ashford chapter in this chronicle raises the first in a series of laments (e.g., "if onlys" and "what ifs"). Whether and how the course of *Cyclospora* history would have been different, if Ashford had chosen a different title or journal for his article or had worked in an ideal world, without real-world constraints, are subjects for fairy tales rather than nonfiction; in fairy tales, pathogens would emerge with passports that included their pedigrees and profiles (e.g., personal and family names, vital statistics, travel histories), as well as high-resolution photographs of their key morphologic features.

The subsequent accomplishments of parasitologists Ortega and colleagues are also remarkable. They surmounted hurdles whose height and importance can be fully appreciated only by parasitologists. In the 1980s and early 1990s, while studying *Cryptosporidium* infection in Peru, they noticed what appeared to be a "big *Cryptosporidium*" species. Fortunately, they were not content with initial impressions (the organism is not a *Cryptosporidium* species), just as Ashford had not been content with best guesses (his best guess about the number of sporozoites per sporocyst would have resulted in misplacement of the microbe in the

[11]The miscount, although understandable (i.e., because of the configuration of the crescent-shaped sporozoites [Figure 3-5]), was not a minor matter. The difference between two sporozoites in each of two sporocysts and four sporozoites per sporocyst represents the difference between the *Cyclospora* and *Isospora* genera, respectively. *Cryptosporidium* species have four naked sporozoites (no sporocysts).

[12]Searching the medical literature for potentially relevant articles about anonymous organisms is difficult.

Isospora genus). Ortega and colleagues were able to demonstrate sporulation/excystation of the structures they noticed and to determine, with confidence, the morphologic features of a sporulated oocyst (Figure 3-5), which enabled them to place the organism in the *Cyclospora* genus and to debunk speculations about its identity (e.g., a cyanobacterium-like body).[13]

They described their observations in 1993, in *The New England Journal of Medicine*, in a seminal article entitled "*Cyclospora* species: A new protozoan pathogen of humans" (Ortega et al., 1993), unaware of Ashford's report 14 years earlier in a tropical medicine journal (Ashford, 1979). Ashford read (detected) Ortega's article in 1993 and realized that it described the organism he had correctly categorized as a coccidian parasite but had been unable to classify by genus. In 1994, in an article in which Ortega and colleagues officially christened the organism as *Cyclospora cayetanensis* (Table 3-3), Ashford's contributions from back in the 1970s, from Papua New Guinea, were cited (Ortega et al., 1994).

The Incalculable Value of Cadres of Experts

The chronicle of the discovery and classification of *C. cayetanensis* underscores the importance of cultivating and retaining cadres of persons with specialized—sometimes seemingly old-fashioned—skills, tools, and depth and breadth of expertise: the expertise includes uncanny abilities to straddle decades, even centuries (e.g., to have historical memory and perspective but not be tethered to the past, and to be comfortable with both morphologic and molecular data); to ponder imponderables; and to see and connect microscopic dots (specks). Protecting and safeguarding brain trusts (i.e., preventing brain drains and diversions) is much easier and wiser than attempting to register and recover lost treasures. The key roles played by parasitologists, skilled in the fine arts of light microscopy and morphologic identification and classification of parasites, exemplified by their predecessor Antoni van Leeuwenhoek,[14] cannot be overemphasized. Their contributions not only were prerequisites for the subsequent advances in the realm of molecular biology (Orlandi et al., 2002, 2003; Relman

[13]Yet another twist in the tale was reported in the mid 1990s. Phylogenetic analyses, based on one gene (i.e., the small subunit ribosomal RNA gene), showed that *C. cayetanensis* is as closely related to some species of a different genus of coccidia—namely, the *Eimeria* genus—as some *Eimeria* species are to each other (Herwaldt, 2000; Relman et al., 1996). The biologic implications of this finding are unknown, but the ramifications for testing environmental samples are clear. Although, to date, no *Eimeria* species have been shown to be human pathogens, because they are prevalent in animals, environmental samples should be analyzed with techniques that distinguish *C. cayetanensis* from *Eimeria* species, not just other *Cyclospora* species. By traditional taxonomic (morphologic) criteria, *Eimeria* oocysts have four sporocysts (*Cyclospora* oocysts have two), each of which contains two sporozoites.

[14]Antoni van Leeuwenhoek (1632–1723), Dutch microscopist extraordinaire.

et al., 1996; Steele et al., 2003; Varma et al., 2003; Verweij et al., 2003) but continue to be essential (e.g., to date, molecular techniques cannot distinguish unsporulated and sporulated oocysts).

Challenges Associated with Detecting and Investigating the First Three Documented U.S. Outbreaks (1990 and 1995)

The accounts of the first three documented U.S. outbreaks of cyclosporiasis, which occurred in 1990 and 1995, underscore the understandable difficulties intrinsic to investigating outbreaks when little is understood about the etiologic agent (e.g., potentially pertinent questions and hypotheses are not considered or rigorously explored). All three of these outbreaks were detected because of unusual circumstances: stool specimens from the index case-patients were examined in clinical microbiology laboratories in which techniques that facilitate detection of *Cyclospora* were used routinely in parasitologic examinations (Table 3-3, Annex 3-1).

The Outbreak in Illinois in 1990: Waterborne or Foodborne?

The first documented U.S. outbreak occurred in a physicians' dormitory in Illinois, in the summer of 1990, before the confusion about the identity of the organism had been resolved. The irresolvable uncertainty about whether the outbreak was waterborne, as it then was thought to be (Huang et al., 1995), or foodborne (Herwaldt, 2000) represents another in the series of laments related to *Cyclospora.* Although the outbreak was exceptional regardless of whether it was waterborne or foodborne, not knowing the mode or vehicle of transmission translates into missed opportunities to generate and explore hypotheses and to distinguish the exceptional that did occur from that which did not.

If the outbreak was waterborne (i.e., associated with fixing a water pump and refilling storage tanks in a penthouse area of the dormitory) (Huang et al., 1995), it represents the only described U.S. waterborne outbreak of cyclosporiasis, the means by which the water supply could have become contaminated are unclear, and the median incubation period (i.e., two days) was uncharacteristically short for common-source outbreaks of cyclosporiasis and enteric protozoan diseases in general (Herwaldt, 2000). If the outbreak was foodborne, it was associated with a meal in late June, the median incubation period was characteristically long (i.e., eight days [Table 3-3, Annex 3-1]), the food vehicle is unknown (details about the ingredients of food items, including a fruit salad, and food-specific attack rates were not obtained), it was the first in a long series of documented U.S. foodborne outbreaks of cyclosporiasis, and it preceded the next described foodborne outbreaks by five years.

The Outbreaks in New York and Florida in 1995: Harbingers of the Subsequent Foodborne Outbreaks?

In 1995, two potentially related outbreaks were detected: one associated with a country club in New York in May–June and the other with two social events in Florida in May (Herwaldt, 2000; Koumans et al., 1998). In retrospect, at least one if not both of these outbreaks in 1995 presaged the raspberry-associated outbreaks that were documented in 1996, 1997, 1998 (Canada), and 2000 (Table 3-4, Annex 3-2; Table 3-5, Annex 3-3) (Herwaldt, 2000). The outbreak in New York in 1995, like the outbreak in Illinois in 1990, was initially thought to be waterborne (i.e., associated with consumption of water from coolers on a golf course). However, reevaluation of the data for the outbreak in New York, prompted by the subsequent foodborne outbreaks, indicated that the outbreak might have been associated with fruit, possibly raspberries (Herwaldt, 2000). Probably not coincidentally, New York and Florida—states with clinicians, laboratorians, and epidemiologists knowledgeable about cyclosporiasis—were the first of the total of 20 states to report cases in the multinational outbreak in 1996 linked to Guatemalan raspberries (Herwaldt, 2000).[15]

Evolving and Persisting Challenges Associated with the Next Era of Outbreaks of Cyclosporiasis: From Harbingers (in 1990 and 1995) to Sonic Booms (1996–2005)

The ongoing saga of cyclosporiasis has evolved from harbingers to serial, large outbreaks, detected during many of the seasons and most of the years in the subsequent decade (1996–2005). Despite the preparedness exercises with the harbinger outbreaks in 1990 and 1995, we[16] knew little about the biology of *Cyclospora* or the epidemiology of cyclosporiasis in 1996, when confronted with a large outbreak (1,465 reported cases), which included 55 clusters of cases (i.e., 55

[15]The positive ripple effects of training received by one person who trains others can continue for years. In Florida, microbiology staff in a community hospital had dutifully examined stool specimens for *Cyclospora* ever since a training course in the spring of 1992 (i.e., before the organism had been christened), despite detecting only two cases of infection, in persons returning from overseas travel, during the ensuing three years (Koumans et al., 1998). In June 1995, the laboratory staff detected and reported the index cases of the outbreak in 1995. The staff subsequently trained laboratorians from other hospitals in the county and a state laboratory to examine stool specimens for *Cyclospora*. The state of Florida added cyclosporiasis to its list of reportable diseases in July 1995. Laboratory and epidemiologic staff in Florida continue to play central roles in detecting and investigating outbreaks of cyclosporiasis associated with imported fresh produce (e.g., mesclun lettuce from Peru in 1997 and basil from Peru in 2005) (Herwaldt, 2000; also see the section in this chapter by R. Hammond and D. Bodager).

[16]The words *we* and *our* are used to include all potentially relevant persons and agencies, without any explicit or implicit focus on the author's roles.

minioutbreaks associated with social and other events). In retrospect, the outbreak in 1996 can be viewed as the first course of what has become an ongoing curriculum of difficult challenges and learning opportunities: a progressive dinner with assorted types of fresh produce, nontraditional exports from several middle-income countries (e.g., raspberries and snow peas from Guatemala, mesclun lettuce from Peru, basil from Peru and Mexico[17]).

Selected details about some of the outbreaks are provided, for illustrative purposes, in the text and tables. As noted in the prologue, Table 3-4 and Table 3-5 provide matrices for listing and dissecting the ingredients of outbreaks and investigations. Examples of challenges, opportunities, approaches, societal contexts and trends, scientific advances, and lessons (re)learned, codified, and yet to be learned are included as well. The outbreaks and their impacts, particularly the series of outbreaks linked to Guatemalan raspberries, are discussed in detail in other articles and case studies (Calvin, 2003; CDC, 1998, 2004; Herwaldt, 2000; Herwaldt et al., 1997, 1999; Ho et al., 2002; Jackson, 2006; Lopez et al., 2001; Powell, 1998; U.S. Senate, 1998).

The Complementary Needs for, and Values of, "One/Few" and "Many": Quality and Quantity

A reverberating theme in this narrative is the potential importance of "one/few" (e.g., one oocyst detected in one stool specimen by one laboratorian; one commonality noted among a few reported cases of infection; one harbinger, clue, or outlier), which can have a positive impact (e.g., the one reported case could be the index case of an otherwise unrecognized multicluster outbreak) or a negative impact (e.g., a red herring misinterpreted as evidence). Missed oocysts and cases translate into missed outbreaks and learning opportunities and into anxious patients with un(mis)diagnosed cases of infection treated with ineffective therapies (Table 3-3, Annex 3-1; Table 3-6, Annex 3-4).

A complementary theme is the value of "many" (e.g., the unmet research need for large quantities of oocysts [Table 3-3, Annex 3-1] and the epidemiologic benefits of outbreaks with many cases and clusters of cases [Table 3-4, Annex 3-2]). Large, multicluster outbreaks, such as the outbreaks in 1996 and 1997—although challenging to investigate and coordinate and potentially devastating for

---

[17]The examples are those that can be provided with confidence (i.e., these vehicles and sources were definitively implicated in investigations of U.S. outbreaks). The evidence for other vehicles and sources (e.g., blackberries from Guatemala, in various years including 1999, and raspberries from Chile, in an outbreak during late December 2001 through early January 2002) was not definitive because of the typical types of constraints (Herwaldt, 2000; Jackson, 2006). For example, only one cluster of cases was documented for the outbreak in the winter of 2001/2002 (i.e., no opportunities to triangulate among clusters were available); the evidence that the raspberries that were eaten—which were grown in Chile—were the vehicle of infection was suggestive but not definitive.

the affected persons, producers, economies, and societies (Table 3-6, Annex 3-4)—can be blessings in disguise. Such outbreaks can translate into opportunities to compile compelling epidemiologic evidence to implicate food vehicles and sources (e.g., Guatemalan raspberries) and, ultimately, to learn to prevent contamination and transmission. Geographically dispersed, multicluster outbreaks provide opportunities (Table 3-4, Annex 3-2; Table 3-5, Annex 3-3), such as:

- to circumvent limitations in knowledge about plausible modes and vehicles of transmission and to overcome limitations of individual clusters of cases (e.g., by triangulating among the clusters and events to identify the common themes in the mixtures of produce vehicles and potential sources);[18]
- to determine where food vehicles became contaminated (e.g., if the source is the only commonality in the distribution system of a widely dispersed vehicle);
- to generate hypotheses about modes by which the vehicle became contaminated at its source (e.g., use of contaminated agricultural water); and
- therefore, to identify and implement potentially effective control measures (i.e., to translate science into action).

Recurrent outbreaks (e.g., the series of outbreaks linked to Guatemalan raspberries), despite of and because of the challenges they pose, also provide opportunities (Table 3-4, Annex 3-2; Table 3-5, Annex 3-3), such as:

- to (re)test hypotheses and to strengthen already compelling epidemiologic evidence (e.g., through the investigation of the raspberry-associated outbreak in the spring of 1997, which was uncannily similar to the outbreak in 1996 [Herwaldt et al., 1997, 1999]);
- to complement compelling epidemiologic evidence with confirmatory laboratory data (e.g., as was done in 2000 in the investigation of the last documented outbreak linked to Guatemalan raspberries because frozen leftovers of the implicated food item—a wedding cake—were found and analytic methods for this complex food matrix were developed [Ho et al., 2002] [Table 3-5, Annex 3-3]); and
- to assess the (in)effectiveness of control measures implemented in the past and to pause to reevaluate how to proceed (e.g., in the spring of 1998, in an inadvertent intervention trial, the United States did not import fresh Guatemalan raspberries, whereas Canada did and experienced an outbreak [CDC, 1998; Powell, 1998] [Table 3-4, Annex 3-2]).

---

[18]Epidemiologic and traceback investigations of produce-associated outbreaks would be greatly simplified, if meals and food items included a maximum of one type of fresh produce, if aliquots of such items were frozen for potential future analytic testing, and all pertinent receipts were saved.

Large and recurrent outbreaks (signals) are blessings in disguise in other ways as well: they get attention in ways that subtle signals do not. Dismissed cases (signals) in distant lands (i.e., cases not considered "our problem") can ultimately translate into sonic booms so loud (U.S. outbreaks so large) that they cannot be ignored (Table 3-4, Annex 3-2). They serve as piercing wake-up calls about the vulnerability of our food supply in general and fresh produce in particular, including the need to bring parasites and parasitologists to the food safety and science tables. These wake-up calls can spur the growth of some good fruits, as discussed below.

Detecting and Classifying Slow-Growing Fruits

Various types of slow-growing fruits pertain to the narrative and illustrate yet again the yin and yang of the chronicle of *Cyclospora*. Certain principles are evident. The unexpected not only occurs but occurs in unforeseen ways and places, at unpredicted times, and with unanticipated effects. The fruits of investments in research, foreign technical assistance, the U.S. public health system, and outbreak investigations might not be evident for years, might not meet expectations (e.g., unfulfilled hopes for trickle-down benefits of investments in particular aspects of the public health infrastructure), or might not resemble the seeds that were intentionally or unwittingly planted.

We remain indebted to the astute scientists whose years of investments yielded timely fruits. Because of them we faced the outbreaks of cyclosporiasis knowing that the etiologic agent is a coccidian parasite, which slowly matures (i.e., has a long extrinsic maturation period), and knowing how to treat cases of cyclosporiasis, which can be slow to resolve (Ashford, 1979; Hoge et al., 1995; Ortega et al., 1993, 1994) (Table 3-3, Annex 3-1). The scientists did not invest in their research activities with foreknowledge that *Cyclospora* would emerge as it did, that the return on their investments would be large, and that U.S. investigators and patients would be among the beneficiaries. The fact that we could pluck the fruits of their years of labors should not be taken for granted.

Some of the U.S. outbreaks of cyclosporiasis, most notably the series of outbreaks associated with Guatemalan raspberries, represent a different type of slow-growing fruit of different types of labors and investments in the 1980s. Unintended fruits of good intentions to address an economic problem (i.e., to strengthen the economies of countries such as Guatemala by decreasing their reliance on traditional export crops) ripened in the 1990s, when markedly increased volumes of raspberries, a nontraditional export crop, were flown from South to North (Herwaldt, 2000; Jackson, 2006; U.S. Senate, 1998). Unintended fruits came in the form of widely dispersed outbreaks of cyclosporiasis, which had economic consequences not only for raspberry growers in Guatemala (i.e., the raspberry business essentially went out of business) but also for collaterally affected growers and suppliers of various types of fresh produce in countries including the United States (Calvin, 2003; Herwaldt, 2000; Jackson, 2006).

It would be overly simplistic to consider the good intentions in the 1980s misguided or shortsighted and to classify the fruits noted in the 1990s and thereafter as bad.[19] The outbreaks and investigations have spurred the growth and maturation of various types of good fruits, with various beneficiaries. Examples of ripening good fruits (Table 3-4, Annex 3-2; Table 3-5, Annex 3-3) include the ongoing processes of:

- increasing knowledge and competence (e.g., increasing understanding of the clinical spectrum and manifestations of *Cyclospora* infection and developing training tools to strengthen capacity related to parasitic diseases in general and cyclosporiasis in particular); and
- developing, using, evaluating, and improving various generic and *Cyclospora*-specific tools (e.g., diagnostic techniques for clinical specimens, analytic methods for food and environmental samples, surveillance systems, epidemiologic survey instruments, protocols for traceback and farm investigations, control measures).

In addition, the translation of the outbreaks into piercing wake-up calls about the vulnerability of our food supply in general and fresh produce in particular has been associated with maturing fruits, with industry-wide ramifications. The outbreaks of cyclosporiasis linked to fresh produce have added to the critical mass of data from other such outbreaks (Table 3-4, Annex 3-2) to help sharpen the focus of the food-safety lens on produce vehicles in the United States and abroad. In short, good science takes time but already has yielded profits that extend beyond this particular unicellular pathogen and include science-grounded food safety guidelines and policies (e.g., "Good Agricultural Practices" for produce).

Epilogue: The Saga Is Ongoing, More Work Needs to Be Done, and the Workers and Resources Are Few

The work is not done just because the organism (i.e., *C. cayetanensis*) has been classified by genus and christened, one highly effective therapy for cyclosporiasis has been identified, our abilities to detect and investigate cases and outbreaks have markedly improved, and specific produce vehicles and sources have been identified in some of the outbreak investigations. *Cyclospora* did not gracefully exit after its dramatic entrance, nor has it fully emerged from obscurity into

[19]In 2004, the saga of cyclosporiasis circled back to Guatemala, when an outbreak was linked to snow peas, another nontraditional export crop (CDC, 2004).

clarity. Despite scientific advances at the margins, *Cyclospora* remains largely veiled in mystery; we remain plagued by fundamental unknowns and by fundamental constraints as we seek to convert unknowns into knowns (Table 3-3, Annex 3-1). Our ability to prevent contamination of produce and thereby to prevent what we have been investigating (i.e., foodborne outbreaks) would be markedly improved by increased understanding of the biology of *Cyclospora* and the epidemiology of cyclosporiasis.

The lack of commitment to and the paucity of resources for the long-term investments—i.e., marathons not sprints—needed to solve the many remaining mysteries are disconcerting, especially because the ramifications of our ignorance and the collateral benefits of the advances to date are palpable. If for no other reason than self-interest (e.g., to avoid the actual and opportunity costs of investigating serial outbreaks), the need to decipher *Cyclospora*'s enigmatic code is evident. Cracking the code of a microbe as hardy and resilient as *Cyclospora*—e.g., identifying decontamination strategies that kill or remove the pathogen without damaging delicate fresh produce—almost assuredly would have far-reaching positive ripple effects for food safety.

One of the reverberating themes in the saga of this parasite is that the investments of "few" (e.g., the parasitologists' mite) can result in large proceeds. Fortunately, some doggedly persistent scientists are continuing to poke and prod *Cyclospora*, despite the paucity of resources and oocysts, with the expectation that ultimately it will excyst its secrets. These resilient investigators emulate the parasite's uncanny abilities to survive in austere microniches and to resist the pressures and stresses in harsh macroenvironments. Relatively few persons deserve the credit for the fact that *Cyclospora* and cyclosporiasis did not emerge in the United States as complete unknowns. In the future, which, by definition, is unknown, relatively few persons may deserve the credit for identifying and implementing an exit strategy for this inscrutable pathogen and for writing the last chapter of the chronicle of cyclosporiasis, which now appears to have no end in sight.

Acknowledgments

I am indebted to the countless persons who have contributed in various ways to the marathon investigations of the U.S. outbreaks of cyclosporiasis. I reluctantly acknowledge that *Cyclospora*, which has defined the seasons of more than a decade of my life, has been a worthy opponent. Special thanks to my CDC colleague, Dr. Dennis D. Juranek, for his innumerable, invaluable insights and for his artistic contributions, most notably to Figure 3-4 and Figure 3-5.

ANNEX 3-1

TABLE 3-3 *Cyclospora cayetanensis* and Cyclosporiasis: Perspectives and Status as of April 2006

Qualifier	Perspective	Comments (related issues are addressed in multiple comments from various perspectives)
No	*No* history (i.e., only a short recorded history)	The parasite *C. cayetanensis* was recently identified (first described in the late 1970s, in Papua New Guinea), classified in the *Cyclospora* genus in 1993, and christened with the species name "*cayetanensis*" in 1994; the name was derived from that of a Peruvian university where key studies about this parasite had been conducted.
	No precedent	*C. cayetanensis* is the first/only species in the *Cyclospora* genus known to infect humans, not merely another species in a genus known to include human pathogens.
	No fulfillment of Koch's postulates	Human volunteer studies have not been successful, nor have attempts to infect animals with homologous spp. (e.g., *Papio anubis* [olive baboon] with *Cyclospora papionis*).[a] *In contrast:* human volunteer studies have been successful for some other enteric protozoa, including *Cryptosporidium* spp.
	No infective oocysts in freshly excreted stool	Infected persons shed immature, unsporulated oocysts, which must sporulate in the environment (i.e., outside the host) to become infective (Figure 3-5; see below regarding extrinsic maturation period). *In contrast:* other protozoa—e.g., oocysts of *Cryptosporidium* spp. and cysts of *G. intestinalis* and *E. histolytica*—are fully mature/infective when shed in stool.
	No risk, if consume noninfective oocysts	Consumption of *Cyclospora* oocysts (e.g., in contaminated food) that have not yet sporulated poses no risk; direct person-to-person (fecal-oral) transmission is highly unlikely.
	No known hosts besides humans	No natural or experimental infection of wild, domestic, or laboratory animals with *C. cayetanensis* per se (versus other *Cyclospora* spp.) has been unequivocally documented; no animal models have been identified (e.g., to study the pathogenesis of infection).
	No means to assess infectivity	No direct methods to assess infectivity of *Cyclospora* oocysts have been identified; sporulation and excystation are indicators of viability and indirect measures of infectivity. The applicability to *Cyclospora* of data about the effects of various conditions/stimuli on other coccidia is unknown (Table 3-5).
	No multiplication, except in infected humans	*C. cayetanensis* oocysts do not multiply in the environment; humans are the only known amplifying hosts, and no *in vitro* cultivation systems have been developed.

	No means to maintain isolates	No means to maintain viable isolates have been identified (e.g., cryopreservation, serial passage in animals).
	No established means for strain differentiation	No PulseNet-equivalent exists (e.g., to link seemingly unrelated cases of infection); potential means for molecular typing/strain differentiation are being explored.
	No treatment alternatives	No highly effective alternatives to trimethoprim-sulfamethoxazole therapy have been identified.
Not	*Not* responsive to empiric antimicrobial therapy	The fact that therapy for cyclosporiasis differs from therapies for amebiasis, giardiasis, cryptosporidiosis, and some bacterial infections underscores the importance of diagnosing infection rather than treating empirically.
	Not included in routine parasitologic testing of stool	Specimens submitted for testing for ova and parasites usually are not examined for *Cyclospora* unless specifically requested.[b]
	Not enough oocysts for research purposes	Acquisition of oocysts is dependent on obtaining stool specimens from infected persons, which is difficult in general, let alone obtaining voluminous fresh stools, with plentiful oocysts, for research purposes. The constraints are compounded by the lack of methods for propagating/maintaining viable oocysts. *Contrast:* The cumulative total number of *C. cayetanensis* oocysts obtained for research purposes is comparable to the quantity of *Cryptosporidium* oocysts shed in a few days by an infected calf.[a]
Long	*Long* extrinsic maturation period in the environment	The process of sporulation of *Cyclospora* oocysts (Figure 3-5) typically requires at least one week under favorable laboratory conditions. The effects of real-world conditions—in micro- and macroenvironments—on the rate of sporulation and on the survival of unsporulated and sporulated oocysts are poorly understood.
	Long survival in the environment	The needs to survive long enough both to sporulate and to be ingested by a susceptible host suggest that *Cyclospora* oocysts are quite hardy. Whether they are even more resistant to environmental stresses than *Cryptosporidium* oocysts, which do not undergo exogenous sporulation, is unknown.
	Long intrinsic incubation period after ingestion of infective oocysts	The median incubation period in common-source outbreaks typically is ~one week (i.e., relatively long, compared with the incubation periods for most nonparasitic enteric pathogens, which adds an insurmountable biologic delay to existing system delays in detecting, reporting, and investigating cases and outbreaks).

continues

TABLE 3-3 Continued

Qualifier	Perspective	Comments (related issues are addressed in multiple comments from various perspectives)
	Long duration of illness in untreated persons without prior exposure to *Cyclospora*	Gastrointestinal illness can be protracted and can wax/wane in intensity, for weeks to months, with substantial weight loss and persistent fatigue (i.e., not a trivial, brief illness). The parasite and host factors that influence the manifestations/severity of infection are poorly understood.
	Long duration of shedding	Even asymptomatic persons can shed oocysts, and shedding can persist >one month after symptoms resolve.
Low	*Low* infectious dose	Although not yet confirmed by human volunteer studies, the infectious dose is presumed to be relatively low, on the basis of data for other protozoa and from outbreak investigations (e.g., seemingly trivial exposures, such as one berry/one bite, have resulted in *Cyclospora* infection).
	Low-level shedding of oocysts, even by ill persons without prior exposure to *Cyclospora*	Low-level shedding (~1–2 logs lower than for *Cryptosporidium* spp.) is common[a] and underscores the utility of sensitive recovery/detection methods (e.g., UV fluorescence microscopy, acid-fast staining, PCR).[b]

[a]M. Arrowood, personal communication, CDC, Division of Parasitic Diseases, February 2006.

[b]Both *Cyclospora* and *Cryptosporidium* oocysts are detectable with acid-fast staining. *Cyclospora* (not *Cryptosporidium*) oocysts are autofluorescent but are not detected by immunoassays for cryptosporidial antigens (Herwaldt, 2000).

SOURCES: Alfano-Sobsey et al. (2004); Ashford (1979); Bern et al. (1999, 2000); CDC (1998, 2004); Connor et al. (1999); Dalton et al. (2004); Dixon (2003); Dubey et al. (1998); Eberhard et al. (1999, 2000); Herwaldt (2000); Herwaldt et al. (1997, 1999); Ho et al. (2002); Hoge et al. (1995); Huang et al. (1995); Jones et al. (2004); Kniel et al. (2002); Koumans et al. (1998); Lee and Lee (2001); Lopez et al. (2001); Orlandi et al. (2002, 2003); Ortega et al. (1993, 1994, 1997); Relman et al. (1996); Robbins et al. (1988); Sathyanarayanan and Ortega (2004); Steele et al. (2003); Varma et al. (2003); Vermeij et al. (2003).

ANNEX 3-2

TABLE 3-4 Characteristics of Foodborne Outbreaks and Investigations: Challenges, Opportunities, Approaches, and Advances, in General and Specific to Outbreaks of Cyclosporiasis Associated with Imported Fresh Produce

	Outbreaks and **investigations** in general *(cluster of cases, epidemic, scourge, plague)* *(evaluation, survey, study, research, inquiry, trial)*	General issues for outbreaks caused by the **etiologic agent** *C. cayetanensis* *(germ, bug, microbe, pathogen, contaminant, adulterant, poisonous/deleterious substance)*	**Food vehicles:** fresh produce (generic and *Cyclospora*-specific issues) *(crop, meal, dish, entrée, ingredient, garnish, agricultural commodity)*	**Food sources: foreign countries** (generic and *Cyclospora*-specific issues) *(garden, plot, farm, cooperative, firm, industry, conglomerate)* *(neighbor, trade partner, competitor, outsider, alien, foreigner)*	Comments (generic and *Cyclospora*-specific issues)
Outbreaks and **investigations** in general	Consume resources Provide opportunities to identify and solve problems (e.g., through control and prevention measures), increase knowledge and expertise, and identify priorities for basic and applied research	Difficult to investigate outbreaks, especially in the mid 1990s, when little was known about biology of *Cyclospora* and epidemiology of cyclosporiasis Cases, clues, harbingers, and outbreaks easily missed, dismissed, and misinterpreted (Table 3-3, Figure 3-5)	Outbreaks of cyclosporiasis have been linked to fresh produce (e.g., raspberries, snow peas, basil, mesclun lettuce). *Context/trends:* Increased consumption of fresh produce (not risk free) and increased proportion of reported U.S. foodborne outbreaks linked to fresh produce	Outbreaks of cyclosporiasis have been linked to foreign sources (e.g., Guatemala, Mexico, Peru). *Context/trends:* Globalization of food supply; perennial fare of produce; decreased reliance of middle-income countries on traditional export crops; and rapid, widespread distribution of perishable food	Local, state, and federal (e.g., CDC, FDA) public health agencies have different (but potentially complementary) roles, responsibilities, capabilities, and cultures with respect to food safety (Table 3-6). Rather than homogenizing the differences into a single institutional approach to complex food safety issues, the power of multifaceted, multiagency collaborations should be harnessed.

continues

TABLE 3-4 Continued

	Outbreaks and **investigations** in general	General issues for outbreaks caused by the **etiologic agent** *C. cayetanensis*	**Food vehicles:** fresh produce (generic and *Cyclospora*-specific issues)	**Food sources: foreign countries** (generic and *Cyclospora*-specific issues)	Comments (generic and *Cyclospora*-specific issues)
Large outbreaks *(important, major, pandemic)*	Difficult to manage ramifications of protracted illness, outbreaks, and outbreak investigations (including actual and opportunity costs)	Even large outbreaks are easily missed (serendipitously detected); if detected, they cannot be ignored (must be investigated), which translates into increased recognition of and knowledge about this obscure pathogen.	Even ostensibly small clues can facilitate identifying vehicle/ source of large outbreaks.	Large outbreaks serve as wake-up calls about vulnerability of food supply. Linkage of implicated food vehicles to foreign sources adds layers of complexity, sensitivity, and skepticism (Table 3-6).	Health professionals should consider that ostensibly isolated or unrelated cases could be part of outbreaks and should notify public health officials. Cyclosporiasis has been placed on the U.S. food-safety agenda and became nationally notifiable in 1998.
Multisite, multicluster outbreaks *(scattered, dispersed, diffuse, extensive, widespread)*	Require multiagency, multidisciplinary collaboration and strong central coordination of the investigations and public health messages Provide opportunities to triangulate among multiple clusters of cases (i.e., to look for commonalities, not just statistical significance), to overcome limitations of individual clusters	Difficult to conduct investigations and coordinate public health messages if sites have disparate levels of expertise about this emerging pathogen and diverse thresholds for making public statements about preliminary data/conclusions	Commonly noted for fresh produce vehicles contaminated where they were grown Opportunities to triangulate particularly helpful, if biologic and epidemiologic plausibility of preliminary findings unknown and if >one type of produce in meal or food item (e.g., in a salad) (Table 3-5)	Provide opportunities to confirm that source is only commonality (e.g., if no commonalities in distribution system) Opportunities to triangulate particularly helpful, if >one possible source of implicated food vehicle (Table 3-5)	Multisite outbreaks of cyclosporiasis spurred development and improvement of various types of tools for conducting and coordinating outbreak and traceback investigations (Table 3-5) and for increasing knowledge and competence related to parasitic diseases (e.g., DPDx, a telediagnosis project initiated in March 1998 by the CDC's of Division Parasitic Diseases [DPD][a]).

Concurrent outbreaks *(simultaneous, synchronized, parallel, separate)*	Provide fertile soil for shortcuts in reasoning (i.e., heuristics), such as presumption that cases/ outbreaks are related	Provide opportunities to identify more vehicle-source combinations, which can translate into clues for hypothesis generation	Can be (and have been) caused by different types of produce	Can be (and have been) caused by same type of produce from different countries	No PulseNet-equivalent exists for *C. cayetanensis* to link seemingly unrelated cases (Table 3-3).
Recurrent outbreaks *(repeated, serial, sequential, frequent, persistent, ongoing, unrelenting)*	Provide fertile soil for heuristics (see above) Provide opportunities to reconsider control measures, to retest hypotheses, and to reevaluate data from current and past outbreaks (with iterative feedback loops and midcourse corrections) to strengthen evidence and conclusions	Provide opportunities to reevaluate data from prior outbreaks, after biologic and epidemiologic boundaries known (e.g., plausible incubation period and modes/ vehicles of transmission)	Can be (and have been) caused by same vehicle/ source (e.g., Guatemalan raspberries), same vehicle/different sources (e.g., basil from Mexico and Peru), and different vehicles/same source (e.g., raspberries and snow peas from Guatemala, mesclun lettuce and basil from Peru)	Strengthened evidence can decrease skepticism about conclusions, especially those derived from epidemiologic data about outbreaks that do not make intuitive sense (e.g., no smoking guns).	Recurrence of outbreak linked to Guatemalan raspberries in 1997 prompted U.S. import alert for spring of 1998; outcome of inadvertent intervention trial (Canada but not the United States imported raspberries and had an outbreak) strengthened conclusions, decreased skepticism, and increased cooperation.
Seasonal outbreaks *(cyclic, periodic, intermittent, regular, predictable)*		No "off season" for U.S. federal-level investigators: relevant season differs among cyclosporiasis-endemic source countries		"Off season" for a particular region provides time to (re)assess risks and control measures.	Seasonality of *Cyclospora* infection provides unexplained clues; in Guatemala, seasonality of infection in humans overlaps with spring export season.

continues

TABLE 3-4 Continued

	Outbreaks and **investigations** in general	General issues for outbreaks caused by the **etiologic agent** *C. cayetanensis*	**Food vehicles:** fresh produce (generic and *Cyclospora*-specific issues)	**Food sources: foreign countries** (generic and *Cyclospora*-specific issues)	Comments (generic and *Cyclospora*-specific issues)
Outbreaks with **high attack rates** (*many hits, strikes, casualties*)	Difficult to identify uninfected persons, whose exposures can be compared with those of infected persons	Common finding for cyclosporiasis; combines two scenarios (i.e., widespread outbreaks *and* local, event-associated clusters of cases with high attack rates)			Repeatedly noting high attack rates in outbreaks of cyclosporiasis has strengthened presumption that infectious dose is relatively low (Table 3-3).

NOTE: In the rows in the left column and in the headings of the other columns, bolded words are sterile words used by investigators and parenthetical italicized words are related words with different denotations and connotations. Although many of the principles are generic (i.e., not *Cyclospora* specific), *Cyclospora* adds layers of complexity to investigations of foodborne outbreaks in general and to those caused by imported fresh produce in particular; lack of familiarity with and knowledge about the pathogen pervades all aspects of investigations, including the implicated source's skeptical reaction to conclusions derived from epidemiologic data. Also see Table 3-5 and Table 3-6.

[a]See link to DPDx: http://www.dpd.cdc.gov/DPDx.

SOURCES: Bern et al. (1999, 2000); Bruzzi (2006); Buchanan (1997); Calvin (2003); CDC (1998, 2004); Fraser (1987); Hall (1997); Herwaldt (2000); Herwaldt et al. (1997, 1999); Ho et al. (2002); Hoffman et al. (2005); Huang et al. (1995); Jackson (2006); Jones et al. (2004); Koumans et al. (1998); Lopez et al. (2001); Novotny (2006); Ortega et al. (1993); Powell (1998); Redelmeier (2005); Sivapalasingam et al. (2004); Sobel et al. (2002); Tauxe (1997).

ANNEX 3-3

TABLE 3-5 Goals of Investigations of Foodborne Outbreaks: Challenges, Opportunities, Approaches, and Advances, in General and Specific to Outbreaks of Cyclosporiasis Associated with Imported Fresh Produce

	Outbreaks and **investigations** in general	General issues for outbreaks caused by the **etiologic agent** *C. cayetanensis*	**Food vehicles:** fresh produce (generic and *Cyclospora*-specific issues)	**Food sources: foreign countries** (generic and *Cyclospora*-specific issues)	Comments (generic and *Cyclospora*-specific issues)
Identify vehicles *(associate, determine, establish, link, implicate, cite, incriminate)*	Can be tedious, resource-intensive process; easy to go astray or reach dead end	Outbreaks of cyclosporiasis have been associated with various fresh produce vehicles, including ones uncommonly linked to bacterial outbreaks (e.g., raspberries, basil).	Notoriously difficult to identify produce vehicle, especially if >one type served and no opportunities to triangulate (Table 3-4); complexities compounded, if served in stealthy, inconspicuous ways (e.g., as garnishes), not noted on menus or in recipes	Demonstration by CDC and FDA of *Cyclospora*/ DNA in frozen leftovers of implicated food (i.e., in food items containing Mexican basil [1999] and Guatemalan raspberries [2000]) added laboratory confirmation to already compelling epidemiologic evidence.	The pertinent pathogen and produce characteristics that, among other factors, account for particular pathogen-produce combinations are unknown. Public health messages must clearly distinguish among types of produce (e.g., the particular type of berry or lettuce).
Identify/ inspect sources (see above; also: *probe, inspect, charge,*	Can be tedious, resource-intensive process; easy to lose trail back to source Even nonimplicated producers (of the same or different types of food) can be spurred to	Outbreaks of cyclosporiasis have been associated with permutations and combinations of vehicles, sources, and seasons.	Perishable food typically is unavailable for analytic testing; even if pertinent food and perfected analytic methods (unfazed by complex matrices) are available, test results	Notoriously difficult to identify source of fresh produce, especially if >one possible source and noopportunities to triangulate (Table 3-4) Food and environmental	The need to retrace the paths of fresh produce all the way back to foreign sources spurred CDC-FDA collaboration to improve and codify epidemiologic-based procedures and protocols for traceback investigations and

continues

TABLE 3-5 Continued

	Outbreaks and **investigations** in general	General issues for outbreaks caused by the **etiologic agent** *C. cayetanensis*	**Food vehicles:** fresh produce (generic and *Cyclospora*-specific issues)	**Food sources: foreign countries** (generic and *Cyclospora*-specific issues)	Comments (generic and *Cyclospora*-specific issues)
incriminate, indict)	improve record keeping (e.g., for tracebacks and traceforwards), to minimize collateral damage.		could be negative because of spotty contamination.	samples obtained during farm inspections might not be helpful/relevant.	farm inspections.
Identify **sites/ modes of contamination**[a]	Contamination of widely distributed vehicles at their source provides opportunities to probe entire food chain and to identify and strengthen weak links.	Ability to trace back to source farms translates into opportunities to generate hypotheses about modes of contamination; use of contaminated water (e.g., in mixtures of substances sprayed onto produce) a strong consideration for at least some outbreaks of cyclosporiasis		U.S. investigators and inspectors need official invitations to access farms in foreign countries; if regulatory decisions are at stake, regulators might have easier access than researchers seeking to explore scientific hypotheses.	Potential interrelationships among food, water, and other elements of the ecosystem, as well as the complexities intrinsic to analytic testing of complex matrices (e.g., food items, environmental samples) underscore need for holistic, multidisciplinary collaborations.

Identify, implement, and evaluate **control measures (interventions and prevention strategies)**[b]	Control measures in acute setting (e.g., to stop transmission) might differ from those for refractory problems and those that can be implemented when insights from risk assessments and scientific advances can be translated into targeted actions.	Constraints related to *Cyclospora* (Table 3-3) have prompted use of other coccidia as potential model systems (e.g., *Toxoplasma gondii*, to assess attachment and survival on various types of berries and response to gamma irradiation, and *Eimeria acervulina*, to study decontamination strategies).	Need increased understanding of pathways by which oocyst-laden feces reach water/food and responses of pathogens, produce, and investigators to various stimuli/stresses	International collaboration essential: entails working with foreign governments, producers, and trade organizations; explaining how and why specific products and sources were implicated; and addressing concerns about trade barriers, blunt (e.g., countrywide) regulatory actions, and criteria for lifting sanctions	Outbreaks of cyclosporiasis have strengthened the precedent to act (e.g., issue import alerts) on basis of compelling epidemiologic data (i.e., spurred the transition from "What is epidemiology?" to "Epidemiologic data can suffice").

NOTE: In the rows in the left column, bolded words are sterile words used by investigators and parenthetical italicized words are related words with different denotations and connotations. Although many of the principles are generic (i.e., not *Cyclospora* specific), *Cyclospora* adds layers of complexity to investigations of foodborne outbreaks in general and to those caused by imported fresh produce in particular; lack of familiarity with and knowledge about the pathogen pervades all aspects of investigations, including the implicated source's skeptical reaction to conclusions derived from epidemiologic data. Also see Table 3-4 (including the parenthetical italicized words in the column headings) and Table 3-6.

[a]NOTE: For the bolded words in this row, the two sets of related words include: (1) problem, oversight, misconception, accident, error, mistake, failure, transgression, violation; and (2) stool, feces, manure, filth, unsanitary conditions.

[b]NOTE: For the bolded words in this row, the two sets of related words include (1) suggestion, recommendation, guidance, standard, warning, alert, requirement, mandate, sanction, regulation, enforcement action; and (2) detain, interdict, refuse entry, embargo, ban.

SOURCES: Bern et al. (1999, 2000); Bruzzi (2006); Buchanan (1997); Calvin (2003); CDC (2004); Dixon (2003); Dubey et al. (1998); Frazer (1987); Hall (1997); Herwaldt (2000); Herwaldt et al. (1997, 1999); Ho et al. (2002); Jackson (2006); Kniel et al. (2002); Koumans et al. (1998); Lee and Lee (2001); Lopez et al. (2001); Orlandi et al. (2002, 2003); Ortega et al. (1993); Relman et al. (1996); Robbins et al. (1988); Sapers (2001); Sathyanarayanan and Ortega (2004); Sobel et al. (2002); Steele et al. (2003); Tauxe (1997); Varma et al. (2003); Vermeij et al. (2003); Wan et al. (1998).

ANNEX 3-4

TABLE 3-6 Factors that Have Complicated Efforts to Communicate About Foodborne Outbreaks of Cyclosporiasis

Factor	Issues, Themes, and Examples
Disparate perspectives about:	
Food	Vehicle for trade/commerce, health/nourishment, or pathogens; something to fertilize, handle, export/import, sell/buy, eat, sample, investigate, or regulate
Fresh produce	Good market, good source of fiber/vitamins, or good vehicle for pathogens; something notoriously difficult to implicate, trace back to its source, and examine (Table 3-5)
Health (poor health)	Well-being (disease), strength (weakness), vitality (lethargy), stability (instability)
Whose matters?	Persons (e.g., patients, field workers), businesses, trading partners, economies, societies
Knowledge (ignorance)	Certainty (uncertainty, doubt), determination (underdetermination, indetermination), truth
Evidence	Anecdote, historical precedent, epidemiologic data, laboratory results (Table 3-5)
Various measures of significance and severity:	
Epidemiologic	Magnitudes of *P* values; widths of confidence intervals; numbers of reported cases in an outbreak and person-hours required to investigate the outbreak
Clinical	Numbers of loose stools and lost days (e.g., days of illness, hospitalization, unemployment, uncertainty about diagnosis, treatment with ineffective medications [Table 3-3])
Commercial	Lost reputation/customers; numbers of unharvested fields and unsold packages of produce
Different interpretations of words/terminologies/messages because of:	
Use of foreign languages	Epidemiology, parasitology, food/environmental science, economics, international law, bureaucratic jargon, idiomatic English, Spanish
Loss of nuances during translation	Distinctions among: impossible, implausible, potential, possible, probable, and proven; and lack of samples, lack of evidence, and evidence of absence (Table 3-5)
Different denotations in different contexts	Culture, media, report, case, power, error, sensitivity, collaboration, gaps/GAPs ("Good Agricultural Practices"), sporulation[a]
Different resonances for diverse audiences	Military metaphors (e.g., food threats/hazards, safety/security, defense/protection, mobilization/fortification, border control/surveillance, silver bullets, smoking guns)

TABLE 3-6 Continued

Factor	Issues, Themes, and Examples
Framing effects	Classification as a "them-versus-us" blame game or a "whodunit" mystery (e.g., a game of "Clue" solved by "disease detectives")
Lack of clarity	What does "thoroughly wash" mean, and what does it accomplish (for contaminated fresh produce in general and *Cyclospora*-contaminated produce in particular)?

NOTE: Also see Table 3-4 and Table 3-5, particularly the examples of sterile words used by investigators and related words with different denotations and connotations.

[a]For coccidian parasites, such as *Cyclospora*: maturation to an environmentally resistant infective stage (Table 3-3, Figure 3-5); for spore-forming bacteria: conversion to an environmentally resistant resting stage.

SOURCES: Baron (1985); Bruzzi (2006); Calvin (2003); Dixon (2003); Fraser (1987); Herwaldt (2000); Jackson (2006); Novotny (2006); Powell (1998); Redelmeier (2005); Sapers (2001); U.S. Senate (1998); Sivapalasingam et al. (2004); Stone (2004); Treadway (2006).

SURVEILLANCE AND INVESTIGATION OF A LARGE STATEWIDE *CYCLOSPORA* FOODBORNE DISEASE OUTBREAK INVOLVING AN IMPORTED STEALTH INGREDIENT

Roberta Hammond, Ph.D.[20] *and Dean Bodager, R.S., D.A.A.S., M.P.A.*[21]
Florida Department of Health

Background

In mid-April 2005, a private laboratory reported a dozen cases of cyclosporiasis to the Florida Department of Health (FDH), Bureau of Epidemiology Surveillance Section. The total number of cases reported in 2004 for Florida was nine. For reporting week 14 ending April 16 (the week the positive results were received from the private lab) the average number of cyclosporiasis cases from 2003 to 2005 was 1.67. The number of cases up to week 14, 2005, was approximately 20 percent higher than normally expected (FDH, 2005a). By reporting week 17, the percent increase was 162 percent, a clear indication of a possible outbreak. Cases were reported from numerous counties with no initial apparent geographical or temporal pattern. This article will discuss the methods of the ensuing complex investigation, epidemiological findings, and recommendations

[20]Statewide Coordinator, Food and Waterborne Disease Program, Bureau of Community Environmental Health.

[21]Central Regional Environmental Epidemiologist, Food and Waterborne Disease Program, Bureau of Community Environmental Health.

for future investigations involving outbreaks of disease resulting from intentional or unintentional contaminants of the United States food supply.

Methods

Epidemiology teams were formed at the state and affected county levels of the FDH. The core statewide team consisted of epidemiologists from the Division of Disease Control and the Division of Environmental Health. A statewide lead investigator was established for this investigation using the established organizational position of Statewide Coordinator of Food and Waterborne Diseases. The statewide team also consisted of information management personnel, public communication experts, and administrators. Each assembled county health department team comprised county epidemiologists, environmental health personnel, and epidemiology nurses. Each of these teams also included regional food and waterborne disease epidemiologists and/or Florida Epidemic Intelligence Service epidemiologists. County health department administrators were also a very supportive part of the county teams. As the investigation progressed, owners and management of the numerous affected food service establishments became integral parts of the investigation, supplying the investigators with critical information pertaining to product and patrons. The FDA, the CDC Division of Parasitic Diseases, the Florida Department of Agriculture and Consumer Services, and the Department of Business and Professional Regulation also provided valuable assistance with consultation, formal traceback, investigation of food service facilities, and farm investigation activities.

Laboratory analysis of clinical specimens originated with private laboratories. Florida has had numerous previous experiences with *Cyclospora* outbreak investigations and, due to prior misidentification issues, understood the necessity of confirming the findings of private laboratories. Table 3-7 depicts a listing of previous outbreaks in Florida, other states, and other countries. Thus a system was set up whereby private laboratory results were sent to a single FDH coordinator. The private laboratories were also asked to send their slides to the FDH Bureau of Laboratories in Jacksonville for confirmation. Laboratory results were provided daily, sometimes up to 30 per day or more. This process also allowed for the opportunity to ensure completeness of information on cases. The FDH's lab confirmation coordinator provided information for out-of-state cases to the CDC laboratory.

A web-based data collection system was inaugurated in order for individual county health department epidemiology staff to directly enter case information into a database for quick, real-time analysis. The web-based system is a module designed for outbreak investigations that is part of Florida's statewide electronic reportable disease management system. The outbreak database included demographic and exposure variables and was monitored in real time by the lead investigator. Florida residents who were confirmed cases and entered into the web-

TABLE 3-7 Selected History, *Cyclospora* Outbreaks, and Vehicles: Florida, National, and International

Year	Location	Vehicle
Florida		
1996	Palm Beach County (primarily), multiple clusters, part of multistate outbreak	Raspberries
1997	Leon County	Mesclun lettuce
1997	Orange County	Mesclun lettuce
1999	Palm Beach County	Undetermined (multiple fruits)
National		
1990	Chicago	Contaminated tap water
1996	Multistate	Raspberries
1997	Multistate	Raspberries
1997	N. Virginia/Baltimore/Washington, D.C.	Fresh basil
2004	Pennsylvania	Snow peas
International		
1992	Nepal	Untreated water
1998	Canada	Raspberries
2005	Canada	Fresh basil

SOURCE: FDH (2004); CDC (1996a,b; 1997a,b; 1998; 2004); Sterling and Ortega (1999).

based outbreak module automatically were also entered into the disease reporting system.

Communication of outbreak investigation progress and current descriptive data were electronically mailed regularly to appropriate FDH administration staff and investigation team members as well as to other state agency partners. Routine and timely updates were also posted on the FDH disease alert notification system, EpiCom, which is accessible by external partners in addition to all department staff. The CDC equivalent system, EpiX, was utilized for solicitation of out-of-state cases and communication nationwide. Press releases were also employed as needed, discussing the statewide number of cases, organism ecology, and methods of reducing risk of illness to the public.

The case definition for this outbreak investigation was a probable or confirmed case of *Cyclospora* infection, using the surveillance case definition, with onset since March 1, 2005, in a resident of or visitor to Florida. The FDH surveillance case defines a confirmed case as a clinically compatible case that is laboratory confirmed; the FDH defines a probable case as a clinically compatible case that is epidemiologically linked to a confirmed case.

Investigation Summary

Dates of exposure in the clustered cases ranged from March 19 to May 15, 2005. Dates of onset in the clustered cases ranged from March 24 to June 24,

2005 (see Table 3-8). Dates of onset of both sporadic and clustered cases ranged from March 1 to July 10, 2005 (see Figure 3-6). Predominant symptoms included diarrhea (78.5 percent), fatigue (64 percent), and abdominal pain (61.8 percent) (see Table 3-8). Over 75 percent of the cases were older than 40 years of age, 81 percent of the cases were Caucasian, 79 percent non-Hispanic, and 57 percent were female. Each case was asked a series of risk factor questions including a long list of various raw fruits and vegetables, other foods, and travel histories. The widespread nature of the cases and the lack of any readily apparent common food item was a strong indicator of a widely distributed food. The only weakly significant preliminary risk factors were iceberg lettuce (OR = 2.94, 95% CI 1.17–7.42; $P < .02$) and limes (OR = 8.54, 95% CI 1.13–64.79; $P < .02$). Initially all the cases appeared to be sporadic, but eventually some clusters emerged (see Table 3-8). Investigation of three of these clusters, from Pinellas, Flagler, and Sarasota Counties were used to determine the implicated food product. The Palm Beach County and the Orange County cluster investigations had inconclusive results.

The first cluster to emerge was the Pinellas County cluster, associated with consuming food at chain restaurant A. In this cluster, there was a total of 42 cases (17 laboratory confirmed, 25 probable). The range of exposures was from April 1 to 2, 2005. The range of dates of onset was March 25–April 23, 2005. The implicated menu item was herb-flavored oil used for bread dipping with the following ingredients: olive oil, fresh basil, Italian parsley, rosemary, and fresh garlic (OR = 52, 95% CI 8.99–300.78; $P < .0000001411$ Fischers exact). During the investigation of the cluster associated with chain restaurant A, another small cluster became apparent at a different chain restaurant owned by the same company. A total of eight cases (four confirmed, four probable) was linked to this second

TABLE 3-8 *Cyclospora* Clusters, Florida 2005: Range of Dates of Exposure, Dates of Onset, Confirmed and Probable Cases

County	Exposure	Onset	Confirmed	Probable
Pinellas # 1	4/1–4/2	3/25[a]–4/23	17	25
Pinellas # 2	4/1–4/9	4/5–4/18	7	7
Flagler	4/1–4/12	4/9–4/21	16	4
Sarasota # 1[b]	3/19–4/17	3/24–4/21	17	78
Palm Beach	4/10	4/13–4/18	4	7
Sarasota # 2	5/5–5/15	5/9–6/24	6	28
Orange	5/2–5/6	5/4–6/8	4	61
Totals	71	210		

[a]The 3/25 case is included due to presumed recall bias by the case as to when symptoms began.

[b]Includes a sporadic, community group that ate at the independent restaurant, plus four subclusters that ate food catered from the same restaurant.

SOURCE: FDH (2005b).

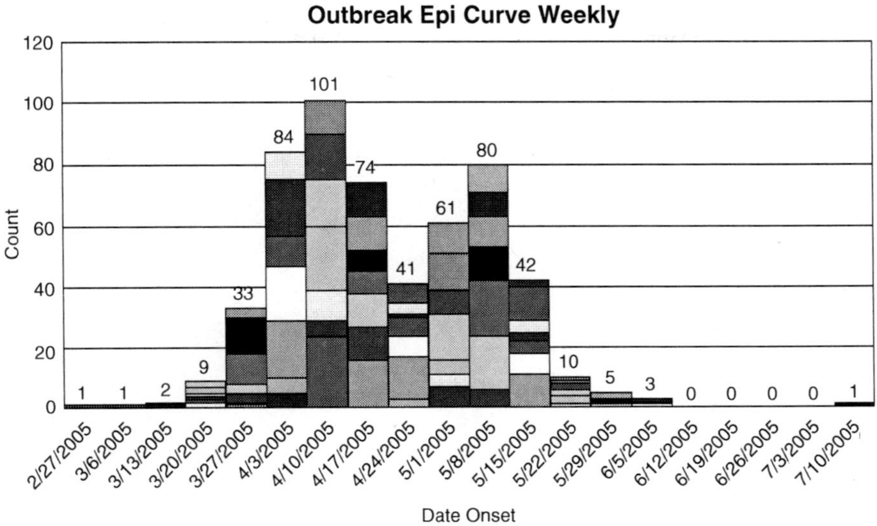

FIGURE 3-6 Epidemiology curve by week of onset, Florida 2005 *Cyclospora* outbreak. NOTE: The epidemiology curve is by week of onset, thus the first case of March 1 occurred during the week of February 27–March 5, 2005.
SOURCE: Florida Department of Health (2005b).

cluster. The implicated item in the second cluster was bread dipping oil mixed with pesto. Both restaurants from different chains receive Italian parsley and fresh basil from the same distributor.

The second cluster, in Flagler County, was associated with consuming food at an independent restaurant. This cluster had a total of 20 cases (16 confirmed, 4 probable) with exposures ranging from April 1 to 12, 2005. The Flagler County cluster investigation also implicated a flavored bread dipping oil with the following ingredients: olive oil, fresh basil, fresh garlic, and parmesan cheese (OR = 27, 95% CI 2.29–534.3; $P = .002$).

The Sarasota County cluster is really five separate doctor's offices whose staffs were provided catered lunches from the same independent restaurant by drug company representatives. There was an additional sporadic group associated with eating at the same independent restaurant. Exposures ranged from March 19 to April 17, 2005, and dates of onset from March 24 to April 21, 2005. While no single, statistically significant food item was identified, an ingredient can be implicated through the food histories. All five medical groups were served a lunch of meat wraps, vegetable wraps, and Greek salad, all with sun-dried tomato vinaigrette. The sporadic cases ate at the restaurant where Greek salad, Moroccan salad, and cucumber salad were on the menu. The Greek salad, meat wrap, and veggie wrap all contained sun-dried tomato vinaigrette with the following ingredients: olive oil, balsamic vinegar, sun-dried tomatoes, fresh onions, salt and pepper, and fresh basil. The inability to generate a statistically significant food is attributed to the lack of controls available for the case-control study, the suspected food ingredient being in multiple menu items and lack of recall for food histories.

A short questionnaire was administered to 35 confirmed *Cyclospora* cases picked at random from the sporadic outbreak cases in various areas of the state to assess fresh basil consumption habits. Five cases were selected from each of seven areas. Questions were asked pertaining to exposure to herbed green salads, basil, herbs, bruschetta, pesto, and pasta salads. There were also three questions related to visiting Italian, Thai, and gourmet restaurants that commonly serve dishes with fresh basil or fresh basil garnish. The frequencies of response to the questions included two questions that had more than 50 percent of respondents answering affirmatively. These were eating at Italian restaurants (64.7 percent) and bread dipped in oil with fresh herbs (68.8 percent). An analysis of these two variables showed significance in going to an Italian restaurant and having bread dipped in olive oil with fresh herbs. The Fisher exact value was $P = .03$. Eighty-one percent of the 31 cases who responded to both questions had visited an Italian restaurant where the practice of dipping bread was customary and where they ate bread in this manner. The FDH, in consultation with epidemiologists at CDC and FDA, requested a formal traceback of the fresh basil based on the significance of the findings of the three disease cluster investigations and the random case-control study.

Results

This disease outbreak was caused by *Cyclospora cayetanensis*, a single-celled protozoan with symptoms of watery diarrhea, nausea, loss of appetite, abdominal pain, fatigue, and weight loss. The case fatality rate is very low. The incubation period is one to seven days, usually about one week, and the ensuing illness can last anywhere from one to three weeks. Typical vehicles include raspberries, basil, lettuce, snow peas, and water. Though water has been implicated, 90 percent of outbreaks of cyclosporiasis are foodborne. Cyclosporiasis is endemic in many developing countries and is often associated with diarrhea in travelers to Asia, the Caribbean, Mexico, and Peru (Heyman, 2004).

The implicated food item in this outbreak was fresh basil imported from Peru, a widely distributed food ingredient used raw in many salads, sauces, and garnishes (Food Track Inc., 2005). It has been called a "stealth" ingredient by many because unless one knows the ingredients of a particular menu item, one might not remember having eaten it. Anecdotal evidence from a visit to the implicated farm in Peru indicates that farm conditions could have been conducive to

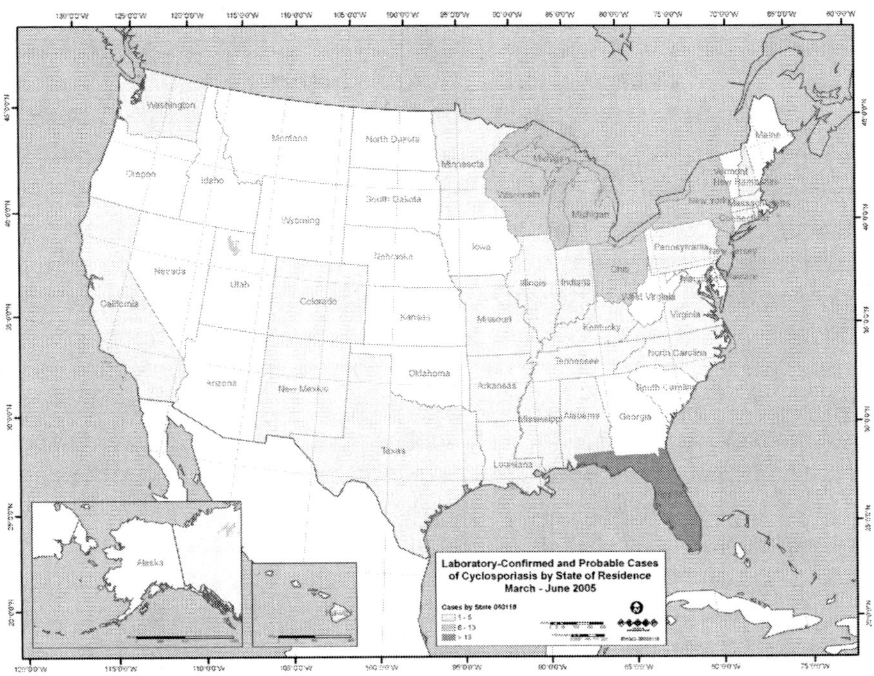

FIGURE 3-7 Laboratory-confirmed and probable cases of cyclosporiasis by state of residence, March–June 2005, *Cyclospora* outbreak, Florida.
SOURCE: FDH (2005b).

opportunities for contamination of the basil. There was a total of 592 cases with 365 confirmed and 227 probable. The investigated illness clusters accounted for 71 confirmed and 210 probable cases (see Table 3-8). A total of 493 cases were residents of Florida with 10 cases in Canadian residents and 89 residents of other states, all having visited Florida during their exposure period. Refer to Figure 3-7 and Figure 3-8 for details on geographical distribution of cases nationwide and in Florida. All out-of-state cases were visitors to Florida who were exposed in Florida during their incubation period.

Conclusion

Due to the nature of this widely distributed stealth ingredient used raw in many common foods, this outbreak was large and diffuse and the investigation thereof was exceedingly complex, involving the entire Regional Environmental Epidemiology Strike Team, the FDH Bureau of Laboratories, staff from the Bu-

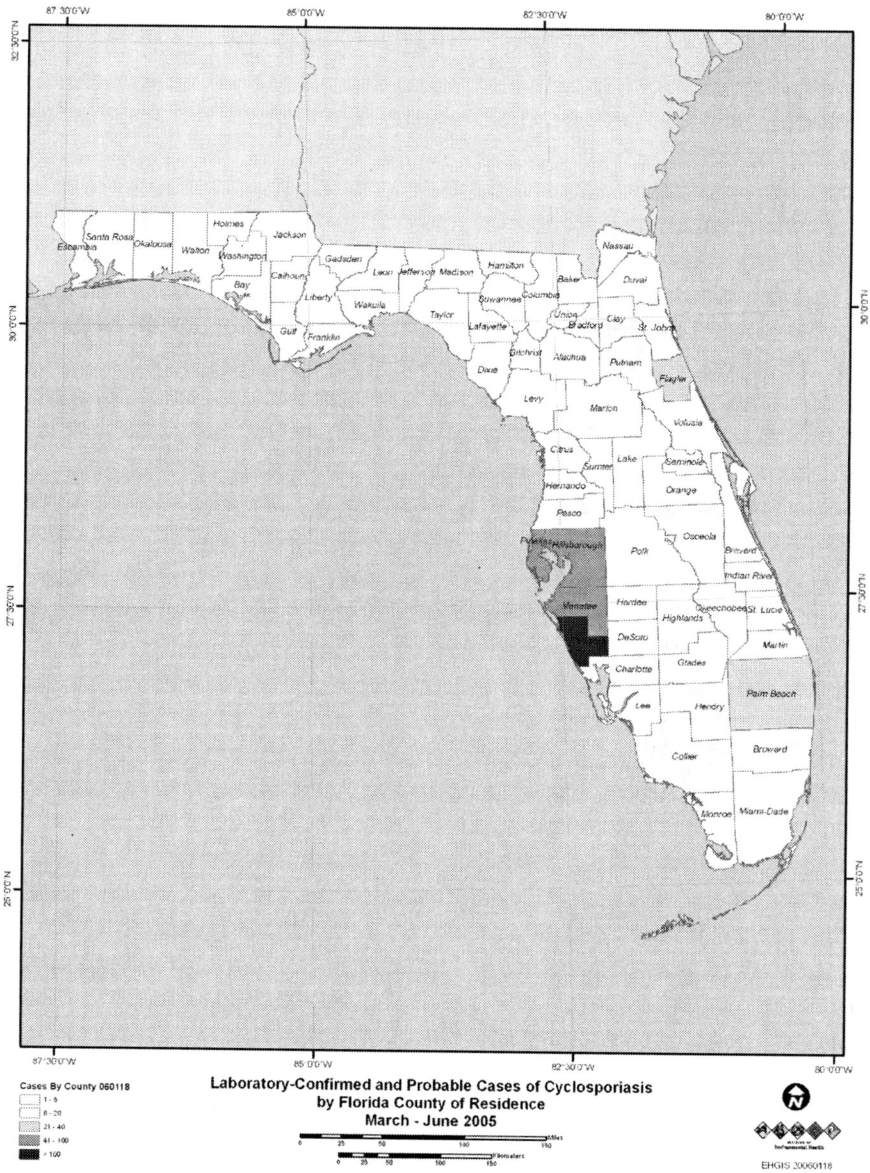

FIGURE 3-8 Laboratory-confirmed and probable cases of cyclosporiasis by Florida county of residence, March–June 2005, *Cyclospora* outbreak, Florida.
SOURCE: FDH (2005b).

reau of Epidemiology and all county health departments who reported cases. The FDH also collaborated with multiple partners in this outbreak investigation including private laboratories who reported cases, the Florida Department of Business and Professional Regulation, the Florida Department of Agriculture and Consumer Services, the FDA, and the CDC's Division of Parasitic Diseases.

It can be expected that similar or more spectacular disease outbreaks will be seen in the future due to increased global distribution of foods (particularly stealth ingredients such as basil), shifts in consumption towards raw consumption of these ingredients, unusual ingredients and recipes, and the increased expectation for availability for out-of-season produce from other countries. The importation of foods from underdeveloped countries possibly with insufficient potable water supplies and processing sanitation standards is also a significant factor in these types of outbreaks. The potential for large outbreaks of this kind is great in Florida, given the large population (18 million) and the estimated annual number of visitors (74.5 million). The FDH continues to conduct surveillance for *Cyclospora* cases along with other emerging and reportable pathogens in order to discover outbreaks early in their occurrence so that their cause can be discovered and further spread of illness can be prevented. FDA continues its ongoing efforts in working with produce-exporting countries to ensure that produce exported to this country is safe and free from disease (FDA, 1998, 2001, 2003c, 2004; DOT and HHS, 1999).

Recommendations

Accurate laboratory analysis is critical in determining the etiological agent and scope of any foodborne outbreak. It should be noted that in this particular investigation only one clinical sample was initially misidentified as a cryptosporidium. It is imperative that public and private laboratories have the capability to accurately detect and quantify emerging pathogens and threats to our food supply as quickly as possible. These analytical and technical capabilities must include all biological, chemical, natural, and intentional threats. Public health laboratory systems need to facilitate and lead in this endeavor. Public funding allocations must reflect these high priorities for detection of food safety threats. It is also important for owners/managers and personnel at private laboratory concerns to be educated on their important role with disease surveillance and outbreak investigations and "buy in" to the investigation and critical communication processes and keep all staff apprised of this responsibility.

While the web-based system used for the data collection for cases for this outbreak investigation was somewhat helpful in rapidly collecting data from a wide geographical area, it was determined to have limited capabilities to collect control data, perform multiple variate analysis easily, and be conducive to easy manipulation of data for analysis. The limited flexibility of the design resulted in duplication of investigation and analytical efforts during some phases of the investigation. When designing and testing such elaborate systems, information technologists and software designers should include epidemiologists and other technical experts on the design and use. Scientists should also welcome and understand that programmers and data system designers should also be a part of the planning process of responding to natural and man-made biological events. Resources also need to be devoted and planned to include training of end users of these types of systems.

It should be noted that Florida was able to successfully investigate this extremely large and complex outbreak using epidemiology, nursing, laboratory, and environmental health personal within the existing organizational structures. Many resources at the county and state level in multiple scientific disciplines have been developed in the past 10–12 years that permitted this to happen. State and local municipalities who have the responsibility to conduct the surveillance, investigation, and reporting of diseases, both natural and intentional, that negatively impact public health must obtain funding to secure the human resources and develop the expertise to respond to large-scale threats to human health.

Acknowledgments

The following people provided their extensive skills and expertise with the successful investigation and reporting of this extremely large foodborne disease outbreak: Kathleen Ward, R.S., M.S.E.H., Bureau of Community Environmental Health; Mike Friedman, M.P.H., Bureau of Community Environmental Health; Robin Terzagian, Bureau of Community Environmental Health; Janet Wamnes, M.S., Bureau of Community Environmental Health; Juan Suarez, Bureau of Community Environmental Health; Carina Blackmore, Ph.D., D.V.M., Bureau of Community Environmental Health; Richard Hopkins, M.D., M.P.H., Bureau of Epidemiology; Joann Schulte, D.O., M.P.H., Bureau of Epidemiology; David Beall, Ph.D., Bureau of Laboratories; Doc Kokol, Public Information Officer; Lindsay Hodges, Public Information Officer; Maria Donnelly, M.S.P.H., Pinellas County Health Department; Sue Heller, R.N., B.S.N., Pinellas County Health Department; Hunter Zager, Pinellas County Health Department; Joe Zwissler, Pinellas County Health Department; Rick Barrett, Pinellas County Health Department; Kelly Granger, M.P.H., Hillsborough County Health Department; Aimee Pragle, M.S., Nassau County Health Department; Andre Ourso, M.P.H., Volusia County Health Department; Quintin Clark, Sarasota County Health Department; K. Eric Stutz, M.P.H., R.S., Sarasota County Health Department; Maria Teresa Bonafonte, Ph.D., Palm Beach County Health Department; Dawn Ginzl, M.P.H., Orange County Health Department; Bill Toth, M.P.H., Orange County Health Department; Barbara Herwaldt, M.D., M.P.H., CDC, Division of Parasitic Diseases.

HEPATITIS A OUTBREAKS FROM GREEN ONIONS

Beth P. Bell, M.D., M.P.H.[22] *and Anthony E. Fiore, M.D., M.P.H.*[23]
Centers for Disease Control and Prevention[24]

During the fall of 2003, several distinct foodborne hepatitis A outbreaks occurred, including the largest such outbreak reported in the United States (Amon et al., 2005; Wheeler et al., 2005). In total, the outbreaks involved over 1,000 cases and at least three deaths. Most cases resulted from exposures in a small number of restaurants, with over 600 cases reported among patrons of a single restaurant in Pennsylvania. In each outbreak, the implicated food item was green onions imported from Mexico. As a result, the FDA imposed an import ban on green onions from the farms potentially implicated in the outbreaks (FDA, 2003a).

The outbreak investigations demonstrate a new use of molecular surveillance for hepatitis A virus (HAV) strains. Although green onions were implicated in each outbreak, the timing of the outbreaks suggested that at least two separate instances of green onion contamination occurred. This was the extent of the information that could be gleaned from the epidemiologic investigation. A more detailed understanding of the relationships among the outbreaks, gained by building on ongoing molecular surveillance, informed the traceback and affected the course of the ongoing investigations.

Features of Hepatitis A Virus Infection

Several key features of HAV infection provide the context for the outbreaks and are relevant to any consideration of prevention strategies (Fiore, 2004). After an incubation period that averages 28 days but can range from 15–50 days, HAV infection can present in a number of different ways, ranging from asymptomatic infection; to nonspecific symptoms such as nausea, abdominal pain, and fatigue; to jaundice and other classical symptoms of acute hepatitis. The likelihood of symptomatic infection and of jaundice is directly related to age; young children with HAV infection are unlikely to have a clinical illness recognizable as acute hepatitis. The period of communicability extends from about two weeks before until about one week after jaundice occurs, and HAV can be excreted in very high concentration in the stool of infected people (e.g., about 1 billion particles per gram). HAV in organic material is stable in the environment at least for a period of weeks.

---

[22]Division of Viral Hepatitis.

[23]Division of Viral Hepatitis.

[24]The findings and conclusions in this manuscript have not been formally disseminated by the CDC and should not be construed to represent any agency determination or policy.

Molecular Surveillance

In the investigations described here, we used molecular subtyping to characterize outbreak-related HAV strains as they became available and to explore their relationship to each other and to strains identified in the context of ongoing molecular surveillance projects in the United States and Mexico. We use nested reverse transcription polymerase chain reaction (RT-PCR) to amplify a 315 nucleotide segment at the VP1-2a junction of strains from persons with hepatitis A onset between January 2002 and August 2003, collected through the six counties comprising the Sentinel Counties Study of Acute Viral Hepatitis, and through the Border Infectious Disease Surveillance (BIDS) Project, which operates along the U.S.-Mexico border (Amon et al., 2005)

At the time the outbreak investigations began, this database included over 100 distinct sequences from over 500 individuals. Approximately 95 percent of the distinct sequences, representing 99 percent of specimens, were genotype 1A (Figure 3-9) (Amon et al., 2005). The majority of these distinct sequences formed a single cluster, in which all sequences were >96 percent similar to each other (cluster X). This cluster included sequences from all individuals identified through the BIDS project, as well as from travelers to Mexico. Particular risk factors predominated in other clusters, such as being a homosexual man or using illicit drugs (Figure 3-9).

Outbreaks in Tennessee, North Carolina, and Georgia

The first series of outbreaks involved over 400 cases and occurred in Tennessee, North Carolina, and Georgia during August to September 2003 (Amon et al., 2005). In Tennessee and North Carolina, investigations indicated that cases were associated with one restaurant in each state, but the restaurants were unrelated to

FIGURE 3-9 Comparison of hepatitis A viral sequences among individuals with hepatitis A from northern Mexico (Border Infectious Disease Surveillance [BIDS] Project), 2002–2003; outbreak-related surveillance, October–December 2003; and six U.S. sentinel county sites, January 2002–August 2003.
NOTE: Numbers in ( ) indicate the number of samples with an identical sequence identified from the same surveillance source. Bars are color coded according to the source of the sample, or, for samples identified through sentinel counties surveillance, by the reported hepatitis A risk factors. Multicolored bars indicate, by the size of each colored segment, the proportion of individuals with an identical sequence reporting a hepatitis A risk factors, or with no identified risk factors. Abbreviations of countries of travel outside of North America: PHI: Philippines; IND: Indonesia; EC: Ecuador; VEN: Venezuela. X represents a cluster of sequences >96 percent similar to one another.
SOURCE: Amon et al. (2005).

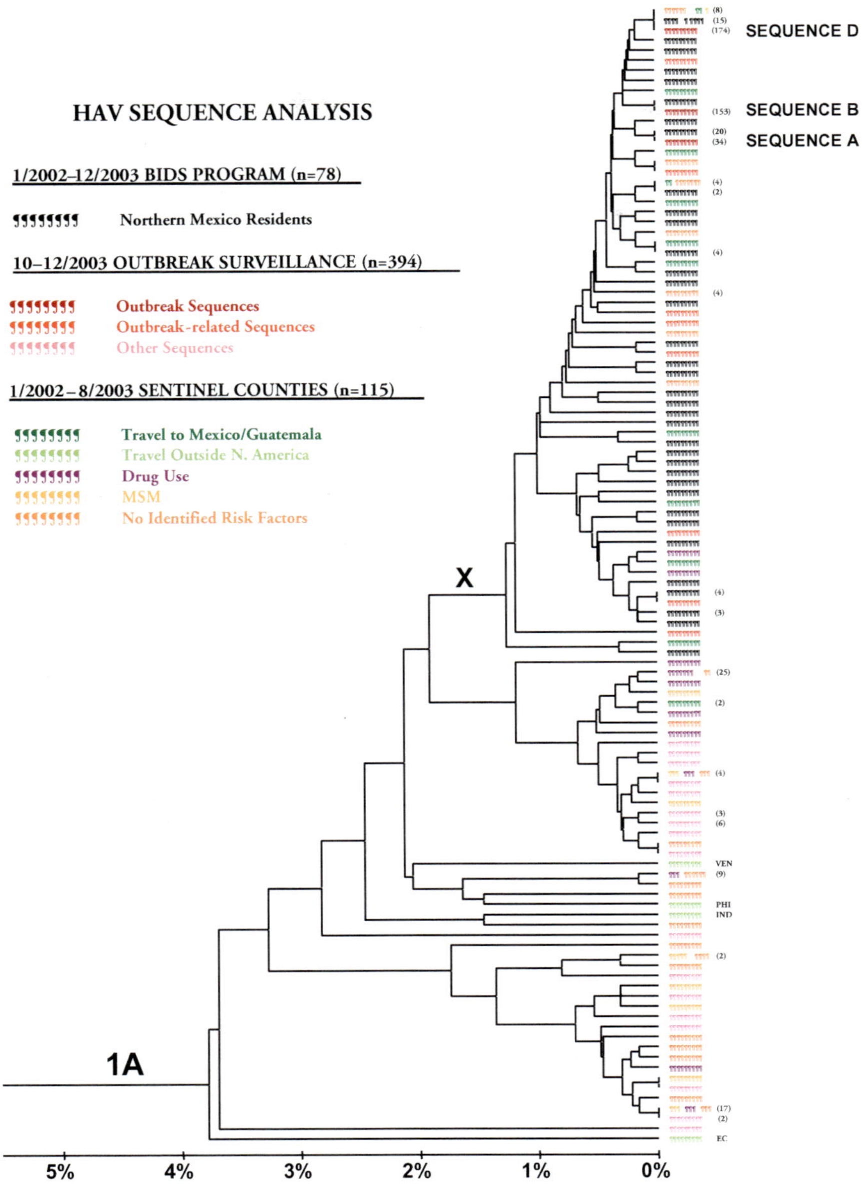
HAV SEQUENCE ANALYSIS
1/2002–12/2003 BIDS PROGRAM (n=78)
Northern Mexico Residents
10–12/2003 OUTBREAK SURVEILLANCE (n=394)
Outbreak Sequences
Outbreak-related Sequences
Other Sequences
1/2002 – 8/2003 SENTINEL COUNTIES (n=115)
Travel to Mexico/Guatemala
Travel Outside N. America
Drug Use
MSM
No Identified Risk Factors
(8)
(15)
(174)
SEQUENCE D
(153)
SEQUENCE B
(20)
(34)
SEQUENCE A
(4)
(2)
(4)
(4)
X
(4)
(3)
(25)
(2)
(4)
(3)
(6)
VEN
(9)
PHI
IND
(2)
1A
(17)
(2)
EC
5%
4%
3%
2%
1%
0%

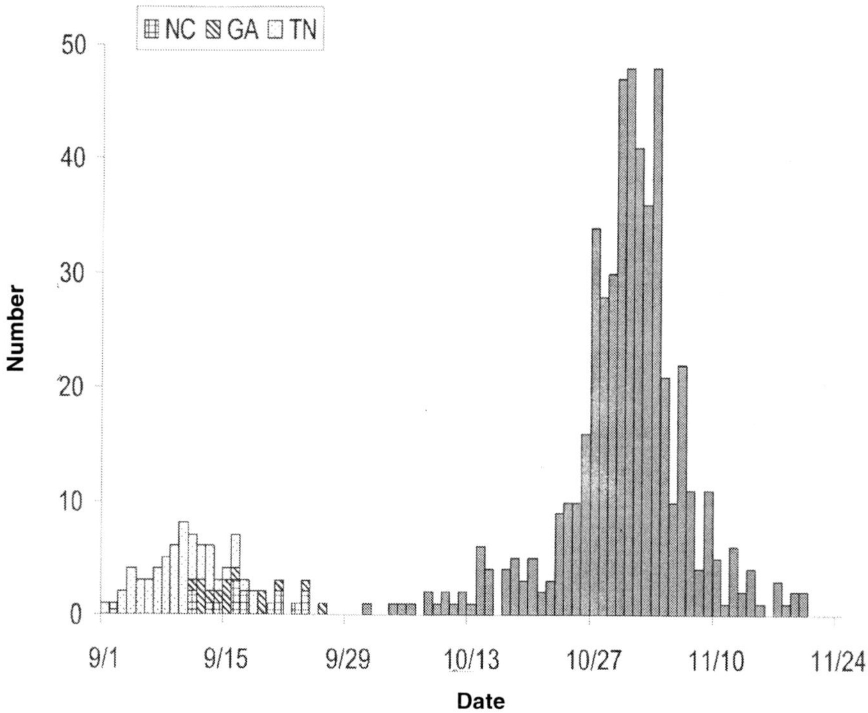

FIGURE 3-10 Date of illness onset among restaurant patrons, September–November 2003; n = 590. The dotted bars represent Tennessee (TN) cases, the hatched bars North Carolina (NC) cases, the diagonal striped bars Georgia (GA) cases, and the solid bars Pennsylvania (PA) cases.
SOURCE: Bell (2005).

each other. Ill food service workers identified in each outbreak had illness onset concurrent with other cases, indicating that they could not have been sources of the outbreaks. Most cases in Tennessee reported an onset of illness during the first week in September. The peak in North Carolina was about a week later. In Georgia, at least three restaurant-associated clusters were identified, but information about many of the cases that shared the outbreak strain was incomplete. An epidemiologic investigation of the largest of these clusters showed that dates of onset were similar to those in North Carolina (Figure 3-10). Exposures at each restaurant occurred primarily during a 10-day period in August, and green onions were implicated as the source in case-control studies among restaurant patrons in each state. In the case-control study in Tennessee, for example, green onions were eaten by 98 percent of 57 case-patients and 46 percent of 204 control subjects (OR = 65.5, 95% CI 8.9–482.5). The epidemiologic investigations were conducted during late September and early October, and the FDA initiated traceback investigations on October 9.

Sera obtained from outbreak-related cases in the three states yielded two distinct outbreak strains (sequence A and B) (Figure 3-9). Sequence A was found among restaurant patrons from Tennessee, and sequence B was found among Georgia and North Carolina cases. Both sequences fell into cluster X, the same cluster of strains that also included most strains identified among persons who acquired illness in Mexico.

Pennsylvania Outbreak

In early November, as the epidemiologic investigations were winding down and the traceback investigations were underway, an outbreak in Pennsylvania occurred, eventually involving a total of more than 600 cases among patrons of a single restaurant in Beaver County, including 13 employees who became ill at the same time as patrons (Figure 3-10) (Wheeler et al., 2005). Over 80 percent of the 425 case-patients who reported eating only once at the implicated restaurant ate there between October 3 and October 6, including 67 percent who dined on October 4 or October 5. The estimated attack rate for the four-day period was 17.9 percent, including an estimated 25 percent of diners on October 4 and 29 percent of diners on October 5.

A case-control study among patrons at the restaurant included 181 cases and 89 controls. Five of the 121 menu items were associated with illness. Mild salsa was eaten by 91 percent of case-patients and 35 percent of controls (OR 19.6, 95% CI 11.0–34.9) and was the only item eaten by more than 25 percent of case-patients. Eating green onions, an ingredient in over 50 menu items, was reported by 98 percent of case-patients and 58 percent of controls and was strongly associated with illness (OR 33.3, 95% CI 12.8–86.2). The final multivariate model included age, eating mild salsa, and eating any other menu item containing green onions.

Green onions arrived at the restaurant in bundles of six to eight onions each, packed on ice in boxes. After unpacking into metal pans, they were stored in the refrigerator for up to five days. When needed, bundles were rinsed with tap water, the rubber band around the bundle was removed, and the onions were chopped using an electric dicer. After chopping, they were refrigerated in plastic containers for up to two days.

Mild salsa, the menu item most strongly associated with infection, was prepared in 40-quart batches. The restaurant prepared up to two batches each day, and stored them for up to three days in the refrigerator. Each quart contained six ounces of raw chopped green onions, equivalent to 10–16 whole green onions.

Of course a pressing question was the relationship, if any, of this outbreak to the outbreaks that had occurred earlier in the fall. Molecular surveillance results obtained to date had pointed to the likelihood of two separate instances of contamination accounting for these earlier outbreaks. The outbreak strain from cases associated with the Pennsylvania outbreak (sequence D, Figure 3-9) turned out to be distinct from but closely related to the other outbreak strains, and fell into the same cluster of Mexico-related strains. These findings established that the four geographically separate but temporally related outbreaks represented at least three distinct events.

Other States

Not all hepatitis A is foodborne, and a common question that arises in the context of many foodborne hepatitis A outbreaks is the extent to which available surveillance methods are sensitive enough such that outbreak-associated cases or small clusters can be distinguished from "background" cases. This is particularly relevant for outbreaks, such as those described here, that are associated with a distributed food item, but in which the majority of cases are associated with exposure at a restaurant. Another "first" accomplished in the context of these investigations was an improvement in the sensitivity of surveillance by incorporating molecular methods. Comparison of strains identified during the outbreak period provided evidence that some apparently "sporadic" hepatitis A cases were indeed foodborne. Specimens were requested from any cases that did not have an identified source of transmission. Of over 50 specimens submitted, a number were identical to outbreak strains (Table 3-9) (Amon et al., 2005).

TABLE 3-9 Source and Distribution of Cluster X Hepatitis A Virus Sequences, September–December 2003 (Outbreak Surveillance Specimens) and January 2002–August 2003 (Sentinel Counties and Mexico [BIDS*] specimens); n = 478

		Cluster X non-A, B, D (n = 73)	Sequence A (n = 54)	Sequence B (n = 154)	Sequence D (n = 197)
Outbreak surveillance	TN	–	32	–	–
	PA/OH/WV	–	–	–	170
	NC	–	–	10	–
	GA	–	1	122	–
	Other	8	1	21	4
U.S. Sentinel Counties	23	–	–	8	
Mexico (BIDS)*	42	20	1	15	

NOTE: TN, Tennessee; PA, Pennsylvania; OH, Ohio; WV, West Virginia; NC, North Carolina; GA, Georgia. *BIDS—Border Infectious Diseases Surveillance System.

SOURCE: Amon et al. (2005).

Investigation of Farms

Findings of molecular surveillance were consistent with sources in Mexico, as sequences matching each of the outbreak strains were identified from among BIDS specimens (Table 3-9). Four farms, all located in northern Mexico, potentially supplied the implicated restaurants, but no single farm could explain all four outbreaks. These traceback results were consistent with the results of sequencing—three distinct strains were identified from outbreak-associated cases in the four states.

Representatives from the FDA and CDC visited the farms in question (FDA, 2003b). The harvesting procedure included a lot of handling of the onions, which were pulled from the ground by hand, after which the outer layer was peeled off, the roots were removed, the onions were cut to a consistent size, and they were banded into bunches. Packing involved spraying bunches with chlorinated water as they passed on a conveyor belt, followed by loading into a cardboard box which was topped with chipped ice. In the distribution network, boxes generally were not handled between the farm and the restaurant destination. A number of conditions on the farm were identified as areas of concern, including poor sanitation, inadequate hand washing facilities, worker health and hygiene, the quality of the water used in the fields at packing sheds, and the ice-making process. However, no single practice or event was identified that could have explained the outbreaks.

Because HAV has no animal host, the original source of green onion contamination was a human infected with HAV and excreting the virus in stool. This fecal contamination could occur in a number of ways. Adults with contaminated hands could have touched the green onions during harvest or processing. Hepatitis A is endemic in Mexico, which means that the vast majority of the population is infected during childhood, and most adults are immune (Tanaka, 2000). Hence the majority of infections at any given time are occurring among children. Thus likely sources of contamination of hands include sewage or feces from workers' HAV-infected children. It is also possible that HAV-infected children were present in the fields and contaminated the green onions directly. Direct contamination of the growing areas by sewage is also possible.

Discussion

The outbreaks described here were investigated rapidly and tracebacks were initiated early. However, a number of features of hepatitis A make detection and control of foodborne hepatitis A difficult, and the results of these investigations illustrate important areas of progress and remaining challenges (Fiore, 2004). Because HAV contamination of foods can be focal and the virus remains viable in the environment for months, cases can be both geographically and temporally dispersed. These investigations demonstrate the benefits of wider and faster use of molecular epidemiologic methods, both in outbreak investigations and in the context of routine hepatitis A surveillance. Viral sequencing showed that four geographically separate outbreaks that occurred in the fall of 2003 represented at least three distinct events. Sequencing activities also improved the sensitivity of surveillance to define the scope of the outbreaks, distinguish outbreak-related from nonoutbreak-related cases, and identify evidence of sporadic unrecognized foodborne transmission. Finally, viral sequencing supported the results of the first traceback investigations and accelerated control efforts related to the outbreak in Pennsylvania.

The investigations also exemplify challenges in foodborne hepatitis A outbreak response that stem from characteristics of routine hepatitis A surveillance and inherent aspects of the infection itself. Because cases reported through routine surveillance are not typically asked about foodborne exposures, the recognition of an unusual increase in the number of cases or of cases occurring among those in an unusual demographic group serves to alert authorities to begin asking about foodborne exposures as one potential common link among cases. However, even with the most rapid response and investigation of clusters of cases, the long incubation period of hepatitis A and inevitable delays in diagnosis and reporting necessitate a considerable lag time between exposure and the earliest possible detection of a foodborne outbreak. For example, the exposure that resulted in the outbreak in Pennsylvania was occurring as cases associated with the previous outbreaks were just being reported in the other states. Thus, even if a farm implicated in the earlier outbreaks had been linked to a farm implicated in the Pennsylvania outbreak, it is unlikely that even the most rapid of responses to the earlier outbreaks could have averted the subsequent outbreak in Pennsylvania.

Green onions are emerging as a potential "problem" food, having been implicated in at least two previous restaurant-associated hepatitis A outbreaks (Dentinger et al., 2001; Datta et al., 2001). The vast majority of green onions consumed in the United States are imported from Mexico, a country in which hepatitis A is endemic (Calvin et al., 2004). They require extensive handling during harvest and may be particularly difficult to clean. A pattern of focal, low-level contamination in which possibly very few bunches were contaminated, may make it difficult to detect transmission when it occurs.

The outbreak in Pennsylvania illustrates how conditions at the point of sale can amplify an outbreak. A combination of factors probably contributed to this outbreak's size and high attack rate. The large number of diners who ate at the restaurant during the days of peak exposure were all offered mild salsa, the food item most strongly associated with illness. Preparation practices, such as rinsing green onions while they are still bundled and chopping and storage methods that allowed for cross-contamination, could also have contributed to the size of the outbreak. Because of the high concentration of HAV in stool and the likely low infectious dose, even a small amount of fecal contamination might result in many hundreds of infectious doses. Although the 2005 Food Code includes a requirement that vegetables that are not subsequently cooked be washed, it does not offer guidance about specific methods to prevent cross-contamination of produce (HHS, 2005).

Progress has been made in developing methods to detect HAV in food, including reproducible methods to detect the virus in "spiked" food samples and produce washes (Shan et al., 2005). Although theoretically attractive, there are a number of difficulties inherent in attempting to detect HAV in produce. The virus does not multiply in foods, and the concentration may be quite low. However, viral culture is not feasible, so there is a need to rely on RT-PCR techniques, which may not perform consistently in the presence of complex food mixtures. Further, RT-PCR cannot distinguish infectious HAV from noninfectious HAV RNA. Even if these technical problems were solved, HAV detection in food is unlikely to be of much practical use in the context of outbreak investigations for a number of reasons. Perhaps most important, particularly in the case of produce, is that the implicated item has almost invariably been consumed or discarded by the time illness is occurring. Further, methods are not at a level of development as of yet such that they can be scaled up to volumes needed to be reasonably sure that contamination is not present, particularly given the low infectious dose. Finally, these currently available methods take days to complete.

Perhaps most important is prevention of HAV (and other enteric pathogens) contamination of produce in the first place by preventing fecal contamination of produce on the farm. Hepatitis A is endemic in Mexico, and while the precise mechanism of transmission in the outbreaks described here could not be determined, control measures can be implemented that could prevent such outbreaks. These include ensuring that field workers are healthy and have access to adequate sanitary facilities and ensuring that water used to irrigate and rinse produce is not contaminated with feces. Children are the source of most transmission of HAV in rural communities in Mexico and much of the developing world, and children should not be present in areas where food is harvested. Reduction in HAV transmission among children in areas where produce is grown would further reduce opportunities for contamination.

REFERENCES

Alfano-Sobsey EM, Eberhard ML, Seed JR, Weber DJ, Won KY, Nace EK, Moe CL. 2004. Human challenge pilot study with *Cyclospora cayetanensis*. *Emerging Infectious Diseases* 10(4): 726–728.

Allos B, Moore M, Griffin P, Tauxe R. 2004. Surveillance for sporadic foodborne disease in the 21st century: The FoodNet perspective. *Clinical Infectious Diseases* 38(Suppl 3):S115–S120.

Amon JJ, Devasia R, Xia G, Nainan OV, Hall S, Lawson B, Wolthuis JS, Macdonald PD, Shepard CW, Williams IT, Armstrong GL, Gabel JA, Erwin P, Sheeler L, Kuhnert W, Patel P, Vaughan G, Weltman A, Craig AS, Bell BP, Fiore A. 2005. Molecular epidemiology of foodborne hepatitis A outbreaks in the United States, 2003. *Journal of Infectious Diseases* 192(30):1323–1330.

APHL (Association of Public Health Laboratories). 2003. *A Recipe for Stronger Food Safety Testing Programs.* [Online]. Available: http://www.aphl.org/docs/foodsafetyreport.pdf [accessed April 12, 2006].

Ashford RW. 1979. Occurrence of an undescribed coccidian in man in Papua New Guinea. *Annals of Tropical Medicine and Parasitology* 73(5):497–500.

Baron RJ. 1985. An introduction to medical phenomenology: I can't hear you while I'm listening. *Annals of Internal Medicine* 103(4):606–611.

Bell B. 2005 (October). *Session III: The Food Supply "Threat Spectrum"—Case Studies: Cyclosporiasis in Imported Produce—Fresh Basil.* Presentation at the Forum on Microbial Threats Workshop Meeting, Foodborne Threats to Health: The Policies and Practice of Surveillance, Prevention, Outbreak Investigations, and International Coordination. Washington, D.C., Institute of Medicine, Forum on Microbial Threats.

Bern C, Hernandez B, Lopez MB, Arrowood MJ, de Mejia MA, de Merida AM, Hightower AW, Venczel L, Herwaldt BL, Klein RE. 1999. Epidemiologic studies of *Cyclospora cayetanensis* in Guatemala. *Emerging Infectious Diseases* 5(6):766–774.

Bern C, Hernandez B, Lopez MB, Arrowood MJ, de Merida AM, Klein RE. 2000. The contrasting epidemiology of *Cyclospora* and *Cryptosporidium* among outpatients in Guatemala. *American Journal of Tropical Medicine and Hygiene* 63(5–6):231–235.

Blaser MJ, Taylor DN, Feldman RA. 1983. Epidemiology of *Campylobacter jejuni* infections. *Epidemiologic Reviews* 5:157–176.

Bruzzi JF. 2006. The words count—radiology and medical linguistics. *New England Journal of Medicine* 354(7):665–667.

Buchanan RL. 1997. Identifying and controlling emerging foodborne pathogens: Research needs. *Emerging Infectious Diseases* 3(4):517–521.

Calvin L. 2003. Produce, food safety, and international trade: Response to U.S. foodborne illness outbreaks associated with imported produce. In: Buzby J, Ed. *International Trade and Food Safety: Economic Theory and Case Studies.* USDA, Economic Research Service, AER-828. Pp. 74–96.

Calvin L, Avendaño B, Schwentesius R. 2004. *The Economics of Food Safety: The Case of Green Onions and Hepatitis A Outbreaks.* [Online]. Available: http://www.ers.usda.gov/publications/vgs/nov04/VGS30501/ [accessed February 24, 2006].

CDC (Centers for Disease Control and Prevention). 1965. *Proceedings:National Conference on Salmonellosis*, March 11–13, 1964, Atlanta, Georgia: U.S. Department of Health, Education and Welfare, Public Health Service, DHEW publication no. (PHS)1262. Pp. 1–217.

CDC. 1996a. Outbreaks of *Cyclospora cayetanensis* infection—United States, 1996. *Morbidity and Mortality Weekly Report* 45(25):549–551.

CDC. 1996b. Update: Outbreaks of *Cyclospora cayetanensis* infection—United States and Canada, 1996. *Morbidity and Mortality Weekly Report* 45(28):611–612.

CDC. 1997a. Update: Outbreaks of cyclosporiasis—United States and Canada, 1997. *Morbidity and Mortality Weekly Report* 46(23):521–523.

CDC 1997b. Outbreak of cyclosporiasis—Northern Virginia-Washington, D.C.-Baltimore, Maryland, metropolitan area, 1997. *Morbidity and Mortality Weekly Report* 46(30):689–691.

CDC. 1998. Outbreak of cyclosporiasis—Ontario, Canada, May 1998. *Morbidity and Mortality Weekly Report* 47(38):806–809.

CDC. 2004. Outbreak of cyclosporiasis associated with snow peas—Pennsylvania, 2004. *Morbidity and Mortality Weekly Report* 53(37):876–878.

CDC. 2005a. Human tuberculosis caused by *Mycobacterium bovis*—New York City, 2001–2004. *Morbidity and Mortality Weekly Report* 54(24):605–608.

CDC. 2005b. *Escherichia coli* O157:H7 infections associated with ground beef from a U.S. military installation, Okinawa, Japan, February 2004. *Morbidity and Mortality Weekly Report* 54(2):40–42.

CDC. 2005c. Preliminary FoodNet data on the incidence of infection with pathogens transmitted commonly through food—10 sites, United States, 2004. *Morbidity and Mortality Weekly Report* 54(14):352–356.

CDC. 2005d. *Foodborne Outbreak Response and Surveillance Unit.* [Online]. Available: http://www.cdc.gov/foodborneoutbreaks/outbreak_satistics/cdc_reported.htm [accessed January 16, 2006].

CDC. 2006a. *FoodNet Homepage.* [Online]. Available: http://www.cdc.gov/foodnet/ [accessed July 7, 2006].

CDC. 2006b. *Electronic Foodborne Outbreak Reporting System (EFORS).* [Online]. Available: http://www.cdc.gov/ [accessed July 7, 2006].

Connor BA, Reidy J, Soave R. 1999. Cyclosporiasis: Clinical and histopathologic correlates. *Clinical Infectious Diseases* 28(6):1216–1222.

Dalton C, Goater AD, Burt JP, Smith HV. 2004. Analysis of parasites by electrorotation. *Journal of Applied Microbiology* 96(1):24–32.

Datta SD, Traeger MS, Nainan OV, et al. 2001. Identification of a multi-state outbreak of hepatitis A associated with green onions using a novel molecular epidemiologic technique [abstract 896]. In: *Program and Abstracts of the 39th Annual Meeting of the Infectious Diseases Society of America.* Alexandria, VA: Infectious Disease Society of America.

Dentinger CM, Bower WA, Nainan OV, Cotter SM, Myers G, Dubusky LM, Fowler S, Salehi ED, Bell BP. 2001. An outbreak of hepatitis A associated with green onions. *Journal of Infectious Diseases* 183(8):1273–1276.

de Wit M, Koopmans M, Kortbeek L, Wannet WJ, Vinje J, van Leusden F, Bartelds AI, van Duynhoven YT. 2001. SENSOR, a population-based cohort study on gastroenteritis in the Netherlands: Incidence and etiology. *American Journal of Epidemiology* 154(7):666–674.

Dixon BR. 2003. The prevalence and control of foodborne protozoan parasites. In: Blais BW, Ed. *Current Challenges in Food Microbiology.* Kerala, India: Trivandrum. Pp. 31–76.

DOT, HHS (Department of the Treasury, Department of Health and Human Services). 1999. *Presidential Initiative—Safety of Imported Food, Status Report, December 11.* [Online]. Available: http://www.foodsafety.gov/~dms/fs-impor.html [accessed April 13, 2006].

Dubey JP, Thayer DW, Speer CA, Shen SK. 1998. Effect of gamma irradiation on unsporulated and sporulated *Toxoplasma gondii* oocysts. *International Journal for Parasitology* 28(3):369–375.

Eberhard ML, da Silva AJ, Lilley BG, Pieniazek NJ. 1999. Morphologic and molecular characterization of new *Cyclospora* species from Ethiopian monkeys: *C. cercopitheci* sp.n., *C. colobi* sp.n., and *C. papionis* sp.n. *Emerging Infectious Diseases* 5(5):651–658.

Eberhard ML, Ortega YR, Hanes DE, Nace EK, Do RQ, Robl MG, Won KY, Gavidia C, Sass NL, Mansfield K, Gozalo A, Griffiths J, Gilman R, Sterling CR, Arrowood MJ. 2000. Attempts to establish experimental *Cyclospora cayetanensis* infection in laboratory animals. *Journal of Parasitology* 86(3):577–582.

ERS (Economic Research Service). 2000. *Economics of Foodborne Disease: Estimating the Benefits of Reducing Foodborne Disease.* [Online]. Available: http://www.ers.usda.gov/briefing/FoodborneDisease/features.htm. [accessed April 13, 2006].

Faruque S, Sack D, Sack R, Colwell R, Takeda Y, Nair G. 2003. Emergence and evolution of *Vibrio cholerae* O139. *Proceedings of the National Academy of Sciences* 100(3):1304–1309.

FDA (U.S. Food and Drug Administration). 1998. *Multi-Year Research Strategy Under the Produce and Imported Food Safety Initiative, September.* [Online]. Available: http://www.foodsafety.gov/~dms/fsrstrat.html [accessed April 13, 2006].

FDA. 2001. *FDA Survey of Imported Fresh Produce, January 30.* [Online]. Available: http://www.cfsan.fda.gov/~dms/prodsur6.html [April 13, 2006].

FDA. 2003a. *Import Alert #25-20: Detention without Physical Examination of Green Onions (Scallions) from Specific Firms in Mexico.* [Online]. Available: http://www.fda.gov/ora/fiars/ora_import_ia2520.html [accessed April 13, 2006].

FDA. 2003b. *FDA Statement: FDA Update on Recent Hepatitis A Outbreaks Associated with Green Onions from Mexico.* [Online]. Available: http://www.fda.gov/bbs/topics/NEWS/2003/NEW00993.html [accessed February 27, 2006].

FDA. 2003c. *FDA and CBP Bolster Safeguards on Imported Food, December 3.* [Online]. Available: http://www.cfsan.fda.gov/~lrd/fpbtamou.html [accessed April 12, 2006].

FDA. 2004. *Prior Notice of Imported Food—Questions and Answers.* 2nd ed. [Online]. Available: http://www.cfsan.fda.gov/~pn/pnqagui2.html [accessed April 12, 2006].

FDH (Florida Department of Health). 2004. *Bureau of Community Environmental Health, Food and Waterborne Disease Program Annual Reports.* [Online]. Available: http://www.doh.state.fl.us/environment/community/foodsurveillance/annualreports.htm [accessed April 13, 2006].

FDH. 2005a. *Bureau of Epidemiology, Weekly Morbidity Report, Week 14, Ending 4/9/05, Selected Diseases and Conditions (Confirmed Cases Only).* [Online]. Available: http://www.doh.state.fl.us/disease_ctrl/epi/Disease_Table/2005_Weeks/dt_Week1420051.HTML [accessed April 13, 2006].

FDH. 2005b. *Statewide Cyclosporiasis Outbreak, Florida, March–June 2005, Final Report.* January 20, 2006.

Finelli L, Swerdlow D, Mertz K, Ragazzoni H, Spitalny K. 1992. Outbreak of cholera associated with crab brought from an area with epidemic disease. *Journal of Infectious Diseases* 166(6): 1433–1435.

Fiore AE. 2004. Hepatitis A transmitted by food. *Clinical Infectious Diseases* 38(5):705–715.

Food Track Inc. 2005 (August 20). Florida outbreak linked to fresh basil from a grower in Peru. Outbreak Bulletin, *Cyclospora*—USA (Florida)—UD#18. *Food Safety & Security Alerts.*

Fraser DW. 1987. Epidemiology as a liberal art. *New England Journal of Medicine* 316(6):309–314.

Frenzen P. 2004. Deaths due to unknown foodborne agents. *Emerging Infectious Diseases* 10(9):1536–1543.

Gerner-Smidt P, Hise K, Kincaid J, Hunter S, Rolando S, Hyytia-Trees E, Ribot EM, Swaminathan B; Pulsenet Taskforce. 2006. PulseNet USA—5-year update. *Foodborne Pathogens and Diseases.* 3(1):9–19.

Griffin PM, Tauxe RV. 1991. The epidemiology of infections caused by *Escherichia coli* O157:H7, other enterohemorrhagic *E. coli*, and the associated hemolytic uremic syndrome. *Epidemiologic Reviews* 13:60–98.

Hall RL. 1997. Foodborne illness: Implications for the future. *Emerging Infectious Diseases* 3(4): 555–559.

Havelaar A, Nauta M, Mangen M-J. 2005. *Costs and Benefits of Controlling Campylobacter in the Netherlands.* Bilthoven, the Netherlands: National Institute for Public Health and the Environment.

Herikstad H, Yang S, Van Gilder T, Vugia D, Hadler J, Blake P, Deneen V, Shiferaw B, Angulo FJ. 2002. A population-based estimate of the burden of diarrhoeal illness in the United States: FoodNet, 1996–1997. *Epidemiology and Infection* 129(1):9–17.

Herwaldt BL. 2000. *Cyclospora cayetanensis:* A review, focusing on the outbreaks of cyclosporiasis in the 1990s. *Clinical Infectious Diseases* 31(4):1040–1057.

Herwaldt BL, Ackers ML, Cyclospora Working Group. 1997. An outbreak in 1996 of cyclosporiasis associated with imported raspberries. *New England Journal of Medicine* 336(22):1548–1556.

Herwaldt BL, Beach MJ, Cyclospora Working Group. 1999. The return of *Cyclospora* in 1997: Another outbreak of cyclosporiasis in North America associated with imported raspberries. *Annals of Internal Medicine* 130(3):210–220.

Heymann, DL. 2004. *Control of Communicable Diseases Manual.* 18th ed. Washington, D.C.: American Public Health Association. Pp. 141–142.

HHS (Department of Health and Human Services). 2005. *Public Health Service Food Code.* [Online]. Available: http://www.cfsan.fda.gov/~dms/fc05-toc.html [accessed February 24, 2006].

Ho AY, Lopez AS, Eberhart MG, Levenson R, Finkel BS, da Silva AJ, Roberts JM, Orlandi PA, Johnson CC, Herwaldt BL. 2002. Outbreak of cyclosporiasis associated with imported raspberries, Philadelphia, Pennsylvania, 2000. *Emerging Infectious Diseases* 8(8):783–788.

Hoffman RE, Greenblatt J, Matyas BT, Sharp DJ, Esteban E, Hodge K, Liang A. 2005. Capacity of state and territorial health agencies to prevent foodborne illness. *Emerging Infectious Diseases* 11(1):11–16.

Hoge CW, Shlim DR, Ghimire M, Rabold JG, Pandey P, Walch A, Rajah R, Gaudio P, Echeverria P. 1995. Placebo-controlled trial of co-trimoxazole for *Cyclospora* infections among travellers and foreign residents in Nepal. *Lancet* 345(8951):691–693.

Hoge CW, Bodhidatta L, Echeverria P, Deesuwan M, Kitporka P. 1996. Epidemiologic study of *Vibrio cholerae* O1 and O139 in Thailand: At the advancing edge of the eighth pandemic. *American Journal of Epidemiology* 143(3):263–268.

Holmes C, Chiller T. 2004. National antibiotic resistance monitoring system for enteric bacteria. *Emerging Infectious Diseases* 10(11):2061.

Huang P, Weber JT, Sosin DM, Griffin PM, Long EG, Murphy JJ, Kocka F, Peters C, Kallick C. 1995. The first reported outbreak of diarrheal illness associated with *Cyclospora* in the United States. *Annals of Internal Medicine* 123(6):409–414.

IOM/NRC (Institute of Medicine/National Research Council). 2003. The science of public health surveillance. In: *Scientific Criteria to Ensure Safe Food.* Washington, D.C.: The National Academies Press. Pp. 28–68.

Jackson GJ. 2006. Inspection and investigation: Tools for detecting sources of food contamination and preventing illness outbreaks. In: Schweitzer G, Zali MR, Jackson G, Eds. *Food Safety and Foodborne Disease Surveillance Systems: Proceedings of an Iranian-American Workshop.* Washington, D.C.: The National Academies Press. Pp. 24–54.

Jones JL, Lopez A, Wahlquist SP, Nadle J, Wilson M. 2004. Survey of clinical laboratory practices for parasitic diseases. *Clinical Infectious Diseases* 38(Suppl 3):198–202.

Kassenborg H, Hedberg C, Hoekstra R, Evans MC, Chin AE, Marcus R, Vugia DJ, Smith K, Ahuja SD, Slutsker L, Griffin PM, Emerging Infections Program FoodNet Working Group. 2004. Farm visits and undercooked hamburgers as major risk factors for sporadic *Escherichia coli* O157:H7 infection: Data from a case-control study in 5 FoodNet sites. *Clinical Infectious Diseases* 38(Suppl 3):S271–S278.

Kniel KE, Lindsay DS, Sumner SS, Hackney CR, Pierson MD, Dubey JP. 2002. Examination of attachment and survival of *Toxoplasma gondii* oocysts on raspberries and blueberries. *Journal of Parasitology* 88(4):790–793.

Kolavic S, Kimura A, Simons S, Slutsker L, Barth S, Haley C. 1997. An outbreak of *Shigella dysenteriae* type 2 among laboratory workers due to intentional food contamination. *Journal of the American Medical Association* 278(5):396–398.

Koumans EH, Katz DJ, Malecki JM, Kumar S, Wahlquist SP, Arrowood MJ, Hightower AW, Herwaldt BL. 1998. An outbreak of cyclosporiasis in Florida in 1995: A harbinger of multistate outbreaks in 1996 and 1997. *American Journal of Tropical Medicine and Hygiene* 59(2): 235–242.

Lee MB, Lee E-H. 2001. Coccidial contamination of raspberries: Mock contamination with *Eimeria acervulina* as a model for decontamination treatment studies. *Journal of Food Protection* 64(11):1854–1857.

LeFebvre B, Diarra M, Giguere K, Roy G, Michaud S, Malouin F. 2005. Antibiotic resistance and hypermutability of *Escherichia coli* O157 from feedlot cattle treated with growth-promoting agents. *Journal of Food Protection* 68(11):2411–2419.

Lopez AS, Dodson DR, Arrowood MJ, Orlandi PA, da Silva AJ, Bier JW, Hanauer SD, Kuster RL, Oltman S, Baldwin MS, Won KY, Nace EM, Eberhard ML, Herwaldt BL. 2001. Outbreak of cyclosporiasis associated with basil in Missouri in 1999. *Clinical Infectious Diseases* 32(7): 1010–1017.

Lopez AS, Bendik JM, Alliance JY, Roberts JM, da Silva AJ, Moura IN, Arrowood MJ, Eberhard ML, Herwaldt BL. 2003. Epidemiology of *Cyclospora cayetanensis* and other intestinal parasites in a community in Haiti. *Journal of Clinical Microbiology* 41(5):2047–2054.

McQuiston J, Parrenas R, Ortiz-Rivera M, Gheesling L, Brenner F, Fields P. 2004. Sequencing and comparative analysis of flagellin genes fliC, fljB, and flpA from *Salmonella*. *Journal of Clinical Microbiology* 42(5):1923–1932.

Mead PS, Slutsker L, Dietz V, McCaig LF, Bresee JS, Shapiro C, Griffin PM, Tauxe RV. 1999. Food-related illness and death in the United States. *Emerging Infectious Diseases* 5(5):607–625.

Novotny TE. 2006. US Department of Health and Human Services: A need for global health leadership in preparedness and health diplomacy [editorial]. *American Journal of Public Health* 96(1):11–13.

Nuorti J, Niskanen T, Hallanvuo S, Mikkola J, Kela E, Hatakka M, Fredriksson-Ahomaa M, Lyytikainen O, Siitonen A, Korkeala H, Ruutu P. 2004. A widespread outbreak of *Yersinia pseudotuberculosis* O:3 infections from iceberg lettuce. *Journal of Infectious Diseases* 189(5): 766–774.

Orlandi PA, Chu D-MT, Bier JW, Jackson GJ. 2002. Parasites and the food supply. *Food Technology* 56(4):72–81.

Orlandi PA, Carter L, Brinker AM, da Silva AJ, Chu D-M, Lampel KA, Monday SR. 2003. Targeting single-nucleotide polymorphisms in the 18S rRNA gene to differentiate *Cyclospora* species from *Eimeria* species by multiplex PCR. *Applied and Environmental Microbiology* 69(8):4806–4813.

Ortega YR, Sterling CR, Gilman RH, Cama VA, Diaz F. 1993. *Cyclospora* species: A new protozoan pathogen of humans. *New England Journal of Medicine* 328(18):1308–1312.

Ortega YR, Gilman RH, Sterling CR. 1994. A new coccidian parasite (Apicomplexa: Eimeriidae) from humans. *Journal of Parasitology* 80(4):625–629.

Ortega YR, Nagle R, Gilman RH, Watanabe J, Miyagui J, Quispe H, Kanagusuku P, Roxas C, Sterling CR. 1997. Pathologic and clinical findings in patients with cyclosporiasis and a description of intracellular parasite life-cycle stages. *Journal of Infectious Diseases* 176(6):1584–1589.

Powell D. 1998. Risk-based regulatory responses in global food trade: Guatemalan raspberry imports into the U.S. and Canada, 1996–1998. Conference on Science, Government, and Global Markets: The State of Canada's Science-Based Regulatory Institutions, Carleton Research Unit of Innovation, Science and Environment, Ottawa, October 1–2, 1998. Pp. 1–15.

Rangel J, Sparling P, Crowe C, Griffin P, Swerdlow D. 2005. Epidemiology of *Escherichia coli* O157: H7 outbreaks, United States, 1982–2002. *Emerging Infectious Diseases* 11(4):603–609.

Redelmeier DA. 2005. The cognitive psychology of missed diagnoses. *Annals of Internal Medicine* 142(2):115–120.

Relman DA, Schmidt TM, Gajadhar A, Sogin M, Cross J, Yoder K, Sethabutr O, Echeverria P. 1996. Molecular phylogenetic analysis of *Cyclospora*, the human intestinal pathogen, suggests that it is closely related to *Eimeria* species. *Journal of Infectious Diseases* 173(2):440–445.

Robbins JA, Sjulin TM, Rasmussen HP. 1988. Scanning electron microscope analysis of drupelet morphology of red raspberry and related *Rubus* genotypes. *Journal of the American Society of Horticultural Science* 113(3):474–480.

Sapers GM. 2001. Efficacy of washing and sanitizing methods for disinfection of fresh fruit and vegetable products. *Food Technology and Biotechnology* 39(4):305–311.

Sathyanarayanan L, Ortega Y. 2004. Effects of pesticides on sporulation of *Cyclospora cayetanensis* and viability of *Cryptosporidium parvum*. *Journal of Food Protection* 67(5):1044–1049.

Schlech WF III, Lavigne PM, Bortolussi RA, Allen AC, Haldane EV, Wort AJ, Hightower AW, Johnson SE, King SH, Nicholls ES, Broome CV. 1983. Epidemic listeriosis—evidence for transmission by food. *New England Journal of Medicine* 308(4):203–206.

Shan XC, Wolffs P, Griffiths MW. 2005. Rapid and quantitative detection of hepatitis A virus from green onion and strawberry rinses by use of a real-time reverse transcriptase-PCR. *Applied Environmental Microbiology* 71(9):5624–5626.

Sivapalasingam S, Friedman CR, Cohen L, Tauxe RV. 2004. Fresh produce: A growing cause of outbreaks of foodborne illness in the United States, 1973 through 1997. *Journal of Food Protection* 67(10):2342–2353.

Slutsker L, Evans MC, Schuchat A. 2000. Listeriosis. In: Scheld W, Craig W, Hughes J, Eds. *Emerging Infections* 4. Washington, D.C.: American Society for Microbiology Press. Pp. 83–106.

Sobel J, Khan AS, Swerdlow DL. 2002. Threat of a biological terrorist attack on the US food supply: The CDC perspective. *Lancet* 359(9309):874–880.

Steele M, Unger S, Odumeru J. 2003. Sensitivity of PCR detection of *Cyclospora cayetanensis* in raspberries, basil, and mesclun lettuce. *Journal of Microbiology Methods* 54(2):277–280.

Sterling CR, Ortega YR. 1999. *Cyclospora:* An enigma worth unraveling. *Emerging Infectious Diseases* 5(1):48–53.

Stone J. 2004. "Gaudeamus Igitur" [poem]. In: Stone, *Music from Apartment 8: New and Selected Poems.* Baton Rouge: Louisiana State University Press.

Swaminathan B, Gerner-Smidt P, Ng LK, Lukinmaa S, Kam KM, Rolando S, Gutierrez EP, Binsztein N. 2006. Building PulseNet International: An interconnected system of laboratory networks to facilitate timely public health recognition and response to foodborne disease outbreaks and emerging foodborne diseases. *Foodborne Pathogens and Diseases* 3(1):36–50.

Tanaka J. 2000. Hepatitis A shifting epidemiology in Latin America. *Vaccine* 18(Suppl 1):S57–S60.

Tappero J, Schuchat A, Deaver K, Mascola L, Wenger J. 1995. Reduction in the incidence of human listeriosis in the United States: Effectiveness of prevention efforts? *Journal of the American Medical Association* 273(14):1118–1122.

Tauxe RV. 1997. Emerging foodborne diseases: An evolving public health challenge. *Emerging Infectious Diseases* 3(4):425–434.

Tauxe RV. 2002. Emerging foodborne pathogens. *International Journal of Food Microbiology* 78(1–2):31–41.

Tauxe RV. 2005 (October 25). *Session II: The Food Supply "Threat Spectrum."* Presentation at the Forum on Microbial Threats Workshop Meeting, Foodborne Threats to Health: The Policies and Practices of Surveillance, Prevention, Outbreak Investigations, and International Coordination, Washington, D.C., Institute of Medicine, Forum on Microbial Threats.

Tauxe RV, Hughes JM. 1996. International investigation of outbreaks of foodborne disease. *British Medical Journal (Clinical Research Ed.)* 313(7065):1093–1094.

Torok TJ, Tauxe RV, Wise RP, Livengood JR, Sokolow R, Mauvais S, Birkness KA, Skeels MR, Horan JM, Foster LR. 1997. A large community outbreak of salmonellosis caused by intentional contamination of restaurant salad bars. *Journal of the American Medical Association* 278(5): 389–395.

Treadway K. 2006. Heart sounds. *New England Journal of Medicine* 354(11):1112–1113.

U.S. Senate, Permanent Subcommittee on Investigations of the Committee on Governmental Affairs. 1998. *The Safety of Food Imports: From the Farm to the Table: A Case Study of Tainted Imported Fruit.* 105th Cong., 2nd Sess., Senate Hearing 105-516 (Part II). July 9, 1998.

Varma M, Hester JD, Schaefer FW, Ware MW, Lindquist HDA. 2003. Detection of *Cyclospora cayetanensis* using a quantitative real-time PCR assay. *Journal of Microbiology Methods* 53(1):27–36.

Verweij JJ, Laeijendecker D, Brienen EAT, van Lieshout L, Polderman AM. 2003. Detection of *Cyclospora cayetanensis* in travellers returning from the tropics and subtropics using microscopy and real-time PCR. *International Journal of Medical Microbiology* 293(2–3):199–202.

Voetsch A, Angulo F, Rabatsky-Ehr T, Shallow S, Cassidy M, Thomas SM, Swanson E, Zansky SM, Hawkins MA, Jones TF, Shillam PJ, Van Gilder TJ, Wells JG, Griffin PM, Emerging Infections Program FoodNet Working Group. 2004a. Laboratory practices for stool-specimen culture for bacterial pathogens, including *Escherichia coli* O157:H7 in the FoodNet sites, 1995–2000. *Clinical Infectious Diseases* 38(Suppl 3):S190–S197.

Voetsch AC, Van Gilder TJ, Angulo FJ, Farley MM, Shallow S, Marcus R, Cieslak PR, Deneen VC, Tauxe RV, Emerging Infections Program FoodNet Working Group. 2004b. FoodNet estimate of the burden of illness caused by nontyphoidal *Salmonella* infections in the United States. *Clinical Infectious Diseases.* 38(Suppl 3):S127–S134.

Vogt DU. 2005. *Food Safety Issues in the 109th Congress.* Washington, D.C.: Library of Congress, Congressional Research Service.

Wan J, Wilcock A, Coventry MJ. 1998. The effect of essential oils of basil on the growth of *Aeromonas hydrophila* and *Pseudomonas fluorescens. Journal of Applied Microbiology* 84(2):152–158.

Wheeler JG, Sethi D, Cowden JM, Wall PG, Rodrigues LC, Tompkins DS, Hudson MJ, Roderick PJ. 1999. Study of infectious intestinal disease in England: Rates in the community, presenting to general practice, and reported to national surveillance. The Infectious Intestinal Disease Study Executive. *British Medical Journal* 318(7190):1046–1050.

Wheeler C, Vogt TM, Armstrong GL, Vaughan G, Weltman A, Nainan OV, Dato V, Xia G, Waller K, Amon J, Lee TM, Highbaugh-Battle A, Hembree C, Evenson S, Ruta MA, Williams IT, Fiore AE, Bell BP. 2005. An outbreak of hepatitis A associated with green onions. *New England Journal of Medicine* 353(9):890–897.

Wick L, Qi W, Lacher D, Whittam T. 2005. Evolution of genomic content in the stepwise emergence of *Escherichia coli* O157:H7. *Journal of Bacteriology* 187(5):1783–1791.

Yazaki Y, Mizuo H, Takahashi M, Nishizawa T, Sasaki N, Gotanda Y, Okamoto H. 2003. Sporadic acute or fulminant hepatitis E in Hokkaido, Japan, may be food-borne, as suggested by the presence of hepatitis E virus in pig liver as food. *Journal of General Virology* 84(Pt 9):2351–2357.

Zhang X, McDaniel A, Wolf L, Keusch G, Waldor M, Acheson D. 2000. Quinolone antibiotics induce Shiga toxin-encoding bacteriophages, toxin production, and death in mice. *Journal of Infectious Diseases* 181(2):664–670.

4

Bioterrorism and the Food Supply

OVERVIEW

Each of the three papers collected in this chapter address a different aspect of a single, highly publicized scenario for foodborne terrorism: the intentional contamination of the U.S. milk supply with botulinum toxin, as described in a May 2005 *New York Times* op-ed essay by Lawrence Wein (Wein, 2005). The article sparked an intense debate about the possible security risk it posed, a controversy that was fueled in subsequent weeks by the delayed publication of a peer-reviewed paper by Wein and a coauthor (Wein and Liu, 2005) in the *Proceedings of the National Academy of Sciences* (Alberts, 2005).

These concerns are expressed in the first part of this chapter by Clay Detlefsen of the International Dairy Foods Association. "Disclosure of information that can be used to harm people needs to be limited except when necessary," he argues, extending the definition of "harm" to include the needless scaring of consumers who might stop buying milk. Indeed, Detlefsen asserts, the dairy industry has been aware for years of the threats described by Wein and has been working with the U.S. government to safeguard its operations and products from bioterrorism. To prevent such efforts from being undermined by the release of sensitive information to potential terrorists and other malefactors, Detlefsen supports the creation of a vetting system as a means to fairly assess and, when appropriate, prohibit the publication of scientific findings that could be used to develop and launch an attack.

As workshop contributor Milton Leitenberg notes in the second contribution to this chapter, considerably less attention has been paid to the questionable validity of Wein's conclusion that milk represents "a uniquely valuable medium for a terrorist" than to its status as a threat to national security. Leitenberg, a senior research scholar at the University of Maryland's Center for International Security Studies at Maryland (CISSM), offers detailed evidence that contradicts key assumptions upon which Wein based his model, most notably the ease by which terrorists could obtain botulinum toxin and use it to launch an attack. More generally, Leitenberg notes that several existing historical reviews of agricultural terrorism contain inaccuracies that serve to inflate the number of instances of actual attacks. As a result, he concludes, U.S. policy has been influenced by "gross exaggeration surrounding the potential for bioterrorism."

Using the controversy over the Wein model as a jumping-off point, Dr. David Acheson, Director of the Food and Drug Administration (FDA) Office of Food Safety, Defense, and Outreach within the Center for Food Safety and Applied Nutrition, outlines the FDA's multifaceted approach to protecting the U.S. food supply from attack in this chapter's final paper. Acheson explains how the agency uses risk management and vulnerability assessment tools to determine which food/agent combinations present the greatest threats to U.S. biosecurity, and in particular how these analyses have raised concerns about the potential consequences of the deliberate contamination of milk with botulinum toxin. He then describes how the FDA addresses such findings through the development of guidance documents and training programs to prevent and mitigate the effects of specific bioterrorism threats.

THE THREAT AGAINST MILK: JUST ONE OF MANY, WITH MORE TO COME

Clay Detlefsen, M.B.A., Esq.[1]
International Dairy Foods Association

After September 11, 2001, leaders in this country vowed that we would never be caught off guard again and began an extensive process by which every imaginable terrorist threat scenario is analyzed. The laudatory goal is to identify reasonable mitigation strategies for any threats within the realm of possibility of being perpetrated. More than four years later, that effort is continuing and expanding. Today, virtually every industry is working with the government to harden itself against a potential terrorist attack. The food industries are no exception, and the dairy industry, in particular, has been quite active and proactive.

I have worked with the government and various industries on food-specific scenarios involving terrorism, and I have participated in government and industry

[1]Vice President for Regulatory Affairs.

exercises to plan for chemical and biological terrorist attacks that had little to do with the food supply. Further, I have brainstormed with government officials as to the private-sector response to a nuclear attack on U.S. soil. Due to the sensitive nature of the exercises and discussions, most of these activities take place with little fanfare or public acknowledgment. In some cases, participants such as myself are required to sign nondisclosure agreements. The bottom line is that the federal, state, and local government agencies and the private sector are working closely together to enhance the public's safety. Being discrete about it is par for the course when dealing with a public safety or national security issue.

Secrecy or discretion is called for in these matters for fundamental reasons. For instance, the general public can scare easily and may then needlessly avoid the subject matter of the concern. This was exemplified by the dramatic downturn in commercial airline travel after 9-11, which lasted, as indicated in Figure 4-1 below, until nearly January 2004.

With respect to food, the 1980s, Alar/apple scare clearly establishes how consumers react when confronted with any implication that a food might present a risk or contain a deleterious substance. This is so even when the risk is only theoretical or otherwise unproven. As author Michael Fumento noted:

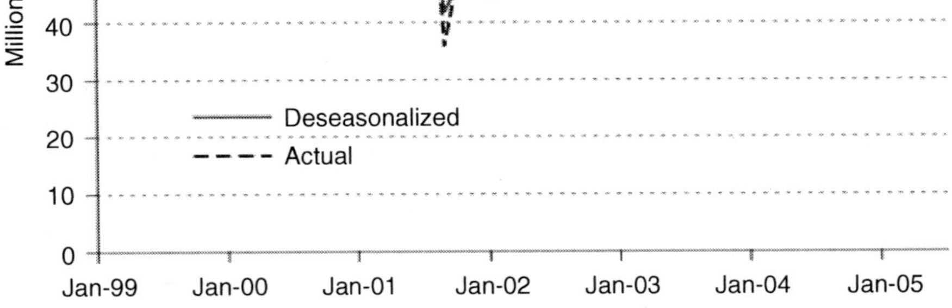

FIGURE 4-1 U.S. domestic airline passengers. These graphs present both actual data, and data that have been seasonally adjusted in order to clarify the trends over time. The data cited in the text represent actual (unadjusted) values.
SOURCE: Bureau of Transportation Statistics (2005).

> Nothing makes Greens—radical environmentalists—turn an angry red faster than invoking the word *Alar* to epitomize bogus environmental scares and imply that a current one is equally phony.
>
> Manufactured by Uniroyal Chemical Co., Alar was commonly sprayed on apples to keep them on trees longer so that fewer would fall and rot before being harvested. The attack on it began in February 1989 when *60 Minutes* reporter Ed Bradley called it "the most potent cancer-causing agent in our food supply."
>
> Bradley's main source was the Natural Resources Defense Council (NRDC), which had decided to scapegoat a single substance to illustrate the horrors of all manmade chemicals. The NRDC had retained a radical environmentalist public relations firm, Fenton Communications, to create a front group called Mothers and Others for Pesticide Limits and place horrifying articles in newspapers and women's magazines.
>
> The result: Terrified mothers threw out their applesauce, poured out their apple juice, and swore off apples entirely for "healthier foods" such as Twinkies. Apple farmers across the nation suffered, and some went bankrupt. Subsequently, articles, monographs, and books peeled the wraps off one of the slickest, most cynical fear campaigns in recent American history (Fumento, 1999).

Although the harm in the above case is significant, it is largely one of economics and is overshadowed by a more significant type of harm—harm that results from a deliberate attack on people and loss of human lives. Disclosure of information that can be used to harm people needs to be limited except where necessary. Too often, the wrong people get their bad ideas from disclosures. The National Academies and many others in the scientific community are aware of the "dual use" problem of attempting to advance science while at the same time running the risk of assisting and aiding terrorists. Unfortunately, the debate seems to end with a statement along the lines "there is nothing new here that terrorists don't already know, so there is no harm in publishing this article." But, a "terrorist" needs to be thought of in a broader way—not just what would traditionally be thought of as a terrorist; but potentially our own misguided or mentally ill citizens, as well. Virtually every law enforcement agency in the nation is aware of, or concerned about, copycat criminal activity. The issue has been debated and discussed on a regular basis for decades. In recent years, a protracted period of carjacking was theorized to have escalated because of media attention:

> Carjacking has always been around, especially in large metropolitan cities, we just rarely read about it. The crime of carjacking "took off" in the 1980s after the media published stories of bizarre situations and the violence associated with the crime. The media coined the phrase "carjacking," and the crime of auto theft took on a new identity. After a rush of publicity, other criminals "copied" the crime of carjacking. These copycat criminals must have said, "Hey, I can steal any vehicle I want without damaging it, I get the car keys, and I can rob the owner too. What a concept!" (McGoey, 2006).

In more recent times, carjacking has largely disappeared and the occurrence of a multitude of Columbine-like school shootings have been theorized to have stemmed from the media attention given to that unfortunate event. A Google internet search of the words *copycat* and *Columbine* yields 44,000 hits, which is a fairly clear indication that some association exists. Further, the mimicking of notorious events is by no means limited to our own domestic criminals. As Florida State University professor Cecil Greek noted in his paper on censorship, the issue is complex and may potentially link to terrorism:

> Ray Surette has done extensive research on copycat crimes since the mid-1980s. He argues that copycat crime is a persistent social phenomenon, common enough to influence the total crime picture, but mainly by influencing crime techniques rather than the motivation to commit a crime or the development of criminal tendencies. A copycat criminal is likely to be a career criminal involved in property offenses rather than a first-time violent offender. The specific relationship between media coverage and the commission of copycat crime is currently unknown, and the social context factors influencing copycat crimes have not been identified. . . .
>
> Surette also noted that copycat crimes . . . seemed to fall into at least four groupings with some overlap. "Mode" copiers were those who already intended to commit a crime and who received a method from the media event. For example, a potential car thief copies the techniques seen on a television police drama for breaking into and hot-wiring a car. "Group" copiers were those who copied acts in groups. In 1995, a group of Tampa, Florida, teens bragged to police they stole cars and shot at robbery victims because earlier in the same week a 12-year-old repeat robber had been granted probation rather than prison. The case had been given major media attention. The other two categories were mentally ill or mentally deficient copiers, and terrorists. Since terrorism is partially driven by media attention, it is not surprising that terrorists choose to repeat methods that have produced high media ratings in the past. This has led concerned media executives to consider carefully how much attention they focus on terrorist acts (Greek, 1997).

Last summer, the dairy industry found itself in the middle of a media flurry over a paper that paints a terrorist scenario about botulinum toxin in milk. The paper, by Dr. Lawrence Wein of Stanford University, described a scenario by which terrorists could poison thousands of people through the U.S. milk supply (Wein and Liu, 2005). Wein's paper was initially withheld at the government's request over fears that it could aid attackers; later, the National Academy of Sciences (NAS) published the paper, insisting that it did not put any new information before terrorists.

Coverage of this issue was widespread, including features in the *New York Times*, *USA Today*, the *Washington Post*, and on major television networks. The story ultimately appeared around the globe in more than 500 newspapers. Today, a Google search of the Internet using the search of the combined words *Wein* and *milk* yields 282,000 hits.

Unbeknownst to most though, the scenario was neither novel nor new. In fact, the industry had been working with the FDA for several years after the FDA brought the matter to industry's attention in 2002. Long before that, the government had theorized about this particular scenario being perpetrated by communists. As early as the mid 1950s government scientists studied the possibility that a variety of beverages, including milk, could be contaminated with botulinum toxin. The report's conclusion was that the threat to the milk supply was negligible because of the nullifying effects of pasteurization on the toxin. In fact, the report concluded that 99 percent of any toxin would be inactivated by pasteurization. This inactivation finding is not consistent with information obtained by Wein that indicated the temperature and time required for inactivation would be much greater. However, the research cited by Wein explored inactivation of toxin in creamed corn, tomato soup, tomato juice, string beans, and canned corn (Woodburn et al., 1979). The research did not include research using milk. The research of the 1950s and more recently conducted research did utilize milk, and those studies are consistent with each other. In fairness to Wein, neither of those studies are publicly available. Curiously, one of the researchers in the 1950s project is one of the researchers of a study cited by Wein.

In addition, what you did not see in the newspaper or on TV were the efforts the dairy industry made behind the scenes to correct the misperceptions we feared the Wein paper might raise, and—more broadly—the extensive work that has already been done to address security issues.

We knew that the Wein paper was flawed in the assumptions it made about the milk supply and about milk processing—I and others pointed those flaws out to Wein himself, who has admitted to shortcomings in his own research. Close scrutiny by a seasoned biosecurity expert—Milton Leitenberg—found that there is "an extraordinary degree of uncertainty associated with Wein's estimates," finding flaws with everything from his mathematical methodology to his assumptions on the production of the necessary toxin.

Moreover, pasteurization steps have been taken within processing plants that substantially eliminate the threat Wein presents. Although Wein was successful in publishing his paper, the International Dairy Foods Association (IDFA) and others have been successful in delivering the facts to government officials—many of whom we have built relationships with since the events of 9-11.

To be clear, the dairy industry welcomes scientific research that is aimed at helping our nation secure its vital systems, including the food supply. But the Wein paper does not fall into that category—and it remains a lesson on how important it is for researchers and security experts to work together with industry in assessing possible terrorist threats.

One area where cooperation is working well is in communication between industry and government. An impressive amount of work has been done cooperatively on security since 9-11. I work closely with officials at the U.S. Department of Homeland Security (DHS), the FDA, the U.S. Department of Agriculture (USDA) and other federal and state government agencies on a daily basis to help evaluate situations and further safeguard the dairy industry. Other individuals in other sectors and industries fill similar roles.

A thorough government analysis of possible threats to the food and dairy supply was completed fairly soon after 9-11. Based on that analysis, the dairy industry has worked diligently, without fanfare, to implement a wide range of measures to secure facilities and the milk supply. For example, based on guidelines prepared by the National Milk Producers Federation and the IDFA, dairy farmers and processors have implemented new standards for sealing milk tankers. Using these new protocols, any unauthorized opening of a tanker before its delivery to a processing plant is immediately evident.

In addition, producers and processors have taken many proactive steps to increase awareness among employees about security measures at the farm and in processing facilities, including increased security of milk storage areas. Dairy plants have secured entry systems and employee screening programs, and have restricted access on the plant floor. And, of course, most packaging operations are already automated, enclosed, and secure.

There is always more we can do as an industry to be vigilant—and we encourage dairy facilities to make every reasonable effort along these lines. But it is also important to realize we have done quite a lot. I expect new challenges to continually emerge between government and industry on security issues. We will never be "done" when it comes to protecting our most valuable attribute—the safety of our products. The good news is that we have good working relationships and valuable new protocols in place.

Our efforts, though, should not be undermined by inappropriate publication of sensitive material that has a potential to be used by foreign or domestic terrorists or criminals. Instead, the scientific community needs to work collaboratively with industry and the government, and this may at times require self-censorship or restraint. The downside of not being cognizant or otherwise ignoring the possibility of harm being perpetrated on the U.S. citizenry can be the loss of human lives, which is clearly unacceptable. We are aware of the scientific community's interest in addressing this important concern, as was recently described by Dr. Brian Gorman in his Yale journal article:

> The open science dilemma has been recognized as a top priority in the scientific and national security communities since the terrorist attacks of 2001. It is undisputed that the fruits of scientific advancements may also be subject to harmful "dual use" by enemy combatants, terrorists, and any number of other malefactors with the necessary skills and resources. The dilemma over open science arises from the incompatibility of restricting access to scientific findings in the interests of public welfare with a notion of public welfare that is itself reliant upon the open exchange of findings and scientific data. Therefore, great care is

needed to avoid remedies that unnecessarily impede the exchange of information between researchers and deter important lines of inquiry. Thus, a carefully crafted remedy is needed to cease "free ride" opportunities available to malefactors interested in misusing scientific advancements without impeding much needed advancements in science interests.

Surprisingly, the most draconian and potentially deleterious remedies to the open science dilemma, to date, come from the scientific community. As of January 2003, over 20 scientific journals adopted a policy calling for the censorship of articles that present unjustifiable risks (Journal Editors and Authors Group, 2003).[2] However, many recognize that censorship is not a guarantee of protection. In October 2002, the former president of the American Society for Microbiology (ASM) warned that, "censorship of scientific communication would provide a false sense of protection" (Greenberg, 2002). Severe measures are of concern because, if carried out, they may discourage research in areas critical to biodefense efforts. Moreover, even if applied sparingly, censorship policies are destined to undermine academic freedom and compromise national security interests.

Unfortunately, there has been little discourse in the literature on specific methods to effectively remedy the problem. While the dilemma clearly calls for "an articulated and uniform practice" to identify and assess sensitive research, efforts to create formal procedures have been abandoned (Cozzarelli, 2003). For example, the journal *Proceedings of the National Academy of Sciences*, which published a sensitive article on the variola virus (Rosengard et al., 2002), abandoned its pursuit for uniform procedures after a self-congratulatory assessment of its ad hoc handling of the article (Cozzarelli, 2003). Despite satisfaction with the "natural" manner in which the article was vetted, flaws remain in the allegedly successful approach. For instance, the national security community was not consulted during a review of the article (Gorman, 2005).

Ultimately, Gorman describes a proposal to pursue a strategy for the creation of a due process vetting system (DPVS). Gorman has clearly given considerable thought to the problem and has proposed a complex, though fair and workable process:

---

[2]On February 20, 2003, *Nature* published an editorial entitled "Statement on the consideration of biodefense and biosecurity" *Nature* 421(6925):771. The editorial described a one-day workshop at the National Academy of Sciences that was attended by representatives of editorial boards, societies (including ASM), and a select group of investigators. The workshop culminated in adoption of four statements pertaining to review and publication of manuscripts that might contain information that could be harmful in the context of bioterrorism. The fourth statement is as follows: "We recognize that on occasions an editor may conclude that the potential harm of publication outweighs the potential social benefits. Under such circumstances, the paper should be modified, or not be published."

> The DPVS is a comprehensive system that enables immediate and informed communication between the scientific and national security communities on new research in line for publication and public release. The rapid communication on potentially sensitive research enables immediate cooperative vetting of flagged articles between the scientific community and the relevant government authority. The DPVS also provides temporary safe harbor for sensitive research by consensus rather than unilateral classification imposed by the government. In the rare occasion when the government needs to classify a research article absent consensus, the government will have notice of the article before it reaches the presses and the scientific community will have ample opportunity to be heard through a fair hearing on the matter if desired. As previously stated, for the purposes of this discussion, the administrative board charged with federal authority will be deemed a new federal agency called the Biologic Regulatory Commission (BRC). . . .
>
> The stakes in this debate could not be higher. The potential showdown between the scientific community and the government on open science, absent goodwill and cooperation, would certainly yield a duel of mutual destruction.
>
> If scientific journals can cooperate by accommodating the parameters of articles in LRC [Least Restrictive Classification] status, and if professional stakeholders agree on fair scaling procedures and joint vetting, the entire field of science can move forward in a safe and efficient manner. The DPVS could provide a superior alternative to the ASM model and ad hoc approaches undertaken by the majority of U.S. bioscience journals. But, the DPVS is just a proposal, and is by no means seen as a comprehensive solution to the debate on open science. It is hoped that the flaws and virtues of this proposal will help inspire a fair and comprehensive approach to sensitive and dual use science that will accommodate the needs of all of the stakeholders in this debate (Gorman, 2005).

Industry and government will continue to work together and we will, as we have in the past, involve the scientific community. It would be foolhardy to think we could cover our security bases without the scientific community. For the sake of the public's safety, we will conduct our activities discretely and cautiously. We have already achieved considerable success with our endeavors and will undoubtedly achieve much more. It is hoped issues involving freedom of the press and censorship will not undermine the efforts that are so vital to the nation's security and the public's safety. I encourage readers in the scientific community not to overlook the dangers associated with our own domestic malefactors, and to, at the very least, read Gorman's paper and consider that as a starting point. No one should ever be put in a position to regret their decision to publish after human lives were lost as a result of such a publication. A robust and systematic approach as outlined by Gorman could obviate such an occurrence.

BOTULINUM TOXIN: THE LINKAGE WITH BIOTERRORISM

Milton Leitenberg, M.S.[3]
University of Maryland

My task was to prepare a paper that brought three subjects together: the traditional biological weapons agent, botulinum toxin; its possible use by bioterrorists; and its dispersion by application to food as the mechanism of such use.

The very opening lines of the guidance document for this conference read as follows:

> In December 2004, at a press conference called to announce his departure as Secretary of the Department of Health and Human Services, Tommy Thompson raised both concern and controversy when he remarked that he could not understand why terrorists had not yet attacked our food supply "because it is so easy to do" (Branigin et al., 2004).[4]

Secretary Thompson's comment is a useful introduction to this paper. In contrast to the expectation that it suggests, one realizes immediately that in the entire period since 1945 there have been only two instances in which any individual or group deliberately added a pathogen or a toxin to the U.S. food supply. The more significant of these was the event in 1984 in The Dalles, Oregon, in which a prepared culture of *Salmonella* was placed on food in a salad bar, resulting in 751 recorded cases of illness (Carus, 2000).[5] Many more people were probably affected, although there was no record of mortality.

In November 2000, Dr. William Fry, a plant pathologist at Cornell University, and an expert on potato late blight in particular (*Phytophthora infestans*), the fungus that caused the historic potato famine in Ireland in 1845–1848, gave an excellent presentation at a conference titled "Agro-Terrorism: What Is the Threat." His assignment for the conference was "Think Like a Terrorist," and he enjoined the conference attendees to do so. Yet his own detailed and thorough presentation repeatedly emphasized the difficulties in producing an artificially caused outbreak of potato blight, to the point of often frustrating the efforts of

---

[3]Senior Fellow, Center for International and Security Studies at Maryland.

[4]The original statement continued with the added words: ". . . and the fact that the United States imports a lot of food products form the Middle East."

[5]It is pertinent to note that the purpose of the Rajneesh use of the biological agent was not "terrorist": It was done covertly and intended to remain covert, and its purpose was a trial run to test its subsequent use intended to cause large-scale public absenteeism from a local election.

In his presentation to the Forum on Microbial Threats, Dr. Robert Tauxe noted that in 20 years there had been 20,000 outbreaks of disease due to food contamination, only two of which were caused by a deliberate act. The second event was the incident in which a laboratory worker in Texas placed *Shigella* into baked goods, which she gave to her colleagues. The organism was obtained from the laboratory in which she worked.

academic researchers when they sought to do so for purposes of their research. He concluded that:

> Devastating crop loss caused by anticrop terrorism is certainly within the realm of possibility, but there are many obstacles to successful implementation. While there are many examples of terrible crop destructions by plant pests, the manipulation of these agents as biological warfare agents to destroy crops on a wide scale by terrorist states or groups faces severe technical challenges. Even if an aggressive plant pathogen can be developed or found, its potential is severely limited by meteorological conditions. Thus, it is difficult to conceive that a biological warfare agent could be used "at will" by a terrorist group or even by a state (Fry, 2003).[6]

But perhaps even more to the point was that while he urged his audience to "think like a terrorist," and many members of the academic and contract analytical community quickly identified ways they thought terrorists could make use of plants or animal pathogens, no real-world terrorist organization had ever done so.

Another guide, in a similar vein to Secretary Thompson's remark, was to be found in the opening line of a report by the Congressional Research Service in August 2004, stating that "The potential of terrorist attacks against agricultural targets (agroterrorism) is increasingly recognized as a national security threat, especially after the events of September 11, 2001" (Congressional Research Service, 2004).[7] At first thought, the statement seems logical: after 9-11, civil authorities looked at every sector of the nation's infrastructure to identify vulnerabilities and points of access by which terrorists could wreck havoc or destruction or injure the public. Nevertheless, the statement is a non sequitur: nothing in the events of 9-11 suggested that any terrorist group intended to attack U.S. agricultural targets or had even considered doing so. The purpose of this study, however, is not to suggest another particular vulnerability. It is rather to attempt a classical threat assessment: an identification and evaluation of real-world entities, their parameters, performance, experiences, and capabilities as regards the potential for terrorist use of botulinum toxin.

Before doing that it would be useful to examine the more general subject of agroterrorism because it serves as an example of what quickly became evident as a major problem in the course of this work. Two tables dealing with historical

---

[6]The last sentence in the quotation implicitly refers to plant pathogens only.

[7]Other reports on agroterrorism that might be of use for the reader are:

- Parker HS. 2002. *Agricultural Bioterrorism: A Federal Strategy to Meet the Threat.* McNair Paper 65. Washington, D.C.: Institute for National Strategic Studies, National Defense University.
- GAO (Government Accountability Office). 2005. *Homeland Security: Much Is Being Done to Protect Agriculture from a Terrorist Attack, but Important Challenges Remain.* GAO-05-214. Washington, D.C.
- GAO. 1999. *Food Safety: Agencies Should Further Test Plans for Responding to Deliberate Contamination.* GAO-RCED-00-3. Washington, D.C.

aspects of agroterrorism prepared by the Center for Nonproliferation Studies of the Monterey Institute of International Studies are posted on their Web site. Both the center and the institute are well known, and their work would ordinarily be considered authoritative and of the highest quality. The first table is titled "Chronology of CBW Attacks Targeting Crops and Livestock 1915–2000" (CNS, 2001). It lists 18 events for the 85-year period. As the title of the table states, all 18 are characterized as "attacks." However, an examination of the 18 entries demonstrates the following:

- Three were false allegations;
- Three others were "threats," and as best as is known, more accurately described, they were bluffs;
- One was an incident in which one man killed his neighbor's animals;
- One was unsubstantiated (Alabama);
- One was a very low-scale "economic" event (Wisconsin);
- Two, both in Israel, were low-scale economic sabotage that could perhaps qualify as "attacks"; and
- One, the U.S. use of a herbicide in the DMZ (demilitarized zone) separating North and South Korea, was done for the purpose of impeding infiltration of North Korean military and security personnel into South Korea. It did not target "crops and livestock" at all.

In sum, 11 or 12 of the 18 events in the table—two-thirds of the entries—are not what they claim to be. They are not "attacks." At a minimum, the title for the table should have read "Attacks, Incidents, False Allegations, and Bluffs."

The second table is titled "Agricultural Bio-warfare: State Programs to Develop Offensive Capabilities" (CNS, 2000). It lists programs for 13 states. The entries for 8 of them need corrections of varying degree:

- Egypt: The claim that Egypt has a dedicated antianimal biological weapons (BW) program is based on a paper that is unreliable and unsubstantiated. The Israeli author, Daniel Shoham, essentially listed any pathogen for which an Egyptian journal publication existed. If the same criterion were applied to Israel, the list of the pathogens would be five times longer than for Egypt. Nevertheless, Israel does not appear in the table at all, even though it maintains an extensive anthrax research program, for example.
- Iraq: Anthrax in the Iraqi BW program was for antihuman purposes, not for use against animals. Studies on camel pox served as a research simulant for smallpox. Finally, contrary to the entry in the table, there was no evidence ever found by the UN Special Commission (UNSCOM), UN Monitoring, Verification, and Inspection Commission (UNMOVIC), or the U.S. postwar Iraq Survey Group to indicate that work on foot-and-mouth disease was ever part of the Iraqi BW program.

- Rhodesia: Regarding the allegation of anthrax use in 1979 during the civil war, the outbreak was almost certainly of natural origin, not due to government action.
- South Africa: The anthrax produced was added to food and cigarettes to produce intestinal or pulmonary anthrax in people; there is no evidence that it was ever intended for or used against animals.
- USSR (Russia, Kazakhstan, Uzbekistan): The facilities and the activities in what became those countries belonged to the Soviet-era BW program. There is no presumption that BW-relevant work continued in them once the two new states became independent in 1992, although the facilities continued to exist. Neither Kazakhstan nor Uzbekistan was an independent entity at the time of the USSR, so there is no justification for listing them.
- North Korea: If North Korea has an offensive BW program, and if that program includes anthrax, it would in all likelihood be intended for antihuman use.
- Syria: The source given is one of the large survey studies by Cordesman; it would have to be checked to evaluate the validity of Cordesman's source.
- UK: The year in which the offensive BW program was terminated is known.

Of the entries for 13 countries, 3 are totally incorrect, 5 others include varying degrees of inaccuracy, and only 5 can stand as the original entries were written.

Literature References to the Production of Botulinum Toxin by Terrorist Groups

References exist for the production of botulinum toxin by two terrorist groups. The first of these was the Red Army Faction, another name of the West German Baader-Meinhof Group.

> A laboratory in a safe house of the Red Army Faction in Paris, France, was found to have made quantities of botulinum toxin; it is believed that none was used (Caudle, 1997).[8]

Allegedly, an Erlenmeyer flask containing the substance had been found in an apartment bathtub. The source for this claim, which allegedly had taken place in 1980, was given as Brad Roberts, *Weapons of the Future?* (Roberts, 1993). The German intelligence agency Bundesnachrichtendienst (BND) had always—privately—said that the story was apocryphal, that is, it was untrue. Nevertheless, numerous U.S. analysts and some U.S. government officials persisted in claiming

---

[8]Douglas and Livingstone, and Kupperman, citing access to classified U.S. government sources, would frequently state the allegation as fact in various seminars in the Washington, D.C., area in the late 1980s and early 1990s.

for two decades that this "event" had occurred. The claim was finally laid to rest in the book edited by Jonathan Tucker in 2000 (Taylor and Trevan, 2000).

The extensive briefing materials prepared in advance of the workshop included two published papers that referred to the production of botulinum toxin by the Japanese Aum Shinrikyo organization or by other unidentified "terrorist" groups. The first was by Sobel, Khan, and Swerdlow, who wrote in *The Lancet* in 2002, "Aum Shinrikyo . . . reportedly had produced stocks of botulinum toxin and other biological agents" (Sobel et al., 2002). Their source for this statement was the chapter by Kadlec, Zelicoff, and Vrtis in Joshua Lederberg's 1999 book, *Biological Weapons, Limiting the Threat* (Kadlec et al., 1999). The source for these authors was in turn Kaplan and Marshall's 1996 book on the Aum, which is inaccurate in virtually all its discussion of the Aum's work on biological agents, except that such work was carried out and that numerous attempts were made by the group to distribute whatever "products" they had made (Kaplan and Marshall, 1996).

The crucial point is that all the biological materials produced by the Aum Shinrikyo group were innocuous, nonpathogenic, and nontoxic. The Aum produced no "stocks" of botulinum toxin. At first it appeared that either they had obtained a strain that produced no toxin, or that they had not succeeded in producing the toxin due to incompetence. It now appears certain that they never obtained a strain of *Clostridium botulinum* at all. This will be discussed further below. The Aum produced no "other biological agents," specifically anthrax, because they only had the Sterne vaccine strain of anthrax, and in addition they did not work with it properly. The Aum had no other biological agents of any kind. By the end of 1999—and therefore certainly by 2002—three publications were available that explained the above as well as additional inaccuracies that by then had appeared in print in every reference to the Aum and BW and which continue to appear in print to this day.[9]

---

[9]A detailed description of the efforts of the Aum group to produce biological agents became available in 1999 and 2000 in three publications by this author:

- Leitenberg M. 1999. Aum Shinrikyo's efforts to produce biological weapons: A case study in the serial propagation of misinformation. *Terrorism and Political Violence* (Special Issue on the Future of Terrorism) 11(4):149–158.
- Leitenberg M. 2000. The experience of the Japanese Aum Shinrikyo group and biological agents. In: Roberts B, Ed. *Hype or Reality: The "New Terrorism" and Mass Casualty Attacks.* Alexandria, VA: Chemical and Biological Arms Control Institute.
- Leitenberg M. 2000. Aum Shinrikyo's efforts to produce biological weapons: A case study in the serial propagation of misinformation. In: Taylor M, Horgan J, Eds. *The Future of Terrorism.* London: Frank Cass.

The second paper was by Arnon et al. in the *Journal of the American Medical Association* (*JAMA*) in 2001:

> Terrorists have already attempted to use botulinum toxins as a bioweapon . . . by the Japanese cult Aum Shinrikyo. These attacks failed, apparently because of faulty microbiological technique, deficient aerosol generating equipment, or internal sabotage. The perpetrators obtained their *C. botulinum* from soil that they collected in northern Japan. . . .
>
> Four of the countries listed by the U.S. government as "state sponsors of terrorism" (Iran, Iraq, North Korea, and Syria) have developed, or are believed to be developing, botulinum toxin as a weapon (Arnon, 2001).[10]

Here, there are several important points to be made. In the statement on the Aum group, both sources used by the authors are not reliable regarding the information that they contain about the Aum and BW. As will be explained below, it appears that the Aum did not succeed in isolating *C. botulinum* from soil or obtaining it in any other way. As regards the other countries, except for Iraq, the U.S. government does not claim to know which specific BW agents the identified countries produced in the past or may be developing (Leitenberg, 1996, 2004). The Russian intelligence agency Federal'naya Sluzhba Bezopasnosti 1993 report, the only publicly available source that could be considered authoritative, does not list botulinum toxin among the four BW agents that it claimed North Korea was working with (Federal'naya Sluzhba Bezopasnosti, 1993). Finally, official U.S. government statements consider it *highly unlikely* that BW or chemical weapons (CW) would be included in state assistance to terrorist groups. It has never happened to date despite four decades of state assistance to terrorist groups by states which do, or may, possess both BW and CW capabilities and which have assisted terrorist groups in every other conceivable manner (Leitenberg, 2004). That includes funding, sanctuary, training, arms, explosives, embassy support, false documents, and other forms of assistance.

A third publication by Roger Shapiro of the Centers for Disease Control and Prevention (CDC), also published in the *JAMA* in 1997, contained the following statements (Shapiro, 1997):

- "Reports that national governments and terrorist groups have stockpiled botulism toxin." However, no "terrorist group" is known to have "stockpiled botulism toxin" to date.
- "As many as 17 countries are suspected of either including or developing biological agents in their offensive weapons program; botulism toxin is frequently

---

[10]The sources given in Arnon et al. for the first quotation are David Kaplan's chapter in *Toxic Terror*, which repeats all the errors in his own book, as well as a *New York Times* article of 1998. The sources for the second quotation are papers by Anthony Cordesman in 1998 and Joseph Bermudez in 2001.

one of these agents." According to official U.S. government tallies, the number has never been alleged to exceed 13. As of mid-2005, it had been reduced by 3 or 4, again according to U.S. government statements. Only Iraq is known to have produced and stockpiled botulinum toxin (Leitenberg 2004, 2005).

- "The Aum Shinrikyo cult in Japan also produced botulism toxin." The Aum group produced no toxin, and they did not have the organism.
- "Instructions for the production of botulism toxin have been broadcast on the Internet as well." Virtually all the "instructions . . . on the Internet" are useless, excluding professional journal papers that may be available online. This will be discussed further below, and an example provided.

What then was the actual experience of the Aum Shinrikyo group and botulinum toxin, and why has misinformation been propagated for all these years? As early as May 24, 1996, the major Japanese daily newspaper, *Asahi Shimbun*, reporting on evidence presented by the Japanese prosecutor, wrote:

> A group led by Seiichi Endo tried to culture botulinum, but failed in isolating the germ. Then . . . Hideo Murai installed a big tank in order to make a large-scale production of the germ. After all, the facility was not accomplished to produce germs.

The decision of the Public Security Commission of the Public Security Investigation Agency (Japan), January 31, 1997, stated that "The Aum had failed to isolate *Clostridium botulinum*."[11] In February 1998, the Chief Toxicologist of Chiba Prefecture, adjacent to Tokyo, told this author that "The group had not been sufficiently competent to succeed [in their effort] to produce biological agents," a statement that referred to their efforts regarding both botulinum toxin and anthrax (personal communication, Chiba Prefecture, February 1998).[12]

In anticipation of this workshop, it nevertheless seemed desirable to revisit this question once again and to try to establish as definitive an answer as possible. I therefore sent a series of very explicit and specific questions to a Japanese academic, Masaaki Sugishima, who had examined the full Japanese prosecutorial record in the Aum Shinrikyo court trials. I asked if the Aum group had acquired a pathogenic strain of botulinum toxin by whatever means. All possible alternatives for acquisition of the organism were explicitly enumerated, and if it had been obtained, whether the group had been able to work with the organism to the point of obtaining the toxin. Box 4-1, below, provides Masaaki Sugishima's response.

---

[11]The full report of the Public Security Commission, *Production of Biological (Bacteriological) Weapons by the Organization*, is classified, but the decision is available.

[12]Translation provided by a Japanese colleague, Dr. Minoru Ouchi, during the conversation.

BOX 4-1

Date: 10/18/2005 8:25:54 AM EDT

Dear Milton,

As far as I know, there is NO publicly available information that the Aum had successfully obtained a strain of *Clostridium botulinum*. You might know, according to the prosecutors' opening statement at Asahara's trial (Tokyo District Court, May 23, 1996).

(1) Tomomasa Nakagawa taught Asahara about the toxicity of botulinum toxin.
(2) Asahara asked Sei-ichi Endo to isolate and cultivate *Clostridium botulinum*.
(3) Endo, together with Kiyohide Hayakawa and Tomomitsu Niimi, went to Hokkaido to collect soil for that purpose.
(4) But Endo FAILED [in] isolating *Clostridium botulinum*.

In this statement, prosecutors have NEVER said that the Aum had successfully obtained (bought, stolen, etc.) a strain of *Clostridium botulinum*.

Best regards,
Masaaki Sugishima
School of Law, Asahi University

In a chapter of his own in a book published early in 2006 Sugishima wrote:

> Endo attempted to isolate *C. botulinum* from soil samples collected in Hokkaido, but there is no evidence that he was successful. Where the strain that was ultimately used came from is unknown, as are its identity and toxigenicity. The fact that multiple dissemination events led to no casualties suggests that the Aum was using an avirulent strain or was unable to cultivate *C. botulinum* properly. Nakagawa told another senior follower that the substance his team produced had proved ineffective in mice (Wheelis and Sugishima, 2006).

The third possibility was more definitively stated above in 1997 by the Japanese Public Security Commission, namely that the group had never isolated any *C. botulinum* at all. Sugishima adds:

> Finally, about a week before the Tokyo sarin incident in 1995, the Aum tried to disseminate botulinum toxin from attaché cases with built-in spray devices. Three such cases were found abandoned at the Kasumigaseki subway station in Tokyo, but nothing harmful was found in them. Endo testified at Asahara's trial

that he had been unable to produce botulinum toxin and had filled the devices with harmless liquid (Wheelis and Sugishima, 2006).[13]

In contrast, the information in Kaplan and Marshall's book on the Aum Shinrikyo and BW derives from three reports by the Japanese National Police Agency dating from 1995 and 1996. These would appear to be based on early statements made to the police by members of the Aum during interrogation rather than on forensic investigation. These were clearly not reliable. All subsequent references in the Western international media as well as in the scientific literature derive in one way or another from the original Kaplan and Marshall book. The information on the Aum and BW in a lengthy report by the two legal counsels to the U.S. Senate Committee on Governmental Affairs in October 1995 is similarly totally incorrect for the same reason (U.S. Senate Government Affairs Permanent Subcommittee on Investigations, 1995).

Botulinum Toxin: A Brief Description

Botulinum toxin is produced by a gram negative spore-forming anaerobe, *Clostridium botulinum*. There are seven distinct serotypes, A through H, and roughly 100 or more available isolates for each serotype.[14] Many of the isolates produce little or no toxin at all. Only serotypes A, B, E, and F are involved in human poisoning and of these, primarily A. The toxin is a single protein with a molecular weight of around 150,000 that acts presynaptically, blocking the release of acetyl choline, and possibly other neurotransmitters, producing a flaccid paralysis (Middlebrook and Franz, 1997).

During the years of the U.S. offensive biological weapons program stretching from 1943 to 1969, hundreds of isolates of *C. botulinum* were tested for toxin production. From these, about a dozen were selected for further research. Those

---

[13]Sugishima supplies the following Japanese-language sources for the material quoted in the text, as well as the paragraph below.

- Police newly identified Aum's microbiological laboratory. 1995 (May 5). *Yomiuri Shinbun*.
- Aum's two scientists were addicted to scientific experiments. 1995 (May 30). *Mainichi Shinbun*.
- Testimony of Endo, January 10, 2005, in Ken-ichi Furihata, *Aum Hotei* [Court Trials of the Aum], vol. 12, Tokyo: *Asahi Shinbun*, 2005, P. 292.

The Aum Shinrikyo group did not lack for financial resources. When Japanese police finally raided the Aum's facility for the first time after the release of sarin by the group in the Tokyo subway, they reportedly found ". . . a glove box, incubator, centrifuge, drier, DNA/RNA synthesizer, electron microscope, two fermenters each having about a 2,000-liter capacity, and an extensive scientific library." Yet the group was not able to obtain or produce any pathogenic agent, demonstrating the point that although equipment is certainly desirable, the key requirements are a culture and competence.

[14]These individual isolates located in various culture collections have at times been referred to as "strains." However, as genomic identification is not available for nearly all of them, it would be better to refer to them as isolates.

in turn were reduced to two, one of which was finally selected for production on the basis of its stability of toxin production, yield, and hardiness of the organism under the condition of large-scale culture (personal communication, Dr. William Patrick, 1988). It took many person-years of work to achieve that result. In 1997 at a NATO Advanced Research Workshop in Budapest, Hungary, Dr. Jerzy Mierzykowski, at that time director of the Polish biodefense laboratory at Pulawy, made an unusual appeal to the researchers present. He was about to retire after a lifetime's work with *C. botulinum*. Nevertheless, he explained, he was unable to obtain repeatable levels of toxin production. He asked the American and the British scientists present to advise him on how one obtained reproducible toxin production.[15] In some months his cultures produced toxin, and in other months they did not. The reason for this is that the structural gene for the toxin appears to vary between chromosomal and extrachromosomal locations in the seven *C. botulinum* serotypes. Some are located in a plasmid, some in a bacteriophage, and some apparently are chromosomally located.

Botulinum toxin—or the group of botulinal toxins—are frequently referred to as the most toxic substances known, with an LD50 of 1 nanogram per kilo of body weight. Although unrelated to botulinum toxin poisoning via ingestion by food, two of the scientific publications referred to earlier, Arnon et al. (2001) and Shapiro (1997), state that one gram of botulinum toxin if distributed as an aerosol would result in the death of "more than one million people," and "at least 1.5 million" people, respectively. All such estimates made on the basis of mathematical extrapolations from LD50 values assume perfect distribution. They are many orders of magnitude from possible realization in the real world. In fact both the United States and later the Soviet offensive BW programs discovered that botulinum toxin did not perform well under aerosol distribution, and both programs lost interest in weaponizing the agent.[16]

Botulinum Toxin Poisoning and the U.S. Milk Supply

On May 25, 2005, the *Proceedings of the National Academy of Sciences* (*PNAS*) announced that it would publish a paper that presented a mathematical model of the possible consequences of deliberate botulinum toxin contamination of the U.S. milk supply. The paper was written by Dr. Lawrence Wein of the Stanford University Graduate School of Business, and Yifan Liu, a graduate stu-

[15]The author was present and contributed a chapter to the book that resulted from the conference. See Geissler E, et al. 1998. *Conversion of Former BTW Facilities*. Dordrecht, The Netherlands: Kluwer Academic Publishers.

[16]Among other problems, the neurotoxin protein must first cross the air-blood barrier in the lungs and then the blood-brain barrier. Other toxins are more effective when delivered by aerosol because they act directly on cells in the lungs.

dent. Stewart Simonson, Assistant Secretary for Public Health Emergency Preparedness at the Department of Health and Human Services requested that the paper not be published on the grounds that it served as a "road map for terrorists," supplied "very detailed information on vulnerability nodes in the cow-to-consumer chain," and that "publication is not in the interests of the United States" (Carr, 2005a,b).[17] *PNAS* editors agreed to a delay in publication. However, a preprint of the paper had been released in advance to journalists, and it was possible to obtain a copy within a day or two.

On May 30, Wein (alone) published an op-ed in the *New York Times* titled "Got Toxic Milk." It presented the conclusions of the unpublished manuscript. This short version included one crucial aspect not contained in the *PNAS* paper: It stated that "a terrorist, using a 28-page manual called *Preparation of Botulinum Toxin* that has been published on several jihadist Web sites and buying toxin from an overseas black market laboratory," could produce "a few grams of botulin" (Wein, 2005). It took a few additional days to obtain a copy of the jihadi manual in question, and to query appropriately informed professional colleagues in Europe as to whether any "overseas black market laboratory"—or overseas black market—for botulinum toxin existed. With these, plus an extensive search of the professional literature dealing with the isolation and purification of botulinum toxin, one was able to try to make sense of the mathematical model in question.[18] *PNAS* duly published the original paper without modification at the end of June 2005 (Wein and Liu, 2005). Comment by the general media as well as editorials and news section reports in journals such as *Nature* and *Science* commented only on the fact that publication of the *PNAS* article had been delayed. None took issue with any aspect of the model itself (Editorial, 2005; Shane, 2005; Weiss, 2005).

Wien's model postulated that contamination of milk with less than one gram of botulinum toxin would cause 100,000 poisoned individuals, and that mortality could be in the range of 400,000 or 500,000 people—"the great majority of 568,000 consumers"—if 10 grams were used. In early seminar presentations of his model at Stanford University, Wien had even posited that the terrorists could have 1 kilogram or more of the toxin (personal communication). His *New York Times* article postulated that a *single* "terrorist" could achieve such levels of toxin production. Some 15 years ago scientists at the Center for Applied Microbiological Research in the United Kingdom had made a few grams of toxin, which served to supply the entire European and U.S. commercial market for a decade. Producing 10 grams—down two orders of magnitude from a kilo—would be a feat for professional scientists.

---

[17]Assistant Secretary Simonson's letter was sent to the head of the National Academy of Sciences, Dr. Bruce Alberts, on May 27, 2005.

[18]Research and part of the writing for this section of the paper were done together with Dr. George Smith. I would also like to thank Dr. Mark Gorwitz and three other anonymous colleagues for assistance in supplying references to relevant literature and other information.

To begin with, the terrorist or terrorists would have to obtain a good producing strain of *C. botulinum*. The jihadi manual begins by extraction from soil. The *deus ex machina* that Wein invoked as an alternative, an "overseas black market lab," apparently does not exist to anyone's knowledge. The 25-page jihadi manual that Wein refers to is in fact a good one: it was composed by splicing together the "Methods" sections of several professional scientific papers. However, applying its directions requires a very long list of reagents and equipment, including a walk-in cold room, a refrigerated vacuum centrifuge, a substantial number of highly specialized reagents, a mouse colony (since the testing for various steps in the isolation of the toxin requires repeated in vivo assays), and, not least substantial, technical skill and experience. Without such knowledge, the manual is useless. None of these are likely to be available in any jihadi terrorist camp, and none of them have ever been found to date in any such location. Annex 4-1 contains excerpts from a far more typical jihadi manual concerning botulinum toxin. They provide an indication of what the knowledge base of such a group is more likely to be.

Alternatively, if the terrorist group obtained the services of a competent trained scientist, or if the terrorist himself had such qualifications as well as access to equipment and facilities (as was apparently the case for the individuals who produced the anthrax used in the United States in October and November 2001), then there is no need to invoke a "jihadi manual." Such an individual would be likely to already have a culture of the organism or to know how to obtain it from nature, know how to produce and purify the toxin, and how to perform the in vivo mouse assays.

Fortuitously, we have the rudiments of a real-world example to measure against. In December 2001, the United States and allied forces overran an al-Qaeda facility in Afghanistan that contained documentary material relating to their program to attempt to produce biological agents. This author obtained the declassification of these materials. They demonstrated that botulinum toxin was one of the agents in which the group was interested (Leitenberg, 2005). A Ph.D.-level Pakistani scientist working in a Pakistani government facility had provided the group with photocopies of papers from the journal literature that Dr. Zawahiri, a senior al-Qaeda official, had requested. However he was not willing to do any laboratory work himself, and as best as is publicly known, he had not provided them with a culture of *C. botulinum*. In addition to journal papers on anthrax, plague, and hepatitis A, the following were the publications that the group possessed that dealt with botulinum toxin:

- Roberts TA. 1965. Sporulation of *Clostridium botulinum* type E in different culture media. *Journal of Applied Bacteriology* 28(1):142–146.
- Hobbs C, Roberts TA, Walker PD. 1965. Some observations on OS variants of *Clostridium botulinum* type E. *Journal of Applied Bacteriology* 28(1):147–152.

- Roberts TA, Ingram M, Skulberg A. 1965. The resistance of *Clostridium botulinum* type E to heat and radiation. *Journal of Applied Bacteriology* 28(1): 125–141.
- A one-page extract of a handbook of gram-positive bacteria, on *Clostridium tetani.*
- A four-page extract of a medical or microbiological handbook on *Clostridium tetani* and *Clostridium botulinum.*

There was no indication that the group had obtained a culture of *C. botulinum* from any source, and there was no indication that it had initiated any laboratory work.

If we return to examining Wein's model, it appears that it was constructed with little knowledge of the relevant literature concerning botulinum toxin. The few sources referenced are of poor quality, inappropriate, or inaccurate. As indicated, the mathematical model is built upon a thin supposition regarding what terrorists can do. Wein starts with the assumption that terrorists can make gram quantities of botulinum toxin. For the *PNAS* publication, the reasoning for this was delivered in a little over a paragraph and based on three citations. The first is an article published in the *Journal of Bacteriology* in 1971. Although it deals with the production of botulinum toxin, it more specifically concerns the preliminary characterization of another protein from the microbe that activates the toxin.

The second citation that Wein used to posit terrorist capability was not from another scientific journal at all but, surprisingly, from a short news piece published by the *New York Times* on April 27, 2003, written by Judith Miller, then embedded with the U.S. Army's Mobile Exploitation Team Alpha in Iraq. It is a very brief interview with a scientist who worked in Iraq's bioweapons program, and it delivers one brief and contextually meaningless claim about the degree of toxin concentration achieved in that country's production of botulinum toxin. It was a simple task to determine that neither UNSCOM, UNMOVIC, nor the Iraq Survey Group inspectors were ever able to verify his statement or find documentary verification for it in any internal Iraqi government report. Even if accurate, the claim could not be expected to reflect an achievement level that a terrorist group might reach. The Iraqi biological weapons program was a national program with access to unlimited resources. Late in 1985, botulinum toxin and anthrax were one of the first two pathogens selected as candidate agents for the Iraqi BW program. Initial production began in 1988, and early in 1989 full-scale production began (United Nations Security Council, 2005). Approximately three full years were thus taken up by Iraqi scientists and technicians in preparatory work, and although UNSCOM inspectors never obtained any of the prepared material to evaluate, they assumed it to have been a relatively crude preparation. Given that this was a state program—in contrast to "a" *single* terrorist postulated by Wein's model—it perhaps offers a more realistic estimate of what might be required.

The third citation was used by Wein to bolster an argument for possible advanced production methods in the hands of terrorists. It too is not from a scientific publication, but is a reference to a "paper for discussion" attributed to Richard Danzig, a former U.S. Secretary of the Navy, which includes the single sentence saying that there are such advanced methods. Of course there are advanced methods for botulinum toxin production; the question is whether they are within the capabilities of terrorists. Finally, the data point used in the model for toxin survival during thermal processing was out of date, and was for canned corn rather than for milk.

But the most critical assessment of the model results from several lines at the very end of Wein's *PNAS* paper:

> In closing, it is important to stress that several elements of the model contain enough irreducible uncertainty to preclude estimating the impact of the attack to within several orders of magnitude. . . .
>
> The dose-response curve, pasteurization inactivation rate, and terrorists' release size capabilities each contain several orders of magnitude of uncertainty. . . . Taken together, we have reasonably accurate estimate of the number of people who could be poisoned, but a very poor estimate of how much toxin is required to cause a large outbreak (Wein and Liu, 2005).

As it turns out, there apparently is variability of three or more orders of magnitude in *each* of the three variables. Taken together, this could result in a possible difference of *nine orders of magnitude* from the numbers presented by Wein. The mortality result could be one billionth of Wein's estimate. Instead of the predicted mortality of half a million people, there might not have been a single death. By definition, Wein could not have had "a reasonably accurate estimate" if the results could vary anywhere over a range of nine orders of magnitude. The first and last lines in the quotation above are contradictory, and the last lines appear to be internally contradictory. The model builder apparently knew little or nothing of the relevant literature on botulinum toxin and nothing at all about the real-world capabilities of would-be bioterrorists and bioterrorism. Intelligence analysis and mathematical modeling share the same classic limitation: faulty assumptions lead to faulty conclusions. A mountain of mathematics, formulas, and curves cannot remedy flawed basic assumptions and inputs. It is difficult to understand how the *PNAS* reviewers and editors let this pass. Finally, Wein had given presentations of his model to public groups and government officials in Washington, D.C., long before the manuscript was submitted to *PNAS* for publication. During both the private and public presentations he had been informed that remedial measures had already been taken by the U.S. milk industry to raise both the temperature and duration of heating during the pasteurization process (personal communication, June 2005). This sharply increased the level of toxin inactivation reached during pasteurization—one of the three variables in question—and concomitantly reduced the amount of inactivated toxin that might remain. Thus one of the two recommendations that Wein suggested at the end of his paper had essentially already been carried out, although not mandated by law.

Although all of the public discussion surrounding the model concerned issues related to the delay in its publication, the far more germane issue appears to be that the model was wrong. At the same time, the episode served as yet another example of the gross exaggeration surrounding the potential for bioterrorism. The most likely outcome of such exaggeration is to prompt would-be terrorists who might not otherwise consider or pursue the development of biological agents to do so because a fictitious simplicity and a fictitious effectiveness was touted. Documentation captured in Afghanistan demonstrated that precisely that occurred in the case of al-Qaeda. On April 15, 1999, the Egyptian-born physician, Dr. Ayman al Zawahiri, deputy to Osama bin Laden, wrote in a message to one of his colleagues:

> We only became aware of them [biological weapons] when the enemy drew our attention to them by repeatedly expressing concerns that they can be produced simply with easily available materials (Leitenberg, 2005).

There was a final coda to the *PNAS* publication, which ironically also concerns publication restrictions. When *PNAS* published the Wein-Liu model, it printed an accompanying lengthy commentary by Dr. Bruce Alberts, then the president of the NAS. In it he noted:

> The Wein and Liu article has been widely circulated in preprint form, generating a great deal of discussion. For this reason, we are already aware of scientists who plan to publish challenges to some of its conclusions. This type of give-and-take lies at the heart of scientific progress and is precisely why scientific analyses are made available in the open literature (Alberts, 2005).

Alberts' reference to "scientists who plan to publish challenges" referred specifically to a very brief critique of the Wein model by this author and Dr. George Smith. It had been submitted to *PNAS* asking if it could be published together with the model. However, Dr. Nicholas Cozzarelli, the *PNAS* editor, had already rejected that suggestion by June 2, a full six weeks earlier, saying "We do not have a letters to the editor section in our journal for what you propose. You are of course free to send in an article that will be subject to our customary peer review."[19] The catch-22 however was that we did not write a scientific paper, only a brief three-page critique very similar to the material presented here. We then submitted the same critique to the *New York Times*. The editor who had published the Wein op-ed replied, "Thank you for your submission. As a matter of policy, we do not publish rebuttals on the op-ed page—that is the job of the letters page. I have taken the liberty of forwarding your article to them."[20] We never heard

[19]Dr. Nicholas Cozzarelli, Editor, *Proceedings of the National Academy of Sciences*, e-mail to the author on June 2, 2005.

[20]David Shipley, op-ed page editor, *New York Times*, e-mail to the author, June 8, 2005. Shipley's statement is factually incorrect, since responses that are functionally "rebuttals" appear relatively frequently on the *New York Times* op-ed page.

from the letter editor. *Nature* had editorialized about the *PNAS* publication delay, and the *Washington Post* had also carried an op-ed on the same aspect. The critique was submitted to both. The *Washington Post* declined to publish it either as an op-ed or as a letter. There was no reply from *Nature*. Despite Albert's generous anticipation, no scientific "give and take" ever appeared in print.

Alberts also claimed that when:

> NAS and *PNAS* representatives met with government representatives to discuss their specific concerns about the Wien and Liu article on June 7 . . . we learned in our discussion with government representatives that a great deal has been done to improve the pasteurization of milk since 9/11 . . . we appear to be considerably safer from an attack than they [Wein and Liu] have calculated (Alberts, 2005).

Although the NAS officials and *PNAS* editors professed not to have previously known what nearly everyone acquainted with the model apparently had heard about, they suggested no revisions in the manuscript as a result of their new knowledge, and it was printed exactly as it had been submitted with its original projections.

A Brief Conclusion

The degree of inaccuracy in information published by members of the scientific community regarding the past record and feasibility of bioterrorism by essentially untrained true terrorist organizations is unbelievably bad. That is a situation that the scientific community should consider impermissible. Any scientist that includes information concerning the record of terrorist interest and experience with biological agents in his papers is responsible to apply the same standards for accuracy to such passages as he does in reporting his own research work.

Much of that same information continues to grossly exaggerate, to misinform, and by suggesting the relative ease and feasibility of producing biological weapon agents, provokes interest among potential actors, state and nonstate, to investigate BW, which they might not otherwise have considered. As was indicated, the al-Qaeda experience is a case in point: it was explicitly provoked by the bioterrorism furor in the United States in 1996–1998. It is legitimate to explore vulnerabilities and to improve defenses, but there is no justification for imputing capabilities to real-world terrorists that they do not possess.

A Single Recommendation

The United States has appropriated $30 billion since FY 2002—in four years—towards bioterrorism prevention. Fiscal year 2005 and 2006 expenditure will amount to $12.7 billion. All further funding for "select agent" programs should be cancelled. Future funding should be split between public health programs such as described in the presentation by Dr. Robert Tauxe to the Forum on

Microbial Threats and to preparations to anticipate an H5N1 pandemic influenza outbreak. The former should include increased earmarked funding for state and county public health agencies to enable them to carry out the specified programs. The latter should include the construction of a National Influenza Vaccine Facility as well as a dedicated national pharmaceutical facility for the production of anti-influenza pharmaceuticals. These two dedicated facilities could be rented to commercial entities in the same way that production facilities for weapon systems were built by the federal government and rented to manufacturers during World War II, and for a very large portion of the post-WWII period. The vaccine facility should be prepared to produce an H5N1 vaccine. In all other years of operation, it could produce the required U.S. quota of influenza vaccine to cover annual needs, so that no shortfalls would continue to occur (annual flu mortality in the United States ranges from 22,000 to more than 80,000) (GAO, 2005a,b). Funds freed up by cancellation of existing and proposed Bioshield legislation for "select agents," as well as the massive spending on infrastructure targeted to work on the same agents would more than suffice for this purpose.

ANNEX 4-1

The Microbe *Clostridium*

The word *clostridium* comes from the Greek word meaning "little spindle." Among its characteristics is the ease with which it can be obtained. It is widely available in the environment, found in water and in soil, especially in areas fertile with the dung of grass-eating animals.

These microbes can have within them organisms, microbes, or bacteria which have potential in nonideal climatic circumstances. At this stage, they are latent and inactive until they get into the right circumstances. At that point, the walls of the bacteria are shed and they become active as deadly microbes. They are freed of the glucose that creates an acidic substance. They are active in the absence of oxygen (anaerobic).

As mentioned these kinds of poisons are of the *Clostridium botulinum* type. They are considered among the most destructive poisons because they act immediately on the nervous system and cause the muscles and respiratory organs to fail. These poisons resist fever to an extent, as well as gastric acid. Their effects are similar to food poisoning. The *Clostridium* microbe multiplies in fresh meat and causes it to rot (the strength of the poison is limited in the presence of heat, which invites the question of how it could survive the heat of an explosion. It might be possible to position the poison somehow away from the heat of the explosion, and transfer the poison onto, for example, legs or shoes in the case of a suicide operation). There may also be a way to specially design something to spit the poison out of the exhaust pipe of a car as an alternative to an aerosol.

Clostridium Bacteria

The bacteria of this microbe is killed in the presence of dry heat above 120 degrees Celsius. Its poison emerges from the cell into the environment. It might work to capture these contents on some of the plants on which the bacteria grows. It might be possible to obtain a lot of the poison available *in the cell, after it has been released*. These poisons have a protein nature such that they lose their poisonous quality if they are exposed to acid (in spite of the fact that they can stand up to gastric acid) or to heat. This microbe is rarely transmitted on tissue, living or dead, but it can be grown inside some cans of food, discharging its lethal poisons. These poisons can lose their effectiveness in temperatures between 61 and 80 degrees Celsius. They causes [sic] food poisoning when food is contaminated with the poisons. However, in observing cases of sickness by the same illness (botulism) occurring as a result of contamination with the microbe, it is my opinion that its usefulness would double in suicide operations. The microbe grows well in regular laboratory cultures under intense anaerobic conditions (meaning its worth as a lethal biological weapon could double.) The ideal temperature for growth is 25 degrees Celsius, but it can grow in temperatures between 20 and 30 degrees Celsius. The bacteria of this microbe are active in anaerobic conditions. The activity causes the microbe to release the poisons.

Properties of the Poisons

They are released after [exposure to] a temperature of 80 degrees Celsius for a period of 30 minutes, or a temperature of 100 degrees Celsius for 10–15 minutes. They are released in acid, but the exception to that is stomach acid. The poisons are divided into six kinds: A, B, C, D, E, F (A, B, and E cause sickness in people, and C and D cause sickness in animals. The sickness in people is also caused by F, which is found in water environments and produces poison symptoms in people and fish). In English: [it is a] "globulin of high molecular weight." The weight of the A part is between 6,000 and 9,000 B. These weights are beneficial in the electronic separation of poisons.

How to Cultivate the Specimen

These bacteria are cultivated in normal cultures in the complete absence of oxygen. This requirement can be met simply by lighting a candle inside the flask containing the microbe after either a rubber stopper or a piece of cotton has closed off the opening. This means: place the specimen contaminated with the microbe—which is a piece of dirt—. . . .

From Where to Obtain the Specimen

From dry dirt. Place some of the dung of grass-eating animals in the dirt. Take the specimens after some days.

The nature of the specimen, as mentioned, is simply dirt. Leave it in anaerobic conditions for a number of days; it will become liquid.

A Section on Poisons

Seeing as bacterial culture contain a number of substances, it is important to use electricity on the poisons. These [processes] are known as electrophoresis and affinity column chromatography. They separate the different materials depending on the differences in their weights (references prior). Admittedly, I do not have details on this point, nor the topics of the concentration and preservation of poisons, may God forgive me.

THE FOOD AND DRUG ADMINISTRATION'S APPROACH TO FOOD DEFENSE

David W. K. Acheson, M.D.[21]
Food and Drug Administration

A Risk-Based Approach to Food Defense

The FDA is pursuing a multipronged approach to food defense. It includes increasing the awareness of the food industry and other stakeholders to critical opportunities for safeguarding the U.S. food supply, developing prevention strategies and building capacity to implement them, and planning for response to and recovery from an intentional food contamination event. There are many foods that could be intentionally contaminated, and one food that has attracted a lot of attention of late is milk and its potential to be deliberately contaminated with *Clostridium botulinum* neurotoxin. Although this scenario is discussed in more detail below, it is important to recognize that this is only one food-agent combination amongst the many that the FDA has focused on.

Finding the Risks

The FDA has adopted a risk-based approach to determine where food defense resources should be applied. Following September 11, 2001, the FDA utilized an approach known as operational risk management (ORM). ORM involves

[21]Chief Medical Officer and Director, Office of Food Safety, Defense and Outreach, Center for Food Safety and Applied Nutrition.

a determination of which combinations of foods and agents, and where on the farm-to-table continuum, constitute the highest risks. The FDA began this process with a list of potential terrorism agents that was developed by the CDC in 2000. The FDA modified the agents' rankings according to a variety of criteria such as the stability of the agent in a food matrix; the effect of the agent on the odor, flavor, or color in a food matrix; the severity of public health outcomes associated with the agent; its oral infective or toxic dose; its availability; and perhaps most important, existing threat intelligence on the use of this agent for foodborne bioterrorism. We then evaluated combinations of these agents with a wide range of foods and food ingredients considered to represent possible targets for foodborne attacks.

The ORM evaluations revealed the probability of contaminating a specific point in the food chain with a specific agent. That information was further enhanced by combining it, in matrix format, with an assessment of the likely severity of outcome, as measured by estimated mortality. The construction of these matrices involved the application of basic science, knowledge of food processing, the food industry, transportation, and logic, but the availability of credible intelligence of a food threat trumped all other factors. We recognize that any food could potentially be contaminated by a determined person or group, thus zero-risk foods do not exist. Higher-risk foods do, however, share several common vulnerability factors: large batch size, which implies a large number of servings; short shelf life, which implies rapid turnaround at retail and rapid consumption; uniform mixing, which would maximize the number of people exposed to an agent; and accessibility of a so-called critical node, defined as a process or activity in the farm-to-table chain during which the agent could be added, undetected, in effective quantities.

Based on this information, the FDA developed guidance documents and training for its staff, state and local regulatory colleagues, and the food industry. This knowledge has also contributed to shaping the agency's considerations of preventive measures, its emergency response planning, and the setting of its research priorities. Because the FDA does not have authority to regulate the security or defense of the food supply, we use this information as we work cooperatively with state and local regulatory officials, the food industry, and other stakeholders in food defense. A For Official Use Only (FOUO) version of the FDA ORM evaluations was prepared and distributed to both industry and states to facilitate a better understanding of where the risks lie.

Following the ORM approach described above, which gave a broad overview of the relative risks, the FDA has also employed a more sophisticated vulnerability assessment tool called CARVER + Shock. CARVER is an acronym for the following factors by which it assesses the vulnerability of a potential food-agent combination as a target for terrorism:

- **C**riticality (public health and economic impacts)
- **A**ccessibility (physical access to the targeted food)
- **R**ecuperability (ability of the affected system/population to recover from the attack)
- **V**ulnerability (ease of accomplishing the attack)
- **E**ffect (losses directly attributable to attack)
- **R**ecognizability (ease of identifying a target)

An additional measure called "shock," which combines the physical, psychological, and economic effects, was also evaluated. This framework allows a far more detailed assessment of the farm-to-table continuum than is possible with operational risk management. For example, we might perform a CARVER + Shock vulnerability assessment of a specific beverage product, having already recognized that the uniform mixing of large volumes of this beverage from different suppliers raises the vulnerability of that commodity to terrorism. For example, for fruit juice production a flow diagram is developed, starting with the fruit on a tree in a growing area in the United States or abroad, and continuing with the worker who picks that fruit, the fruit storage facilities on the farm, transport to the dock, shipping and transport from the docks to the warehouse, every processing step through blending and pasteurization, packaging, distribution, and retail. Initially the FDA undertook CARVER + Shock determinations within the federal government only. The results of this process were classified documents that could not be readily shared and thus had the distinct disadvantage of not being readily available to the industry. To address this shortcoming the FDA worked with a number of industries to train them in CARVER + Shock methodology so they could perform their own assessments. With that information, food industries can make the best use of limited resources for food defense.

The current approach for vulnerability assessments is a joint approach led by FDA, USDA, DHS, and the Federal Bureau of Investigation (FBI), and is known as the Strategic Partnership Program Agroterrorism (SPPA) initiative. The SPPA was launched in July 2005 and solicits industry and state volunteers to undertake locally based vulnerability assessments on a variety of food commodities. By being locally based these assessments not only address a specific food commodity but also facilitate local interactions between the very federal, state, and local officials that would have to deal with a deliberate attack on the food supply.

Deliberate Contamination of Milk with Botulinum Toxin

Vulnerability assessments such as the ORM and CARVER + Shock methods discussed above indicate certain foods of higher concern. One of these foods is fluid milk and the specific example of botulinum toxin in milk is frequently raised, since milk production is a significant industry, both in terms of the volume of product consumed and its importance to the U.S. economy.

After the milking process, milk is typically stored in a tank on the farm that may hold up to 500 gallons until it is transported to the dairy in a 5,000-gallon tanker. At the dairy, milk received from several such tankers is held in bulk tanks of up to 60,000 gallons before it is pasteurized and packaged. Packaged milk is distributed first to a warehouse and then to a retail outlet. Milk has many of the common vulnerability factors mentioned above. The same conclusion was reached in an FOUO report prepared by the U.S. Department of Transportation's Volpe National Transportation Systems Center in 2004, which was intended to inform the dairy industry about vulnerabilities in the milk supply and ways to address them.

In response to the results of this report, and continuing discussions with the dairy industry, changes have been made by individual milk producers and the dairy industry as a whole that have improved the security of the U.S. milk supply.

There are multiple points along the farm-to-table continuum where food may be vulnerable, and it is critical that the approach to this problem be multifaceted. To this end, the FDA has produced a series of guidance documents, one of which is targeted at the dairy industry and outlines an array of possible steps that can be taken to minimize the chance of a deliberate attack on the food supply (CFSAN, 2003).

Fluid milk is not the only food commodity that may be subject to a deliberate attack, and to that end the FDA produced guidance documents directed toward a variety of other industries. These include the following:

- Retail food stores and food service establishments: www.cfsan.fda.gov/~dms/secgui11.html
- Food producers, processors, and transporters: www.cfsan.fda.gov/~dms/secguid6.html
- Importers and filers: www.cfsan.fda.gov/~dms/secguid7.html
- Cosmetics processors and transporters: www.cfsan.fda.gov/~dms/secgui10.html

Each one of these documents provides general guidance as well as more focused messages directed toward the specific industry groups.

Research Questions

During the vulnerability assessment process, whether it be ORM or CARVER + Shock, a number of questions typically arise that require research. FDA has undertaken a food defense research strategy that is focused on a number of areas. These include work on the behavior of select agents in certain food matrices, the value of specific mitigation approaches, sensitive and specific detection methods that are rapid, and dose-response relationships with select agents that may be added to food.

Mitigation of Botulinum Toxin in Milk

Specific steps to mitigate the intentional contamination of milk with botulinum toxin are also being researched. The toxin is sensitive to the effects of heat, and thermal destruction of the toxin occurs in foods that are heated to certain temperatures for long enough times. Milk that is shipped in interstate commerce has to be pasteurized using a minimum temperature of 161° Fahrenheit for 15 seconds. Consideration was therefore given to the impact of pasteurization of milk at higher temperatures and/or for longer times. Basic research was undertaken to address this question and the results shared with the milk industry. However, a number of other issues have to be taken into account if higher pasteurization temperatures or longer times are considered. Such things include the economic impact of heating, then cooling the milk, the increase in plate fouling that occurs at higher temperatures, as well as any possible affect to milk's taste and color, and potential reductions in its nutritional value.

Another research question that has arisen is whether testing for botulinum toxin in milk provides an alternative to raising pasteurization temperatures. Testing could potentially be performed at various points from farm to table, and depending on a variety of factors such as the sensitivity, specificity, cost, and assay speed it could be a useful addition to other mitigation strategies. Issues such as sensitivity are critical as approximately one million milk tanker trips occur annually in the United States, a test yielding a one percent false positive rate (e.g., an Enzyme Immuno Assay) would falsely identify 10,000 positive tankers holding a total of 500,000 gallons of milk each year. Dealing with such false positives in a timely way could become complex and time consuming.

Although tests for botulinum toxin currently exist, they are not necessarily appropriate for mass testing because of cost or time required to conduct the assay and so on. Toward the goal of a rapid, sensitive, specific, and cost effective assay, a DHS initiative is currently funding the first phase of a program for a rapid (less than 20 minute turnaround), sensitive, specific (less than one per million false positives), simple (could be performed by someone with a high school education), and cost-effective test for botulinum toxin in food. The eventual objective of this project is to develop a platform that could be adapted to detect multiple agents in different food matrices.

At the end of the day, the most important message regarding mitigation strategies is not to rely on a single strategy alone to produce adequate protection. Rather put in place as many different strategies at different points on the farm-to-table continuum that will, overall, minimize the chances of a successful attack on the food supply.

Preparatory Measures

Being prepared for an attack on the food supply is a very important aspect of the FDA's work. To that end, in 2004 the FDA initiated a series of assignments that were associated with special security events and focused on ensuring the safety and defense of the nation's food supply. These assignments involved activities associated with the G8-Summit, as well as the Democratic and Republican National Conventions. These special event assignments were, however, regional and limited in scope. Based on heightened security during the national election in November 2004, the FDA determined that it was appropriate to issue a broader nationwide food defense assignment. The first assignment of this nature was issued in 2003 during Operation Iraqi Freedom under Operation Liberty Shield. In October 2004, the FDA initiated a new assignment (FDA Security Surveillance Assignment [FSSA]) that, while similar to the Liberty Shield assignment, was designed to involve federal, state, local, and industry partners to a greater extent than was done in Operation Liberty Shield and to better evaluate our national preparedness capabilities. The primary goals of this national assignment are as follows:

1. Deter intentional contamination of food through heightened and targeted preventive activities at various points in the chain of supply; and
2. Exercise the planning and implementation of the system for responding to a period of increased food security risk to identify and address gaps in the system.

The food items selected to be part of the assignment were based on the ORM vulnerability assessments undertaken previously by the FDA. This process allowed the FSSA to focus the limited federal, state, and local public health resources on those food commodities with the highest potential for intentional contamination (CFSAN, 2005). The FSSA was designed to test the FDA's ability to respond to a threat to the food supply, and as such FDA inspectors entered the premises of domestic firms that produced certain foods to discuss food security and food defense issues with their managers. They also took samples of foods in the above categories, which were tested for a variety of chemical (e.g., cyanide) and microbiological (e.g., botulinum toxin) agents using the Food Emergency Response Network (FERN) laboratories. In addition, the FDA conducted an electronic vulnerability analysis of registrations for imported foods in the above categories; it identified 38 "suspicious" products that were subsequently tested using the FERN laboratories.

Response and Recovery

It is likely that a successful attack on the food supply would be detected first at a local level, most likely due to the detection of a sick animal or a sick human, so an effective response requires close coordination with local public health officials. Key aspects of such a response is containment of the threat and communication with the public. Achieving recovery from such an attack requires the means to demonstrate that the food supply is safe, as well as to decontaminate and dispose of potentially large amounts of tainted food—including food in the homes of consumers—and processing equipment. Once again, good communication with consumers is critical to the success of a recovery program to reassure the public of when a particular food is safe to consume.

Food Safety vs. Food Defense

Although the discussion in this chapter has been focused on food defense, it is imperative that we do not lose sight of the importance of food safety. A deliberate attack on the food supply is plausible and potentially catastrophic both economically as well as in loss of life. However, foodborne illness due to unintentional events is an ongoing and real everyday event resulting in sickness and death. As we continue to move forward in meeting our food defense goals by increasing preparedness, developing response plans and ensuring we have the tools to facilitate recovery, we must also integrate these approaches into our ongoing food safety work. In this context, we are talking about the same foods in the same farms, manufacturers, warehouses, and so on, as well as the same set of inspectors at the local, state, and federal level, and in some instances even the same agents. The overlap is huge and obvious, and the same resources are used for both. Food safety and food defense are here to stay, and it is critical they be integrated to the maximum extent possible to ensure the most efficient use of resources as well as optimizing response to an event.

REFERENCES

Alberts B. 2005. Modeling attacks on the food supply. *Proceedings of the National Academy of Sciences* 102(28):9737–9738.

Arnon SS. 2001. Botulinum toxin as a biological weapon: Medical and public health management. *Journal of the American Medical Association* 285(3):1059–1070.

Branigin W, Allen M, Mintz J. 2004. Tommy Thompson resigns from HHS: Bush asks Defense Secretary Rumsfeld to stay. *Washington Post.* [Online]. Available: http://www.washingtonpost.com/wp-dyn/articles/A31377-2004Dec3.html [accessed April 13, 2006].

Bureau of Transportation Statistics. 2005 (December). *Issue Brief: U.S. Airline Travel Since 9/11.* U.S. Department of Transportation, Research and Innovative Technology Administration. [Online]. Available: http://www.bts.gov/publications/issue_briefs/number_13/pdf/entire.pdf [accessed July 18, 2006].

Carr R. 2005a (June 21). Government request stops publication of article about terror threat to milk. *New York Times Washington Wires.*

Carr R. 2005b (June 26). Publication heeds U.S., pulls terror article: Professor speculates about attack. *Atlanta Journal-Constitution.* [Online]. Available: http://www.ajc.com/print/content/epaper/editions/sunday/news_24ebc541731e70fe0050.html [accessed April 13, 2006].

Carus SW. 2000. The Rajneeshees (1984). In: Tucker JB, Ed. *Toxic Terror: Assessing Terrorist Use of Chemical and Biological Weapons.* Cambridge, MA: MIT Press. Pp. 115–137.

Caudle LC. 1997. The biological warfare threat. In: Sidell FR, Takafuji ET, Franz DR, Eds. *Medical Aspects of Chemical and Biological Warfare.* Washington, D.C.: Walter Reed Army Medical Center. P. 463.

CFSAN (Center for Food Safety and Applied Nutrition). 2003 (July 11). *Dairy Farms, Bulk Milk Transporters, Bulk Milk Transfer Stations and Fluid Milk Processors Food Security Preventive Measures Guidance.* [Online]. Available: http://www.cfsan.fda.gov/~dms/secguid8.html [accessed July 10, 2006].

CFSAN. 2005. *Summary Report FDA Security Surveillance Assignment October–November 2004.* [Online]. Available: http://www.cfsan.fda.gov/~dms/fssarpt.html [accessed July 10, 2006].

CNS (Center for Nonproliferation Studies). 2000. *Agricultural Biowarfare: State Programs to Develop Offensive Capabilities.* [Online]. Available: http://cns.miis.edu/research/cbw/agprogs.htm [accessed April 13, 2006].

CNS. 2001. *Agroterrorism: Chronology of CBW Attacks Targeting Crops and Livestock 1915–2000.* [Online]. Available: http://cns.miis.edu/research/cbw/agchron.htm [accessed October 1, 2005].

Cozzarelli NR. 2003. PNAS policy on publication of sensitive material in the life sciences. *Proceedings of the National Academy of Sciences* 100(4):1463.

CRS (Congressional Research Service). 2004 (August 13). *Agroterrorism: Threats and Preparedness.* RL 32521. Washington, D.C. P. 1.

Editorial. 2005. Risks and benefits of dual-use research. *Nature* 435(7044):855.

Federal'naya Sluzhba Bezopasnosti. 1993 (March 5). *Proliferation Issues: A New Challenge After the Cold War, Proliferation of Weapons of Mass Destruction.* JPRS-TND-9-3-007. Russian Federation Foreign Intelligence Report [translation]. Joint Publications Research Service. JPRS-TND93-007. P. 29.

Fry WE. 2003. Technical feasibility of anti-crop terrorism. In: Pate J, Cameron G, eds. *Agro-Terrorism: What Is the Threat.* CGSR-03-01. Livermore, CA: Lawrence Livermore National Laboratories. Pp. 69, 74.

Fumento M. 1999. Greens still trying to salvage their Alar-stained reputation. *Outlook Magazine.* [Online]. Available: http://www.junkscience.com/jun99/salvage.htm [accessed April 12, 2006].

GAO (Government Accountability Office). 2005a. *Influenza Pandemic: Applying Lessons Learned from the 2004–05 Influenza Vaccine Shortage.* GAO-06-221T. [Online]. Available: http://www.gao.gov/docdblite/details.php?rptno=GAO-06-221T [accessed April 14, 2006].

GAO. 2005b. *Influenza Vaccines: Shortages in 2005–05 Season Underscore Need for Better Preparation.* GAO-05-984. [Online]. Available: http://www.gao.gov/docdblite/details.php?rptno=GAO-05-984 [accessed April 14, 2006].

Gorman BJ. 2005. Balancing national security and open science: A proposal for due process vetting. *Yale Journal of Law and Technology.* [Online.] Available: http://research.yale.edu/lawmeme/yjolt/files/20042005Issue/3_Gorman_052005.doc [accessed April 12, 2006].

Greek C. 1997. Copy-cat crimes. In: Rasmussen RK, Ed. *Ready Reference: Censorship.* Pasadena, CA: Salem Press.

Greenberg DS. 2002. Self-restraint by scientists can avert federal intrusion. *Chronicles of Higher Education* 49(7):B20.

Journal Editors and Authors Group. 2003. Statement on the consideration of biodefense and biosecurity. *Nature* 421(6925):771.

Kadlec RP, Zelicoff AP, Vrtis AM. 1999. Biological weapons control: Prospects and implications for the future. In: Lederberg J, Ed. *Biological Weapons: Limiting the Threat.* Cambridge, MA: MIT Press. Pp. 95–111.

Kaplan DE, Marshall A. 1996. *The Cult at the End of the World.* New York: Crown.

Leitenberg M. 1996. *Biological Weapons Arms Control: Project on Rethinking Arms Control.* PRAC Monograph 16. College Park, MD: Center for International and Security Studies. Pp. 39–51.

Leitenberg M. 2004. *The Problem of Biological Weapons.* Stockholm: The Swedish National Defense College. Pp. 12–19.

Leitenberg M. 2005. *Assessing the Biological Weapons and Bioterrorism Threat.* Carlisle, PA: Strategic Studies Institute.

McGoey CE. 2006. *Carjacking Facts, Robbery Prevention Advice.* [Online]. Available: http://www.forcedignition.com/Articles/carjacking_facts.htm [accessed April 12, 2006].

Middlebrook J, Franz DR. 1997. Botulinum toxin. In: Sidell F, Takafuji ET, Franz DR, Eds. *Medical Aspects of Chemical and Biological Warfare.* Washington, D.C.: Office of the Surgeon General, Department of the Army. Pp. 643–654.

Roberts B, ed. 1993. *Biological Weapons: Weapons of the Future?* Washington, D.C.: Center for Strategic and International Studies. CSIS Significant Issues Series Vol. 15(1).

Rosengard AM, Liu Y, Nie Z, Jimenez R. 2002. Variola virus immune evasion design: Expression of a highly efficient inhibitor of human complement. *Proceedings of the National Academy of Sciences* 99(13):8808–8813.

Shane S. 2005 (June 29). Paper describes potential poisoning of milk. *The New York Times.*

Shapiro R. 1997. Botulism surveillance and emergency response: A public health challenge for a global challenge. *Journal of the American Medical Association* 278(5):443–435.

Sobel J, Khan AS, Swerdlow DL. 2002. Threat of a biological terrorist attack on the US food supply: The CDC perspective. *Lancet* 359(9309):874–880.

Taylor T, Trevan T. 2000. The Red Army Faction (1980). In: Tucker JB, Ed. *Toxic Terror.* Cambridge, MA: MIT Press. Pp. 107–133.

United Nations Security Council. 2005. Appendix: Biological Weapons Programme of Iraq. In: *Twenty-Second Quarterly Report on the Activities of the United Nations Monitoring, Verification and Inspection Commission in Accordance with Paragraph 12 of Security Council Resolution 1284(1999).* S/2005/545. New York: United Nations. Pp. 5–15.

U.S. Senate, Government Affairs Permanent Subcommittee on Investigations. 1995. *Global Proliferation of Weapons of Mass Destruction: A Case Study of the Aum Shinrikyo.* Staff Statement. Washington, D.C.: U.S. Government Printing Office. Pp. 47–102.

Wein LM. 2005 (May 30). Got toxic milk? *The New York Times.* [Online]. Available: http://www.nytimes.om/2005/05/30/opinion/30wein.html?ex=1275105600&en=e5692b8396d5681e&ei=5090&partner=rssuserland&emc=rss [accessed April 25, 2006].

Wein LM, Liu Y. 2005. Analyzing a bioterror attack on the food supply: The case of botulinum toxin in milk. *Proceedings of the National Academy of Sciences* 102(28):9984–9989.

Weiss R. 2005 (June 29). Report warns of threat to milk supply, release of study citing vulnerability to bioterrorism attack was opposed by U.S. officials. *The Washington Post:* A 08.

Wheelis M, Sugishima M. 2006. Terrorist use of biological weapons. In: Wheelis M, Rozsa L, Dando M, Eds. *Deadly Cultures: Biological Weapons Since 1945.* Cambridge, MA: Harvard University Press. Pp. 296–297.

Woodburn MJ, Somers E, Rodriguez J, Schantz EJ. 1979. Heat inactivation rates of botulism toxins A, B, E and F in some foods and buffers. *Journal of Food Science* 44: 1658–1661.

5

Surveillance of the Food Supply

OVERVIEW

The search for the organisms that cause foodborne disease—both before and after people consume them—involves a constellation of overlapping information networks, none of which constitutes a complete surveillance system. As John Besser of the Minnesota Department of Health notes in the first paper of this chapter, the scores of existing food surveillance programs can be reduced to two basic types: food monitoring (the direct detection of microbial pathogens along the food chain) and disease surveillance (the collection of human or animal disease data, followed by analyses of case clusters and disease trends). He describes and compares various strategies and methods of both food monitoring and foodborne disease surveillance, noting their strengths and limitations as currently practiced.

Although food monitoring is theoretically capable of providing primary prevention against foodborne disease, Besser finds that such systems seldom meet this standard because of the technical complexity of the task (which can only be addressed at considerable expense). However, another workshop participant, Robert Buchanan of the Food and Drug Administration (FDA) Center for Food Safety and Applied Nutrition (CFSAN), observed that food monitoring plays an important role in verifying the effectiveness of food safety systems (see Summary and Assessment, p. 15). Although Buchanan acknowledged the many technical challenges associated with the detection of disease-causing microbes in food—from the collection of samples to the detection of tiny populations of bacteria in food that are nevertheless capable of producing severe disease if ingested—he also provided several examples of recent technological advances that have enabled researchers to identify food contaminants in "real time" (a relative term in the food industry, measured by the length of time the monitoring agency has to act upon detecting contamination), as well as targeted sampling techniques that can boost the efficiency of food safety systems.

Besser, by contrast, concludes that while microbial monitoring has its place, particularly in high-risk situations (e.g., botulinum toxin in milk; see Chapter 4), a better return on investment is likely to be achieved through increased funding of foodborne disease surveillance programs. Notable among these is PulseNet, which tracks diseases through standardized pulsed-field gel electrophoresis (PFGE) protocols (see Tauxe in Chapter 3 for descriptions of PulseNet and other foodborne disease surveillance programs). Another source of information on foodborne disease is captured by the U.S. Department of Agriculture (USDA) Consumer Complaint Monitoring System (CCMS), and is described in the second contribution to this chapter by Kimberly Elenberg and Artur Dubrawski. CCMS uses an algorithm-based tool that organizes and analyzes data concerning food-associated symptoms or foreign objects present in food in real time in order to provide early warning of a foodborne threat. The database is used to record, evaluate, and track all consumer food complaints involving meat, poultry, and egg products. Based on its proven ability to detect low-amplitude signals amid noisy data, CCMS appears poised to join the "network of networks" that constitute the U.S. foodborne disease surveillance system.

SYSTEMS TO DETECT MICROBIAL CONTAMINATION OF THE FOOD SUPPLY

John M. Besser, M.S.[1]
Minnesota Department of Health

Increasing concern about threats to our food supply caused by microbial contamination, either intentional or accidental, has resulted in the establishment of many local, national, and global networks to address the problem, each with its own function and acronym (GAO, 2003, 2004), as shown in Table 5-1. Although none of these networks by itself constitutes a complete surveillance system, each serves some part of a broader food surveillance effort. Such surveillance efforts fall into two main categories: (a) those involving direct detection of microbial pathogens in food ingredients, products, or production environments (referred to as food monitoring); and (b) those involving the collection of human or animal foodborne disease data to identify problems in the food supply through analyses

[1]Clinical Laboratory Manager, Public Health Laboratory.

TABLE 5-1 Networks and Resources for Food Safety

Acronym	Program Name
Biosense	Biosense (CDC)
CAHFSE	Collaboration in Animal Health and Food Safety Epidemiology (USDA; APHIS, ARS, FSIS)
CaliciNet	CaliciNet (CDC)
eFORS	Electronic Foodborne Outbreak Reporting System (CDC)
eLEXNET	Electronic Laboratory Exchange Network
eLRN	Environmental Laboratory Response Network
Epi-X	Epidemic Information Exchange
Essence	Electronic Surveillance System for Early Notification of Community-based Epidemics
FERN	Food Emergency Response Network
FoodNet	Foodborne Disease Active Surveillance Network
GEMS	Global Environmental Monitoring System
Global Salm-Surv	Global Salmonella Survey (WHO)
GOARN	Global Outbreak Alert and Response Network
GPHIN	Global Public Health Intelligence Network
HAN	Health Alert Network
ICLN	Integrated Consortium of Laboratory Networks
IDSA-EIN	Infectious Disease Society of America Emerging Infections Network
INFOSAN	International Food Safety Authorities Network
LRN	Laboratory Response Network
NAHSS	National Animal Health Surveillance System
NARMS	National Antibiotic Resistance Monitoring System
NEDSS	National Electronic Disease Surveillance System
NETSS	National Electronic Telecommunications System for Surveillance
NPDN	National Plant Diagnostic Network
NRDM	National Retail Data Monitor
PulseNet	PulseNet (CDC)
RASFF	Rapid Alert System for Food and Feed
RODS	Real-time Outbreak and Disease Surveillance
TEPHINET	Training Programs in Epidemiology and Public Health Interventions Network
UNEX	Unexplained Death and Serious Illness

SOURCE: Besser (2005).

that detect clusters of cases and disease trends (referred to as disease surveillance). Within each of these two broad categories, various approaches are used, each with strengths and limitations.

The ultimate goal of all food safety programs is to prevent contaminated products from reaching the consumer. Since the 1950s, Hazard Analysis Critical Control Point (HACCP) programs have attempted to achieve this by identifying, monitoring, and correcting hazards that may occur anywhere in the farm-to-table continuum. Although HACCP programs have been useful, no prevention program can be 100 percent effective. These efforts are challenged by the complexity and ever-changing character of food production and distribution systems, by the limitations of human behavior, and, most recently, by the potential threat of intentional attacks on the food supply. Consequently, there is an increasing demand to identify and close gaps in food safety by microbiological testing. Choosing the best strategy to accomplish this, however, is difficult. Inherent limitations of methods to detect microbial contamination make strategic choices complex and less intuitive.

Strengths and Limitations of Food Monitoring

Direct testing of food prior to consumption is currently used primarily to monitor the efficacy of HACCP programs. Examples of monitored processes includes oyster farming (beds monitored for fecal contamination), milk production (monitored for somatic cell counts as a check on herd health), and ready-to-eat meat and poultry product production. Lot-by-lot testing as a means of assuring food safety is restricted to a few high-risk foods. Effluent from sprout farms is monitored for *Salmonella* and *E. coli* O157:H7, and some beef trim is monitored for *E. coli* O157:H7 before being made into hamburger. The use of lot-by-lot microbial monitoring to protect food is attractive because, unlike disease surveillance, food monitoring can potentially prevent initial cases. This may be the only option for high-risk situations where initial cases are intolerable from a societal point of view. For example, Wein et al. described a model to predict what might happen if 10 grams of botulism toxin was introduced into a milk tanker or silo (Wein and Liu, 2005). Even with optimum disease surveillance, hundreds of thousands of people would be expected to get sick or die by the time the problem was identified and corrected. Food monitoring may add a layer of protection as part of a comprehensive biosecurity plan assuming the basic limitations of food monitoring can be overcome.

Intrinsic limitations of food monitoring are related to sampling and testing (see Table 5-2). Of these, sampling issues represent the greatest challenge. Because the denominator of potential food vehicles could be the total amount of food available for consumption, that amount could be more than 350 billion pounds per year, as estimated by the USDA in 1997 (Kantor et al., 1997). Additionally, microbial contamination of food can be introduced with or without amplification by bacterial growth at any step between production and consumption. Consequently, the potential units to be analyzed include separate food plants, individual animals, all process lots, individual servings, and everything in between. Furthermore, while grossly contaminated food may be easily detected by discoloration, odor, or other manifestations of degradation, most types of microbial contamination with infectious agents leave no visual, olfactory, or tactile clues. Recognition of such microbial contaminates requires direct detection or isolation by growth in culture. But the sampling of food for this purpose is highly problematic. The distribution of microbial contaminates in a product is usually

TABLE 5-2 Comparison of Food Monitoring and Disease Surveillance

	Food Monitoring	Disease Surveillance
Prevention potential	Prevention of initial cases possible	Secondary prevention only
Speed of detection	Potentially fast	Generally slower
Testing		
Sampling Issues		
Denominator (United States)	356 billion lbs food/year (U.S.)[a]	281 million people (U.S.)[b]
Sample selection	By risk or control point	Self-selection
Agent distribution in sample	Uneven	Generally homogenous
Contamination introduction points	Many	Mouth
Testing Issues		
Pathogen load	Generally low	Generally high
Matrices	Complex, varied	Predictable
Damaged cells	Common	Less common (prior antibiotic use)
Inhibitory substances	Common	Rare
Predictive value of broad surveillance (monitoring)	Low	High
Cost of broad surveillance (monitoring)	Very high	Relatively low

[a]Kantor et al. (1997)
[b]2000 U.S. census data.

SOURCE: Besser (2005).

uneven, making sampling decisions critical to success. This may be especially true for pathogens introduced intentionally and sporadically into the food supply. Finally, the amount of confidence in the safety of food screened by testing is proportional to the amount of sampling done and inversely proportional to the prevalence of the pathogen. High levels of assurance require high sampling and expense rates, especially for rare pathogens.

In addition to the limitations imposed by sampling issues, the actual sensitivity of testing methods greatly impacts the usefulness of food monitoring. Under some circumstances microbes may exist in food in very small quantities and still cause significant problems when consumed by a large number of people. For instance, in the 1994 nationwide ice cream-associated outbreak of *Salmonella enteritidis*, less than six organisms per serving were found in contaminated lots, which is far below the standard infective dose and detection limit of most tests. Nevertheless, the wide distribution of the product caused an estimated 224,000 people to become ill (Hennesey et al., 1996). The sensitivity of laboratory tests can be increased by increased sampling. However, the cost of testing and the cost of food lost to testing increases proportionately. Bacterial amplification occurs in improperly prepared or stored food, and during refrigeration of products contaminated with psychotrophic bacteria such as *Listeria monocytogenes*. In these instances, bacteria or their toxins may be present in large quantities and are relatively easy to detect. This is not the case with foods contaminated during production, storage, transport, or preparation that have been otherwise handled properly, or with foods contaminated by viruses and parasites, such as *Norovirus* or *Cyclospora cayetanesis*, which do not amplify in food. In addition, microbial cells tend to become damaged in food, and many food matrices (a food matrix represents the components of food as consumed) interfere with testing procedures. Damaged cells may readily revive under the perfect culture conditions of the human body, but fare less well under the relatively harsh conditions of *in vitro* culture. The problems of food testing are exemplified by the 1996 *E. coli* O157:H7 outbreak in Japan where, despite excellent epidemiological evidence linking 6,000 cases of disease to radish sprouts, pathogens could not be recovered from products after extensive screening (Michino et al., 1999). On the other side of the equation, pathogens found in food may or may not pose a threat to public health. For instance, not all *Listeria monocytogenes* found in food are likely to cause disease in people (Jacquet et al., 2004), but discovery of nonvirulent microorganisms by food monitoring may lead to unnecessary and expensive regulatory action.

New technology has lowered the threshold for food monitoring utility. Nucleic acid-based assays such as polymerase chain reaction (PCR) can in theory solve in vitro viability issues of microorganisms in food and improve test sensitivity and specificity. However, the technology does not change basic issues related to sampling, low pathogen load, and test interpretation. Also, nucleic acids typically survive microbial inactivation procedures such as pasteurization (Hilfenhaus et al., 1997), and PCR reactions are inhibited by substances in many food matrices, adding new interpretive challenges. Biosensor technology, while still in its infancy, holds potential for real-time monitoring of foods (Anderson and Taitt, 2005). Future developments may improve biosensor detection limits and specificity, which are currently inadequate for most analytes. Although encouraging in terms of potential throughput and per-sample cost, biosensor technology has many of the same theoretical limitations described for nucleic acid and conventional technology.

The sum of sampling and sensitivity issues make food monitoring impractical as a broadly applied tool for protecting the food supply. Mass food testing would be extremely expensive and would have very low predictive values. Lot-by-lot testing may be considered if (1) the risk cannot be reduced by process changes or engineering controls, (2) if a test is available that can detect the contaminant at suitably low levels, (3) if the test turnaround time does not interfere unduly with product requirements, and (4) if the cost to the consumer is justifiable.

Strengths and Limitations of Disease Surveillance

One hundred percent of food consumed by humans is essentially subject to a natural bioassay in the consumers. Each case of disease represents some failure of our food protection systems that can potentially be corrected. Disease surveillance is the collection of information that can, in theory, detect problems anywhere in the food supply chain. The denominator for U.S. disease surveillance is 281 million discrete individuals (2000 census data). Unlike food products, people can announce that they have been contaminated by presenting themselves to their physician or by calling a foodborne disease complaint line. Microbial pathogens tend to be evenly distributed through specimens such as feces due to extended mixing in the digestive tract.

Pathogen load is not generally an intrinsic limiting factor in foodborne disease surveillance, as microbial amplification is part of the pathogenesis of most foodborne infections. There are exceptions to this generalization, such as hepatitis A or hemolytic uremic syndrome due to *E. coli* O157:H7 where presenting symptoms are secondary to primary acute infections, and occur at a point in the disease during which pathogen numbers are declining and may limit detection. Detection is also a problem for many enterotoxins, heavy metals, and other foodborne toxins. Test specificity is less of a problem in disease surveillance than food monitoring as established pathogens detected in ill humans or animals are highly correlated with disease.

Foodborne disease surveillance also has inherent limitations. The time interval between a contamination event and a surveillance signal may be considerable. The process can involve many sequential steps. At a minimum, disease surveillance requires (1) exposure, (2) incubation, and (3) presentation to a physician or other notification. In addition, pathogen specific surveillance may also require (4) collection of specimens, (5) diagnostic laboratory testing, (6) reporting to public health authorities, (7) submission of samples to public health laboratories, (8) further laboratory characterization and reporting, (9) analysis of surveillance data, (10) interview of patients, (11) outbreak investigation, (12) case-control study, and (13) national reporting. As a result, detection and investigation of outbreaks can be a lengthy process. In addition, foodborne disease surveillance cannot by definition prevent initial cases.

Although disease surveillance cannot prevent initial cases, it has been very effective at (1) preventing ongoing transmission, (2) identifying unforeseen problems in the food and water supplies, and (3) identifying trends in foodborne disease that can guide public health policy (Besser et al., 2003). For instance, between 1997 and 2004 PulseNet and associated disease surveillance activities played a prominent role in the recall of millions of pounds of contaminated food withdrawn from U.S. markets. Examples of outbreak investigations that uncovered unsafe practices include the 2003 outbreak due to vacuum-packed blade-tenderized steaks allowed identification of the manufacturing process that rendered the product unsafe under current cooking recommendations (Laine et al., 2005) and the 2005 nationwide outbreak of *S. typhimurium* associated with the use of uncooked potentially contaminated products in finished ice cream leading to changed use recommendations (Center for Food Safety and Applied Nutrition, 2005). Changes in the U.S. regulatory policy occurred after *Listeriosis* outbreak investigations highlighted the problems associated with hot dogs (Mead et al., 2006) and turkey deli meat (Gottlieb et al., 2006). Finally, disease surveillance facilitates discovery of significant trends, such as increasing fluoroquinolone resistance in human infections caused by the use of agricultural antibiotics (Smith et al., 1999) or problems associated with increasing importation of fresh produce (Naimi et al., 2003). As much as we may want to prevent initial cases through food monitoring, humans are the best possible culture media and bioassay for detection of human disease agents, and disease surveillance will likely remain our most powerful detection tool for detecting problems in the food supply for years to come.

Types of Foodborne Disease Surveillance Programs

The three most common foodborne disease surveillance strategies, complaint or notification systems, pathogen-specific surveillance, and syndromic surveillance, differ in their application and limitations (see Table 5-3). Complaint and notification systems use a wide variety of factors to link cases of disease. State or local governments, industry, or institutions gather reports of diarrheal illnesses possibly linked to foodborne exposure. The typical scenario is recognition among attendees at a church potluck of group illness or a physician noticing a cluster of cases with some commonality, such as a similar syndrome. Because these systems do not rely on identification of specific pathogens, they can potentially detect a disease cluster caused by any disease agent, including unknown or modified agents, in a relatively short time. This makes complaint systems a valuable adjunct to pathogen-specific surveillance. The information most often used to

TABLE 5-3 Comparison of Disease Surveillance Approaches

	Pathogen-specific Surveillance	Notification/ Complaint	Syndromic Surveillance (nonspecific health data)
Timeliness	Relatively slow	Fast	Fast
Sensitivity of cluster detection	High	Intermediate	Low
Types of agents	Standard agents under surveillance only	Standard or unconventional	Standard or unconventional
Strengths	Detection of widespread outbreaks	Detection of local outbreaks	Detection of large, local outbreaks

SOURCE: Besser (2005).

link cases is personal recognition, which is a useful method for detection of local events but by itself is less valuable for detection of low-level widespread contamination events. However, outbreaks identified through complaint systems may be linked together to detect widespread events. This can be accomplished through disease communication systems such as Epi-X, reporting systems such as eFORS, or through pathogen-specific systems such as PulseNet, once an agent has been identified. All of these mechanisms were used to detect the 1998 international outbreak of *Shigella sonnei* and enterotoxigenic *E. coli* caused by contaminated parsley (Naimi et al., 2003).

Salmonella surveillance is one of the oldest pathogen-specific surveillance systems. Routine collection of information about *S. typhi* began in 1912 and was expanded to include all *Salmonella* in 1942. Serotype-specific *Salmonella* surveillance began in 1963 (Swaminathan et al., 2006). Refinement of the case definition due to the more specific serotype information causes outbreak cases to stand out from background sporadic cases and strengthens the association between illness and a common source. Over the years *Salmonella* serotype surveillance has uncovered diverse problems in the food supply that might not have otherwise been discovered, such as persistent low-level contamination of shell eggs (St. Louis et al., 1988), recurring contamination of pasteurized ice cream during transport (Hennesey et al., 1996), and problems with sprout production (CDC, 2002a). In 1997 Bender et al. showed that the benefits of increased specificity of *Salmonella* serotype surveillance could be extended to *E. coli* O157:H7 through the routine use of PFGE (Bender et al., 1997). The Centers for Disease Control and Prevention (CDC) expanded this capability nationwide with the creation of PulseNet USA in 1998 (Swaminathan et al., 2001) and globally with PulseNet International. The primary factors used to link cases to each other are disease agent and time rather than personal recognition. This dramatically lowered the number of reported cases needed to detect widespread outbreaks. A good example is the 2003 outbreak of vacuum-packed blade-tenderized steaks, which was initially detected by two cases with unique PFGE subtypes and resulted in the recall of 739,000 pounds of potentially contaminated product distributed in multiple states (Laine et al., 2005). Although very sensitive and specific, by definition pathogen-specific surveillance only works for those agents under surveillance. Acts of bioterrorism or naturally occurring outbreaks caused by agents not under surveillance would not be detected by this mechanism nor would outbreaks due to unknown agents. Eighty-two percent of cases of foodborne illnesses are thought to be due to unrecognized agents (Mead et al., 1999). Although pathogen-specific surveillance samples only a small percentage of total foodborne disease cases, it nevertheless has been one of the most robust indicators of problems in the food supply.

Syndromic surveillance is the third type of disease surveillance that could potentially be applied to detection of problems in the food supply. In recent years, this term has generally applied to broad monitoring of nonspecific health data such as diarrheal illness or markers of illness, such as Imodium sales. This is in contrast to complaint or notification systems described above which, while utilizing nonspecific health data such as diarrheal illness, are narrowly focused on recognized clusters or specific complaints. Several large networks have been established to conduct syndromic surveillance, such as BioSense, the Electronic Surveillance System for Early Notification of Community-based Epidemics (ESSENCE), and National Retail Data Monitor (NRDM). Potential outbreaks are detected by spikes in the incidence of common syndromes or surrogate indicators rather than agent or personal recognition, so in theory these systems should be able to detect problems due to known or unknown agents. The primary problem with syndromic surveillance is an unfavorable signal-to-noise ratio. The number of cases needed to trip the system is inversely proportional to the specificity. Thus, syndromic surveillance based on nonspecific health data is useful for detecting very large local events but is very insensitive to small or widespread events. One of the nation's largest systems was established in New York City (NYC) in 2001 (Das et al., 2005; Heffernan et al., 2004). In one year of surveillance involving 2.5 million patient records, the NYC surveillance system had 18 spikes in reports of diarrhea and vomiting syndromes clustered in three outbreak periods. One of the spikes was followed by five institutional outbreak investigations (detected by other mechanisms), but it is unclear whether the surveillance data itself would have been of sufficient specificity to identify the outbreaks.

Surveillance for specific rare syndromes such as hemolytic uremic syndrome or Guillain-Barre syndrome resembles pathogen-specific surveillance more than syndromic surveillance in terms of sensitivity and specificity. Surveillance for unexplained death or critical illnesses with possible infectious etiology is a particularly important type of surveillance. Although postmortem diagnosis of illness can be problematic, unexplained death and critical illnesses may be the only clue that a major foodborne or other type of bioevent has occurred. Surprisingly, only three such programs in the United States exist.

Existing Networks

A large array of acronyms are used to describe existing networks that play serve some role in protecting the food supply (see Table 5-1). Included are communication networks (HAN, Epi-X, INFOSAN, RASFF), surveillance data management systems (NETSS, NEDSS), syndromic surveillance projects and tools (Biosense, UNEX, ESSENCE, NRDM, RODS), a surveillance system designed to determine the burden of foodborne disease (FoodNet), outbreak response and reporting networks (eFORS, GOARN), animal surveillance networks (NAHSS, CAHFSE), an enteric disease antibiotic-resistance monitoring network (NARMS), laboratory data handling networks (eLEXNET, PulseNet, Global Salm-Surv, CaliciNet), and laboratory response networks (LRN, FERN, NAHSS, NPDN, eLRN, ICLN). Laboratory response networks such as LRN and FERN have protocols for testing suspect food items but currently have no role in primary detection of problems in the food supply. Current food-monitoring programs are designed to support HACCP programs or monitor for specific pathogens in high-risk foods but play little role in broad monitoring for unexpected introduction of contaminants into the food supply. Outbreak reporting systems such as eFORS and GOARN can potentially detect national or international outbreaks by linking local outbreaks without previously recognized connection. PulseNet and associated foodborne disease surveillance programs are currently the most sensitive methods for detecting unforeseen problems in the food supply.

Successes, Problems, and Promises of PulseNet and Associated Foodborne Disease Programs

Since its inception in 1998, PulseNet has been a key tool in the detection of a wide range of problems in the food supply, such as *Listeria monocytogenes* in luncheon meat; *Shigella sonnei* in imported parsley; *E. coli* O157:H7 in meats, unpasteurized juices, and produce; and *Salmonella* in almonds and custom ice cream. Estimating cost and benefits of surveillance programs is difficult and rare, but it is becoming clear that prevention benefits of PulseNet and associated activities far outweigh its costs. Bell and colleagues estimated that 800 cases of disease were prevented by the recall of 250,000 hamburgers after detection of the 1993 *E. coli* O157:H7 outbreak on the West Coast of the United States, which occurred prior to development of PulseNet (Bell et al., 1994). Since that time, PulseNet findings have directly or indirectly led to the recall of many times that amount of contaminated products and enabled continuing contamination problems to be detected and rectified. In 1997, PulseNet enabled the Colorado Department of Health to detect an outbreak caused by potentially contaminated beef that led to the recall of 25,000,000 pounds of beef, and 18,600,000 pounds in 2002 (CDC, 2002b). Elbasha et al. estimated that the Colorado PulseNet system would recover all costs if only five cases per year were prevented (Elbasha et al., 2000). A single case of hemolytic uremic syndrome caused by *E. coli* O157:H7 can cost up to $453,675 in medical costs alone (Buzby et al., 1996).

The PulseNet system is currently used to track nine diseases by use of standardized PFGE protocols, but potentially can be used to track any infectious disease confirmed by detection of a specific microorganism. It increases the inherent sensitivity of disease surveillance by refining the case definition and provides a platform for rapid communication and comparison of results. More specific case definitions improve the signal-to-noise ratio, and permits small, yet significant events to be detected. PulseNet has recently bridged the gap between food monitoring and disease surveillance data by incorporating data from the USDA and FDA monitoring and investigation programs. An outbreak of *Salmonella* Kiambu associated with beef jerky in 2003 was detected by linking PFGE patterns from food monitoring to disease surveillance patterns, resulting in the recall of 22,000 pounds of contaminated product. PulseNet International has expanded the network worldwide and has already had early successes at tracing an international outbreak of shigellosis associated with airline meals (Gaynor et al., 2004) and an outbreak associated with ground beef from a U.S. military installation (CDC, 2004). In spite of its history of successes and awards, PulseNet operates unevenly around the country, with most activity associated with a small number of states. Surveys by the Association of Public Health Laboratories and Council for State and Territorial Epidemiologists found important deficits in the nation's capacity to detect, investigate, and respond to food safety problems (Association of Public Health Laboratories, 2003; Council of State and Territorial Epidemiologists, 2004). Most laboratory and epidemiology programs are understaffed and underfunded, leaving many food safety problems undetected and unresolved. As a result of these issues, PulseNet operates at only a fraction of its potential, with its greatest promise yet to be exploited.

Other Potential Systems

Although PulseNet is the most developed system for detection of problems in the food supply, it is not the only useful approach. Clusters of notifiable disease can potentially be detected through analysis of data from the Public Health Laboratory Information System, and widespread events have been detected using the CDC's Electronic Outbreak Reporting System (eFORS) and Epi-X postings. Because the etiology of outbreaks reported through eFORS or Epi-X can be known or unknown, these systems can capture complaint data not associated with a nationally notifiable pathogen. Like PulseNet, eFORS is not being used to its full potential. Resource limitations at the state and local level limit detection and reporting of outbreaks. Completion of the National Electronic Disease Surveillance System (NEDSS) will provide a backbone for national surveillance, but the lack of standard forms for interviewing cases will continue to limit outbreak detection in the absence of specific agent information.

Surveillance for unexplained death and serious illness caused by possible infectious etiology has significant potential for use in detecting serious problems in the food supply, such as intentional tampering. As much as we would like to prevent death, it is not possible to anticipate every possible mode by which pathogens could be intentionally or unintentionally introduced into the food supply. It seems that at a minimum we should be able to know that such an event is occurring so that appropriate control measures can be instituted to prevent additional cases. Investigation of unexplained death possibly caused by infectious causes is expensive and difficult. Nevertheless, national resources dedicated for this purpose is very limited and includes only small CDC-funded programs in California, Minnesota, and Connecticut.

Conclusions

Targeted microbial monitoring of selected high-risk foods and processes plays an important role in protecting the food supply. Expansion of monitoring activities may be justified in situations where initial cases cannot be tolerated. However, broadly applied food-monitoring programs are likely to be costly and insensitive due to intrinsic sampling and testing limitations. Foodborne disease surveillance programs cannot prevent initial cases, but are nevertheless the most sensitive method for detecting unrecognized problems in the food supply. Current foodborne disease surveillance programs, such as PulseNet, are operating at only a fraction of their potential, largely because of underfunding. Disease surveillance programs have a high benefit-to-cost ratio and represent a basic function of public health. Real-time foodborne disease surveillance at the state, federal, and international levels is an achievable, relatively inexpensive goal that would have an immediate, positive impact on food safety.

THE CONSUMER COMPLAINT MONITORING SYSTEM: ENHANCING DISCOVERY AND MITIGATION OF FOODBORNE THREATS TO HEALTH THROUGH PATTERN SURVEILLANCE AND MULTIPLE-ATTRIBUTE ALGORITHMS

CDR Kimberly Elenberg, M.S., R.N.[2] *and Artur Dubrawski, Ph.D.*[3]

The Consumer Complaint Monitoring System (CCMS), owned by the Food Safety and Inspection Service (FSIS) of the USDA, is a database used to record, evaluate, and track all consumer food complaints involving meat, poultry, and egg products. It has assisted public health professionals with evaluating approximately 4,000 consumer complaints since January 2001.

Consumer complaints are received through phone calls to the USDA field compliance officers, and through the toll-free phone number of the Meat and Poultry Hotline. Adverse food event reports can also be received and managed for imported products and school lunch products distributed through USDA's Food and Nutrition Service. Complaints typically involve reports of illness, injury, foreign objects, contamination (including chemical contamination), allergic reactions, and improper labeling.

To further improve food safety and security, FSIS' Office of Public Health Science developed the Consumer Complaint Monitoring System II (CCMS II). CCMS II complements the existing foodborne threat surveillance systems Pulse-

[2]Food Safety Inspection Service, United States Department of Agriculture; Office of Food Defense and Emergency Response until June 2006, currently Commander, Director of Medical Readiness, USPHS.

[3]Carnegie Mellon University; Auton Lab, The Robotics Institute.

Net and FoodNet (see Summary and Assessment and Tauxe in Chapter 3). Although PulseNet and FoodNet actively track pathogen strains isolated from humans with foodborne disease, CCMS employs a form of passive surveillance to provide the earliest possible warning of a wide variety of foodborne threats. This system rapidly organizes and analyzes the incoming complex, multivariate data from consumer complaints concerning such adverse events as food-associated symptoms or foreign objects present in food.

As other contributors to this workshop have noted, the possible sources of foodborne contamination are extremely vast. Although using adverse food reports to assess possible foodborne threats presents the considerable challenge of discerning significant trends against a background of random noise, this approach also offers several benefits. Unlike FoodNet and PulseNet, CCMS is not limited to assessing known pathogens, which account for a minority of foodborne illness; unknown agents account for 81 percent of U.S. foodborne illnesses and hospitalizations and 64 percent of deaths (Mead et al., 1999). In addition to tracking possible emerging foodborne pathogens, including intentionally modified organisms, CCMS examines chemical and foreign object contaminants in food (the latter is the subject of 80 percent of all adverse food reports received by USDA).

Finding Patterns in Consumer Complaints

Surveillance activities involving CCMS are conducted by both the FSIS Office of Public Health Science and the FSIS Office of Food Defense and Emergency Response. The analytical component of CCMS, called Emerging Patterns in Food Complaints (EPFC), developed in collaboration with Artur Dubrawski's group at Carnegie Mellon University, employs computational methods, including multiple-attribute algorithms and Bayesian probability models, to detect patterns in complaints received by CCMS—data that are too voluminous and complex for the human mind to grasp. Public health analysts examine the resulting patterns and assess the likelihood that they represent material foodborne threats. CCMS tracks several variables associated with each report, including the date, time, and location of the event; associated symptoms and their onset times or descriptions of foreign objects; and the type and purchase origin of the suspected product.

When two or more similar complaints are received within a reasonably close time span (the particular range of interest varies depending on the shelf life of the involved food), the EPFC statistically quantifies their relatedness. It compares the group of variables that makes up each consumer complaint with a database of approximately 4,000 past cases and also with a series of 42 causal models we have developed based on passive surveillance records of adverse food events. The results that public health analysts receive indicate the most similar past cases, the likeliest causal scenarios, and the most probable case-cause combinations matching the complaints under investigation. For example, EFPC comparisons might find matches between the symptoms and locations associated with two contemporary cases, but little similarity between the product sources; when these results are in turn compared with the range of causal models, the best match is with a community illness not related to a specific product. If CCMS continued to receive similar complaints, we would alert the appropriate state health department to investigate likely causes of community illness, such as water contamination. By contrast, a series of closely timed complaints with high similarity and a common causal scenario would signify a foodborne outbreak; in that situation, investigators would pursue this hypothesis by testing the suspected product(s) and comparing the results with the PulseNet database. To date, the system has recognized several outbreaks: of *Salmonella*, *Listeria monocytogenes*, and *E. coli* O157:H7.

In addition to providing investigators with valuable leads for tracing the origin of suspected and confirmed contaminants, CCMS can further aid such management decisions as the identification of an emergency response that is appropriate to the nature, location, and extent of a threat. CCMS data can also be used to alert food producers to more general food safety issues associated with specific processes and/or plants. For example, a large number of apparently diverse complaints associated with products from a single company might reflect on overall condition, such as substandard sanitation. When many complaints point to a single causal model (for example, a metal foreign object in a specific product), EPFC analysis can pinpoint the source of the problem and lead to its solution (routinely inspect the product with a metal detector). This process can occur rapidly. For example, within 30 minutes of a report of students being injured with glass in their school lunches, CCMS can identify and investigate the implicated food commodities and, if necessary, communicate with the affected schools to ensure that foods containing the product are removed from cafeteria lines immediately.

Future Expansion of CCMS

Based on the demonstrated ability of the analytical component of CCMS to detect interesting, low-amplitude signals in sparse, noisy data, further expansion of the system is warranted. Although currently operated on a state-by-state basis, CCMS will soon permit state public health officials to track pathogens and contaminants beyond their borders and to view a national "snapshot" of adverse food events in real time. Data from earlier points in the farm-to-table continuum, which would be especially valuable in identifying patterns associated with zoonotic disease, could be analyzed in conjunction with consumer complaints as part of an integrated national biosurveillance system. As CCMS grows in importance and visibility, it will be important to establish surge capacity to deal with the expected high volume of complaints that could arise during a foodborne outbreak.

Early detection is the key to mitigating the consequences of foodborne illness. Improving the timeliness of data collection, pattern detection, and communication of information about adverse food events using CCMS and related passive surveillance technologies requires better tools as well as changes in the way these events are reported. Finally, because tools such as CCMS are only as effective as the humans who use them, we must educate everyone who plays a role in food safety, and encourage collaboration at all levels.

REFERENCES

Anderson GP, Taitt CR. 2005. Biosensor-based detection of foodborne pathogens. In: Fratamico PM, Bhunia A, Smith JL, Eds. *Foodborne Pathogens: Microbiology and Molecular Biology.* Wymondham, UK: Academic Press.

APHL (Association of Public Health Laboratories). 2003. *A Recipe for Stronger Food Safety Programs.* Washington, D.C.: Association of Public Health Laboratories.

Bell BP, Goldoft M, Griffin PM, Davis MA, Gordon DC, Tarr PI, Bartleson CA, Lewis JH, Barrett TJ, Wells JG, Baron R, Kobayashi J. 1994. A multiple outbreak of *Escherichia coli* O157:H7-associated bloody diarrhea and hemolytic uremic syndrome from hamburgers: The Washington State experience. *Journal of the American Medical Association* 272(17):1349–1353.

Bender JB, Hedberg CW, Besser JM, Boxrud DJ, MacDonald KL, Osterholm MT. 1997. Surveillance for *Escherichia coli* O157:H7 infections in Minnesota by molecular subtyping. *New England Journal of Medicine* 337(6):388–394.

Besser J. 2005 (October 25). *Session IV: What Are the Tools and Technologies for "Real Time" Surveillance of the Food Supply for Conventional and Unconventional Adulterants?* Presentation at the Forum on Microbial Threats Workshop Meeting, Foodborne Threats to Health: The Policies and Practices of Surveillance, Prevention, Outbreak Investigations, and International Coordination, Washington, D.C., Institute of Medicine, Forum on Microbial Threats.

Besser J, Beebe J, Swaminathan B. 2003. Investigation of foodborne disease outbreaks. In: Pfaller MA, Ed. *Manual of Clinical Microbiology.* 8th ed. Washington, D.C.: American Society for Microbiology Press.

Buzby JC, Roberts T, Lin JC-T, MacDonald JM. 1996. *Bacterial Foodborne Disease: Medical Costs and Productivity Losses.* Agricultural Economics Report No. 741. Washington, D.C.: Department of Agriculture.

CDC (Centers for Disease Control and Prevention). 1997. *Escherichia coli* O157:H7 infections associated with eating a nationally distributed commercial brand of frozen ground beef patties and burgers—Colorado, 1997. *Morbidity and Mortality Weekly Report* 46(33):777–778.

CDC. 2002a. Outbreak of *Salmonella* serotype *kottbus* infections associated with eating alfalfa sprouts—Arizona, California, Colorado, and New Mexico, February-April 2001. *Morbidity and Mortality Weekly Report* 51(1):7–9.

CDC. 2002b. Multistate outbreak of *Escherichia coli* O157:H7 infections associated with eating ground beef—United States, June-July 2002. *Morbidity and Mortality Weekly Report* 51(29): 637–639.

CDC. 2004. *Escherichia coli* O157:H7 infections associated with ground beef from a U.S. military installation—Okinawa, Japan, February 2004. *Morbidity and Mortality Weekly Report* 54(2): 40–42.

Center for Food Safety and Applied Nutrition. 2005 (August 19). *Bulletin to the Food Service and Retail Food Store Industry Regarding Cake Batter Ice Cream and Similar Products.* [Online]. Available: http://www.cfsan.fda.gov/~ear/ret-batt.html [accessed April 10, 2006].

Council of State and Territorial Epidemiologists. 2004. *National Assessment of Epidemiological Capacity: Findings and Recommendations.* Washington, D.C.

Das D, Metzger K, Heffernan R, Balter S, Weiss D, Mostashari F. 2005. New York City Department of Health and Mental Hygiene. Monitoring over-the-counter medication sales for early detection of disease outbreaks—New York City. *Morbidity and Mortality Weekly Report* 54(Suppl):41–46.

Elbasha EH, Fitzsimmons TD, Meltzer MI. 2000. Costs and benefits of a subtype-specific surveillance system for identifying *Escherichia coli* O157:H7 outbreaks. *Emerging Infectious Diseases* 6(3):293–297.

FAO (Food and Agriculture Organization of the United Nations). 2004. *International Cooperation on Food Contamination and Foodborne Disease Surveillance*. Second FAO/WHO global forum of food safety regulators. [Online]. Available: http://www.fao.org/docrep/meeting/008/ae163e.htm [accessed February 1, 2006].

GAO (General Accountability Office). 2003. *Bioterrorism. A Threat to Agriculture and the Food Supply.* [Online]. Available: http://www.gao.gov/new.items/d04259t.pdf [accessed April 10, 2006].

GAO. 2004. *Emerging Infectious Diseases: Review of State and Federal Disease Surveillance Efforts.* [Online]. Available: http://www.gao.gov/new.items/d04877.pdf [accessed April 10, 2006].

Gaynor K, Kanenaka B, Colindres R, Mintz E, Kalluri P, Kitsutani P, Nakata M, Wedel S, Boxrud D, Jennings D, Yoshida H,Tosaka N, Park SY, Effler PV. 2004 (August). International Outbreak of Shigella sonnei among Airline Passengers—Honolulu, Hawaii. Presentation abstract, Session C, 54th Annual Epidemic Intelligence (EIS) Conference, April 11–15, Atlanta, GA.

Gottlieb SL, Newbern EC, Griffin PM, Graves LM, Hoekstra RM, Baker NL, Hunter SB, Holt KG, Ramsey F, Head M, Levine P, Johnson G, Schoonmaker-Bopp D, Reddy V, Kornstein L, Gerwel M, Nsubuga J, Edwards L, Stonecipher S, Hurd S, Austin D, Jefferson MA, Young SD, Hise K, Chernak ED, Sobel J. 2006. Listeriosis Outbreak Working Group. Multistate outbreak of listeriosis linked to turkey deli meat and subsequent changes in US regulatory policy. *Clinical Infectious Diseases* 42(1):29–36.

Heffernan R, Mostashari F, Das D, Besculides M, Rodriguez C, Greenko J, Steiner-Sichel L, Balter S, Karpati A, Thomas P, Phillips M, Ackelsberg J, Lee E, Leng J, Hartman J, Metzger K, Rosselli R, Weiss D. 2004. New York City syndromic surveillance systems. *Morbidity and Mortality Weekly Report* 53(Suppl):23–27.

Hennessy TW, Hedberg CW, Slutsker L, White KE, Besser-Wiek JM, Moen ME, Feldman J, Coleman WW, Edmonson LM, MacDonald KL, Osterholm MT. 1996. A national outbreak of *Salmonella enteritidis* infections from ice cream. The Investigation Team. *New England Journal of Medicine* 334(20):1281–1286.

Hilfenhaus J, Groner A, Nowak T, Weimer T. 1997. Analysis of human plasma products: Polymerase chain reaction does not discriminate between live and inactivated viruses. *Transfusion* 37(9): 935–940.

Jacquet C, Doumith M, Gordon JI, Martin PM, Cossart P, Lecuit M. 2004. A molecular marker for evaluating the pathogenic potential of foodborne *Listeria monocytogenes*. *Journal of Infectious Diseases* 189(11):2094–2100.

Kantor LS, Lipton K, Manchester A, Oliveira V. 1997. Estimating and addressing America's food losses. *Food Review* 20(1):2–12. [Online]. Available: www.ers.usda.gov/publications/foodreview/jan1997/jan97a.pdf [accessed April 10, 2006].

Laine ES, Scheftel JM, Boxrud DJ, Vought KJ, Danila RN, Elfering KM, Smith KE. 2005. Outbreak of *Escherichia coli* O157:H7 infections associated with nonintact blade-tenderized frozen steaks sold by door-to-door vendors. *Journal of Food Protection* 68(6):1198–1202.

Mead PS, Slutsker L, Dietz V, McCaig LF, Bresee JS, Shapiro C, Griffin PM, Tauxe RV. 1999. Food-related illness and death in the United States. *Emerging Infectious Diseases* 5(5):607–625.

Mead PS, Dunne EF, Graves L, Wiedmann M, Patrick M, Hunter S, Salehi E, Mostashari F, Craig A, Mshar P, Bannerman T, Sauders BD, Hayes P, Dewitt W, Sparling P, Griffin P, Morse D, Slutsker L, Swaminathan B. 2006. Nationwide outbreak of listeriosis due to contaminated meat. *Epidemiology and Infection* 134(4):744–751. Epub December 1, 2005:1–8.

Michino H, Araki K, Minami S, Takaya S, Sakai N, Miyazaki M, Ono A, Yanagawa H. 1999. Massive outbreak of *Escherichia coli* O157:H7 infection in schoolchildren in Sakai City, Japan, associated with consumption of white radish sprouts. *American Journal of Epidemiology* 150(8):787–796.

Naimi TS, Wicklund JH, Olsen SJ, Krause G, Wells JG, Bartkus JM, Boxrud DJ, Sullivan M, Kassenborg H, Besser JM, Mintz ED, Osterholm MT, Hedberg CW. 2003. Concurrent outbreaks of *Shigella sonnei* and enterotoxigenic *Escherichia coli* infections associated with parsley: Implications for surveillance and control of foodborne illness. *Journal of Food Protection* 66(4):535–541.

Smith KE, Besser JM, Hedberg CW, Leano FT, Bender JB, Wicklund JH, Johnson BP, Moore KA, Osterholm MT. 1999. Quinolone-resistant *Campylobacter jejuni* infections in Minnesota, 1992–1998. Investigation Team. *New England Journal of Medicine* 340(20):1525–1532.

St. Louis ME, Morse DL, Potter ME, DeMelfi TM, Guzewich JJ, Tauxe RV, Blake PA. 1988. The emergence of grade A eggs as a major source of *Salmonella enteritidis* infections. New implications for the control of salmonellosis. *Journal of the American Medical Association* 259(14): 2103–2107.

Swaminathan B, Barrett TJ, Hunter SB, Tauxe RV. 2001. CDC PulseNet Task Force. PulseNet: The molecular subtyping network for foodborne bacterial disease surveillance, United States. *Emerging Infectious Diseases* 7(3):382–389.

Swaminathan B, Barrett TJ, Fields P. 2006. Surveillance for human *Salmonella* infections in the United States. *Journal of AOAC International* 89(2):553–559.

Wein LM, Liu Y. 2005. Analyzing a bioterror attack on the food supply: The case of botulinum toxin in milk. *Proceedings of the National Academy of Sciences* 102(28):9984–9989.

6

Reporting Foodborne Threats: The Case of Bovine Spongiform Encephalopathy (BSE)

OVERVIEW

The rapid reporting of foodborne threats is essential to reducing the burden of foodborne illness, but it also carries direct and indirect costs to individuals, communities, industries, and national economies. The balance of costs and benefits associated with reporting foodborne threats is clearly illustrated by the world's recent and ongoing experience with bovine spongiform encephalopathy (BSE, or mad cow disease). A series of workshop presentations by contributors to this chapter explored the biology of BSE and its implications for food safety, international perspectives on BSE surveillance and prevention, and public health lessons learned from this disease and its consequences.

A member of the family of diseases known as transmissible spongiform encephalopathies (TSEs; also known as prion diseases), BSE was first identified in 1986 in the United Kingdom and has since been detected in 26 countries (GAO, 2005). In the early 1980s, Stanley Prusiner, the author of this chapter's first paper, proposed that the pathogens that cause two TSEs—Creutzfeldt-Jakob disease (CJD) and scrapie, a disease of sheep—consist entirely of an infectious form of protein that he termed the *prion*; in 1997, he was awarded the Nobel Prize in Physiology and Medicine for his work on prion biology. Researchers have since learned that in addition to scrapie and CJD, prions cause BSE and its human variant, vCJD, as well as chronic wasting disease in deer and elk.

Prusiner presents experimental evidence for the prion model of TSE and describes the etiology and diagnosis of vCJD and other human prion diseases. He emphasizes the differences between prion and viral illnesses—most notably, that prions can arise spontaneously—and observes that the mistaken equation of the two can impede the development of effective preventions against invariably fatal prion diseases. "The only rational strategy is to test all cattle for prions and eliminate those harboring prions from the food supply," Prusiner concludes.

The second paper, by Steven Collins, codirector of the Australian National CJD Registry, describes his country's approach to TSE surveillance in both animals and humans. The vast majority of CJD cases in the Australian Registry are sporadic; no cases of vCJD or endogenous cases of either BSE or scrapie have been reported to date in the country. Collins recounts the range of measures Australia has adopted to protect commercial livestock from BSE and scrapie, which include bans on the importation of meat and bone meal and of live cattle from any country reporting BSE, as well as the prohibition of ruminant-to-ruminant feeding of meat and bone meal.

Maura Ricketts, who has directed prion disease surveillance and research for Health Canada and the World Health Organization (WHO), discusses BSE and vCJD from a public health perspective in the chapter's third paper. After defining and applying relevant core principles of public health, Ricketts identifies and explores key issues that underlie the development and implementation of health policy to address BSE and vCJD. She concludes with an overview of possible public health actions that reflect the importance of controlling the risk of BSE exposure.

In the chapter's final contribution, Wil Hueston of the Center for Animal Health and Food Safety at the University of Minnesota shares insights gained from 16 years of involvement with BSE and the interface between animal and human health. He distills this experience into seven lessons that lead to a series of key actions that could be taken to address key issues raised by BSE and, more generally, to improve the response to infectious disease.

PRIONS AND THE SAFETY OF THE FOOD SUPPLY

Stanley B. Prusiner, M.D.[1]
University of California San Francisco

In December 2003, mad cow disease made its U.S. debut when federal officials announced that a Holstein cow from Mabton, Washington, had been stricken with bovine spongiform encephalopathy (BSE). Although the U.S. government acted surprised by the finding, they should have expected such cattle based on the biology of the prion diseases. Perhaps the novel principles of disease that have emerged over the past two decades from investigations of prions (Prusiner, 2004b) are still too new and different for many people to grasp easily the implications of this discovery. Prions are unprecedented infectious pathogens that are composed

[1]Institute for Neurodegenerative Diseases, Departments of Neurology and of Biochemistry and Biophysics.

solely of protein; they are devoid of nucleic acid—DNA and RNA. The absence of a nucleic genome sets prions apart from all other infectious pathogens including viruses, viroids, bacteria, fungi, and parasites.

Because prions multiply and cause disease in the host, scientists thought for many years that prions must be slow-acting viruses. Moreover, the identification of varieties or strains of prions made the argument that prions must be viruses even more appealing. Because so many attempts to detect a prion-specific nucleic acid genome failed (Alper et al., 1967; Bellinger-Kawahara et al., 1987a,b; Safar et al., 2005b), some scientists argued that the nucleic acid must be quite small (Bruce and Dickinson, 1987; Chesebro, 2004; Kimberlin, 1982; Weissmann, 1991). Although the identification of micro RNAs has given new life to such arguments in recent years, the production of synthetic prions from recombinant prion protein (PrP) is likely to end the quest for an auxiliary molecule within the prion (Legname et al., 2004, 2005).

Based on a wealth of data including the production of synthetic prions in mammals and fungi, it is reasonable to define prions as infectious proteins. Prions multiply by forcing the precursor protein to acquire a second conformation. Different conformations of proteins in the prion state encipher distinct strains and are prone to aggregation. In mammals, prions accumulate to high levels in the nervous system where they cause dysfunction and fatal degeneration.

Both mammalian and fungal prions have been produced in cell-free systems (Brachmann et al., 2005; Maddelein et al., 2002; Sparrer et al., 2000; Tanaka et al., 2004). Synthetic PrP peptides and recombinant PrP fragments have been used to form mammalian prions, and N-terminal regions, called *prion domains*, that are rich in glutamine and asparagine have been used to form fungal prions.

In mammals, prions cause a group of invariably fatal, neurodegenerative diseases. No human or animal has ever recovered from a prion disease once neurologic dysfunction has manifested. Prion diseases may present as genetic, infectious, or sporadic disorders, all of which involve modification of normal, cellular PrP, designated PrP^C. The tertiary structure of PrP is profoundly altered as prions are formed, and as such, prion diseases represent disorders of protein conformation. In the sporadic and genetic forms of prion disease, prions arise spontaneously. In contrast, infectious prion diseases result from exposure to an exogenous source of prions. Although the incidence of sporadic prion disease in humans is low (1–5 cases per 10^6 people), it is the most common form, accounting for approximately 90 percent of all cases. The genetic, or inherited, forms of prion disease account for approximately 10 percent of all human cases and the infectious forms for less than 1 percent. Whether or not the infectious forms of human prion disease are underestimated and low levels of animal prions in the food supply are responsible for 10–20 percent of the sporadic cases is unknown.

The prion diseases in humans include CJD, which generally presents as a progressive dementia, as well as kuru and Gerstmann-Sträussler-Scheinker disease (GSS), both of which frequently present as ataxic maladies. Like kuru and

GSS of humans, scrapie of sheep and BSE of cattle usually manifest as ataxic illnesses. Deer, elk, and moose with chronic wasting disease (CWD) appear emaciated and ataxic.

In these diseases, mammalian PrP^C is recruited and converted into the disease-causing isoform (PrP^{Sc}). PrP^C has a high α-helical content and little β-sheet structure, whereas PrP^{Sc} has less α-helical structure and a high β-sheet content. Comparisons of secondary structures of PrP^C and PrP^{Sc} were performed on proteins purified from Syrian hamster (SHa) brains (Pan et al., 1993). Limited proteolysis of PrP^{Sc} produces a protease-resistant core, designated PrP 27–30, which retains prion infectivity; under these conditions, PrP^C is completely hydrolyzed.

Prion Disease Paradigm

Despite some similarities between prion and viral illnesses, these disorders are very different. Viral diseases are infectious illnesses that begin with infection by exogenous virions. In contrast, the vast majority of prion diseases are initiated from within the host, in which prions arise spontaneously. Often the term *prion infection* is used synonymously with *prion disease* because once prions are formed spontaneously they can be transferred to another host and thus, are infectious. Unlike viral infections, no host defenses are mounted in response to prion infection: no humoral immunity, no cellular immunity, and no interferons are elicited to the replicating prion.

Molecular genetic studies have been crucial in deciphering the novel features of the prion disease paradigm. In the sporadic form of prion disease, the sequence of the PrP gene is wild-type (wt); whereas, in the inherited prion diseases, the sequence of the PrP gene harbors a nonconservative substitution or insertion. Generally, the PrP genes of humans and animals with infectious prion disease are wt.

Before the discovery of mutations in the PrP gene as the cause of familial prion disease, geographic clusters of prion disease were thought to be due to common source exposures to exogenous prions. For example, Libyan Jews with a very high incidence of CJD were thought to have contracted the disease by eating lightly cooked sheep brains (Alter and Kahana, 1976). Molecular genetic investigations showed that every Libyan Jew developing prion disease carried a PrP gene mutation resulting in an E→K substitution at position 200 (Goldfarb et al., 1991; Hsiao et al., 1991). Risk analysis studies revealed that every Libyan Jew carrying the E200K mutation would eventually develop prion disease if he or she did not die of some other illness (Chapman et al., 1994; Spudich et al., 1995).

Synthetic Prions and Spontaneous Disease

Investigations of humans with PrP gene mutations were extended to transgenic (Tg) mice harboring the analogous mutation causing GSS in humans. Tg mice expressing high levels of MoPrP(P101L) developed neurodegeneration spontaneously (Hsiao et al., 1990; Telling et al., 1996). Extracts prepared from the brains of these mice transmitted disease after approximately 250 days to other Tg mice (designated Tg196) expressing low levels of MoPrP(P101L) (Hsiao, 1994). Subsequently, a synthetic PrP peptide of 55 residues carrying the P101L mutation, designated MoPrP(89–143,P101L), was produced and inoculated into the Tg196 mice (Kaneko et al., 2000). The Tg196 mice developed central nervous system (CNS) dysfunction approximately one year after inoculation, and brain extracts from the ill mice were found to produce disease on serial passage (Tremblay et al., 2004). The MoPrP(89–143, P101L) peptide produced disease in the Tg196 mice only if it was folded into a β-rich conformation (Kaneko et al., 2000).

An approach similar to the one used in the studies with MoPrP(89–143,P101L) peptide was employed with wt PrP. In those studies, wt MoPrP(89–230) was produced in *E. coli*, purified by chromatography, and polymerized into amyloid fibrils (Legname et al., 2004). The amyloid fibrils were injected into Tg mice expressing MoPrP(89–231) and produced neurodegeneration after approximately 500 days. Brain extracts from the ill Tg mice contained protease-resistant PrP^{Sc} and produced disease on subsequent passage into both wt and Tg mice (Legname et al., 2005). These studies demonstrated that only PrP is required to generate prion infectivity, and as such, spontaneous forms of prion disease can occur in any mammal as PrP^{C} seems to be ubiquitous among this class of vertebrates.

Spontaneous prion disease contrasts with viral disorders, for which exogenous infection is required except in the case of latent retroviral genomes. For example, after infection with exogenous HIV, the virus may disappear but often its RNA genome has been reverse-transcribed into DNA, and the DNA copies may remain dormant for years.

The dramatically different principles that govern prion biology from those underpinning the viral diseases are frequently misunderstood. This lack of understanding has led to some regrettable decisions of great economic, political, and possibly public health importance. For example, scrapie and BSE have different names, yet they are the same disease in two different species. Scrapie and BSE differ in only two respects: first, the PrP sequence in sheep differs from that of cattle at seven or eight positions of 270 amino acids (Goldmann et al., 1990, 1991), which results in different PrP^{Sc} molecules. Second, most scrapie strains of prions seem to be different from the BSE strains.

The Mad Cow Epidemic

The world awoke to the dangers of prion disease in cows after the BSE outbreak began ravaging the British beef industry in the mid-1980s. The truly novel concepts emerging from prion science forced researchers and society to think in unusual ways and made coping with the epidemic difficult. Investigators eventually learned that prions were being transmitted to cattle through meat-and-bone meal (MBM), a dietary supplement prepared from the parts of sheep, cattle, pigs and chickens that are processed, or rendered, for industrial use. High heat eliminated conventional pathogens, but PrP^{Sc} survived and went on to infect cattle.

As infected cattle became food for other cattle, BSE began appearing throughout the UK cattle population, reaching a high of 37,280 confirmed fied cases in 1992 (Phillips, 2000). The British authorities instituted some feed bans beginning in 1989, but it was not until 1996 that a strict ban on cannibalistic feeding finally brought BSE under control in the United Kingdom; the country saw 612 cases in 2004. Overall, the United Kingdom has identified approximately 180,000 mad cows, and epidemiologic models suggest that another 1.9 million were infected but went undetected (Anderson et al., 1996).

For many people, the regulations came too late. Despite the British government's early assurances to the contrary, mad cow disease proved transmissible to humans. In March 1996, Robert Will and his colleagues reported that 11 British teenagers and young adults had died of a variant of Creutzfeldt-Jakob disease (vCJD) (Will et al., 2004, 1996). In these young patients, the patterns of PrP^{Sc} deposition in the brain differed markedly from that found in typical CJD patients.

Many scientists, including myself, were initially dubious of the presumed link between BSE and vCJD. I eventually changed my mind, under the weight of many studies. The most compelling of these studies used Tg mice genetically engineered to resemble cattle, at least from a PrP point of view. These mice became ill approximately 250 days after receiving injections of prions either from cattle with BSE or people with vCJD, and the resulting disease looked the same whether the prions originated from diseased cows or vCJD patients (Scott et al., 1999).

Since the detection of mad cow disease in the United Kingdom, two dozen other nations have uncovered cases. Canada and the United States are the latest entrants to the list of countries affected. On May 20, 2003, Canadian officials reported BSE in an eight-year-old cow that had spent its life in Alberta and Saskatchewan. (The country's only previous mad cow had arrived as a UK import 10 years earlier.) Although the animal had been slaughtered in January 2003, slow processing meant that officials did not test the cow remains until April. By then, the carcass had been turned into pet food and exported to the United States.

Seven months later, on December 23, 2003, the U.S. Department of Agriculture (USDA) announced the country's first case of BSE in Washington state. The six-year-old dairy cow had entered the United States at the age of four. The discovery meant that U.S. officials could no longer labor under the misconception that the nation is free of BSE. Like Canada, U.S. agricultural interests want the BSE problem to disappear. Financial woes stem primarily from reduced beef exports: 58 other countries are keeping their borders shut, and a $3 billion export market has largely evaporated. At the time of writing, six more cases of BSE in Canada and two additional cases in the United States have been reported.

Infectious Human Prion Diseases

Prions from different sources have infected humans. Human prions have been transmitted to others both by ritualistic cannibalism and iatrogenic means. Kuru in the highlands of New Guinea was transmitted by ritualistic cannibalism, as people in the region attempted to immortalize their dead relatives by eating their brains (Alpers, 1968; Gajdusek, 1977; Glasse, 1967). Iatrogenic transmissions include prion-tainted human growth hormone (HGH) and gonadotropin, dura mater grafts, and corneal transplants from people who died of CJD. In addition, CJD cases have been recorded after neurosurgical procedures in which ineffectively sterilized depth electrodes or instruments were used.

Variant Creutzfeldt–Jakob Disease (vCJD)

The first cases of vCJD in teenagers and young adults were identified in Great Britain in 1994 (Will et al., 1996). More than 170 teenagers and young adults have died of vCJD in Britain, France, Ireland, Italy, Japan, Portugal, and the United States. Although the average age of vCJD patients is 26 years of age, the youngest patient was 12 years old and the oldest was 74 years of age (Spencer et al., 2002). The median duration of the illness is 13 months, with the range from 6 to 69 months.

In addition to the young age of these patients (Bateman et al.,1995; Britton et al., 1995), vCJD is characterized by numerous PrP amyloid plaques surrounded by a halo of intense spongiform degeneration in the brain (Ironside, 1997). These unusual neuropathologic changes have not been seen in CJD cases in the United States, Australia, or Japan (CDC, 1996; Ironside, 1997). Both macaque monkeys and marmosets developed neurologic disease several years after inoculation with bovine prions (Baker et al., 1993), but only the macaques exhibited numerous PrP plaques similar to those found in vCJD (Lasmézas et al., 1996).

The majority of vCJD patients present with psychiatric symptoms, including dysphoria, withdrawal, anxiety, insomnia, and loss of interest (Spencer et al., 2002; Will et al., 2004). Generally, neurologic deficits do not appear until at least four months later; these neurologic changes consist of memory loss, paresthesias, sensory deficits, gait disturbances, and dysarthria. Most vCJD cases have been reported from Britain, and 10 have been found in France. The one U.S. case was a 23-year-old woman, who is thought to have been exposed to bovine prions while living in Britain during the first 12 years of her life. From both epidemiologic and experimental studies, the evidence is quite compelling that vCJD is the result of prions being transmitted from cattle with BSE to humans through consumption of prion-contaminated beef products.

Transmission of vCJD Prions by Blood Transfusion

vCJD has been identified in two patients who received blood transfusions from donors that later died of vCJD. In one case, the recipient was a 69-year-old male who was transfused 6.5 years before the onset of neurologic dysfunction (Llewelyn et al., 2004). Many details of the second case are not published, but the patient is known to have died of a nonneurologic disease (Peden et al., 2004). Although vCJD prions were found in the spleen and cervical lymph nodes of this patient, none were found in the brain.

A glimpse of future vCJD cases caused by prion-tainted transfused blood may come from a survey of tissues collected during appendectomies and tonsillectomies. Such a survey from the United Kingdom reports that of the 12,674 appendectomy specimens examined, three were positive for PrP^{Sc} by immunohistochemistry (IHC) (Hilton et al., 2004). This finding argues that as many as 3,800 people in the United Kingdom may be replicating vCJD prions in their lymphoid tissues. Considering that immunohistochemistry (IHC) is considerably less sensitive than the conformation-dependent immunoassay (CDI), the number of Britons harboring vCJD prions in their lymphoid tissues may approach 20,000 (Safar, 2005a).

Approaches to Prion Diseases

Because prion diseases have aspects that resemble illnesses caused by viruses as noted above, many people use analogies to viruses when thinking about prions. But these analogies can sow confusion. One example is the presumed origin of the mad cows in Canada and the United States. Although it is true that BSE first appeared in the United Kingdom and then spread elsewhere through exported prion-contaminated feed, approaches from a traditional bacterial or viral epidemic are only partly helpful. In such situations, quarantines or bans can curb the spread of disease. But prions can arise spontaneously, which is an extremely important characteristic that distinguishes prions from viruses. In fact, any mammal is capable of producing prions spontaneously.

Spontaneous prion disease is thought to have triggered the epidemic of kuru, which decimated a group called the Fore in New Guinea in the past century. According to one theory, sporadic (s) CJD occurred in an individual whose brain was then consumed by his or her fellow Fore in a funerary rite involving cannibalism. The continued practice created a kuru epidemic. Ceasing the practice of this funerary rite also resulted in the decreased incidence of kuru.

Similarly, a feed ban that prevents cattle from eating the remains of other animals is crucial in containing BSE. But such bans will not eliminate the presence of mad cows when pathogenic prions arise spontaneously. If every year, 1–5 people per million spontaneously develop prion disease, why not the same incidence for cows? Indeed, I suspect that the North American BSE cases are likely to have arisen spontaneously and that afflicted animals have occasionally appeared unrecognized in herds ever since humans started cattle ranching. We have been extraordinarily lucky that a spontaneous case did not trigger an American BSE epidemic. Or perhaps small epidemics did occur but were undetected.

Still, many prefer the idea that the mad cows in North America acquired prions from their feed. Such reasoning allows people to equate prions with viruses—that is, to think of prions only as infectious agents (even though most of time, they arise spontaneously)—and to offer a seemingly plausible plan to eradicate BSE by quarantining herds. But ignoring the revolutionary concepts that govern prion biology can only hamper efforts at developing an effective program to protect the American public from exposure to these deadly agents. We must think beyond quarantine and bans, and test for prions even in the absence of an epidemic.

Diagnosis of Prion Diseases

The clinical diagnosis of human prion disease is often difficult until the patient shows profound signs of neurologic dysfunction (Roos et al., 1973; Will et al., 2004). In humans with sCJD, the most common clinical presentation is a progressive dementia. Approximately 10 percent of sCJD patients present with a progressive ataxia.

It is widely accepted that the clinical diagnosis must be provisional until a tissue diagnosis either confirms or rules out the clinical assessment. Prior to the availability of antibodies to PrP, a tissue diagnosis was generally made by histologic evaluation of neuropil vacuolation. IHC using anti-glial fibrillary acidic protein antibodies in combination with hematoxylin and eosin (H&E) staining preceded the use of anti-PrP antibody staining.

Postmortem Tissue Detection of Prions

The role of IHC in the diagnosis of scrapie was challenged after a study of the brains from eight clinically affected goats inoculated with the SSBP1 prion isolate (Foster et al., 2001). Thalamic samples taken from seven of eight goats with scrapie were positive for PrP^{Sc} by Western blotting but negative by IHC. The eighth goat was negative by both Western blotting and IHC. Consistent with these findings in goats are the results of a study of humans who died of sCJD or familial (f) CJD. In this study, IHC of formalin-fixed, paraffin-embedded human brain samples was substantially less sensitive than the conformation-dependent immunoassay (CDI) (Safar, 2005a).

The CDI detected PrP^{Sc} in all regions of the brain that were examined in 24 sCJD and 3 fCJD(E200K) cases. Comparative analyses demonstrated that the CDI was vastly superior to both histology and IHC. When 18 regions of 8 sCJD and 2 fCJD(E200K) brains were compared, it was discovered that both histology and IHC were unreliable diagnostic tools except for samples from a few brain regions. In contrast, the CDI was a superb diagnostic procedure as it detected PrP^{Sc} in all 18 regions in 8 of 8 sCJD and 2 of 2 fCJD(E200K) cases (Safar, 2005a).

Concerned that limited digestion with proteinase K (PK) was hydrolyzing some or even most of the PrP^{Sc}, the CDI was developed so as not to require PK digestion to detect PrP^{Sc}. The CDI revealed that as much as 95 percent of PrP^{Sc} is protease sensitive ($sPrP^{Sc}$) and thus was being destroyed during limited proteolysis used to hydrolyze PrP^{C}. $sPrP^{Sc}$ comprises 80–95 percent of the PrP^{Sc} found in the frontal lobe and in the white matter of CJD patients (Safar, 2005a).

The CDI detected $HuPrP^{Sc}$ with a sensitivity comparable to the bioassay for prion infectivity in Tg mice expressing chimeric human-mouse PrP. The high sensitivity achieved by the CDI is due to several factors including the use of phosphotungstic acid (PTA) that specifically precipitates $sPrP^{Sc}$ and $rPrP^{Sc}$ (Lee et al., 2005; Safar et al., 1998, 2005a). PTA has also been employed to increase the sensitivity of Western blots, enabling the detection of $rPrP^{Sc}$ in human muscle and other peripheral tissues (Glatzel et al., 2003; Wadsworth et al., 2001). A comparison between the CDI and Western blotting on brain samples from sCJD and vCJD patients showed that the CDI is 50- to 100-fold more sensitive (Minor et al., 2004).

The CDI has also been used to study GSS caused by the P102L mutation. In mice expressing the GSS mutant PrP transgene, the CDI detected high levels of $sPrP^{Sc}$(P101L) as well as low levels of $rPrP^{Sc}$(P101L) long before neurodegeneration and clinical symptoms occurred (Tremblay, 2004). $sPrP^{Sc}$(P101L) as well as low concentrations of $rPrP^{Sc}$(P101L) previously escaped detection (Hsiao et al., 1994).

BSE Testing

The transmission of kuru prions to more than 2,500 Fore people in the highlands of New Guinea and the transmission of BSE prions to more than 170 teenagers and young adults who died of vCJD argues that oral prion infection can occur. The recognition that patients with vCJD were infected with BSE prions from cattle (Bruce et al., 1997; Collinge et al., 1996; Scott et al., 1997, 2005) prompted the European Union to institute testing of all cattle over 30 months of age at the time of slaughter. Currently, both Western blotting and ELISA tests for $rPrP^{Sc}$ are being used on brainstems from cattle (Grassi et al., 2001; Kübler et al., 2003). The CDI test, which measures both protease-sensitive and protease-resistant PrP^{Sc}, has been adapted for bovine brainstems and is available for testing cattle.

The recent identification of BSE-positive cattle in Canada and the United States has prompted increased surveillance in these countries, but the number of cattle tested remains less than 2 percent of the annual slaughter (Prusiner, 2004a). Despite the small number of cattle being tested, new cases of BSE are being found. These new cases are attributed to tainted feed by agriculture authorities, who continue to think of prion diseases as being similar to infectious illnesses caused by viruses or bacteria. These officials want to believe that BSE will disappear once the consumption of ruminant-derived feed ceases. They refuse to entertain the idea that most cases of prion disease are likely to be sporadic once contaminated feed is eliminated from the food supply. In Japan, 4 million cattle have been tested over the last four years, and close to 20 cases of BSE have been identified. One Japanese cow was 21 months old and another 23 months old (Yamakawa et al., 2003), younger than the animals tested in the European Union. It seems likely that most or all of these young animals developed sporadic BSE.

Determining how early in the incubation period BSE prions can be detected by bioassay is now possible due to the construction of Tg mice expressing bovine PrP, designated Tg(BoPrP)*Prnp*$^{0/0}$ mice (Buschmann et al., 2000; Scott et al., 1997, 1999). Prior to the production of Tg(BoPrP)*Prnp*$^{0/0}$ mice, cattle were used for bioassays of bovine prions. In a limited study using cattle bioassays, bovine prions were undetectable in the obex of the bovine brainstem until 26 months after oral inoculation (Wells, 2002). In these studies, prion infectivity was detected much earlier in the lymphoid tissue of the distal ileum.

Prions in Muscle

Animal meat products consumed by humans are predominantly muscle tissue. For many years, muscle tissue was thought to be devoid of prions. In studies of the hind limb muscles of mice, prions were found at a level of 5 percent of that in brain (Bosque et al., 2002); other muscle groups also had prions but at lower levels. PrP^{Sc} was found in virtually all muscles after prions were fed to hamsters (Thomzig et al., 2003). Investigations of prions in the tongue have shown high levels of both PrP^{Sc} and prion infectivity (Bartz et al., 2003). PrP^{Sc} was identified in the muscles of 25 percent of the sCJD patients analyzed (Glatzel et al., 2003). In livestock, PrP^{Sc} was found in myocytes of the fore and hind limbs of sheep with both natural and experimental scrapie (Andreoletti et al., 2004), and prion infectivity was reported recently in extracts prepared from the muscle of BSE-infected cattle. In the latter studies, prions were detected by transmission to Tg mice expressing bovine PrP (Buschmann and Groschup, 2005).

The Only Rational Strategy

The only rational strategy is to test all cattle for prions and eliminate those harboring prions from the food supply. No reasonable human would knowingly expose himself or herself to prions as prion diseases are invariably fatal.

In Europe, a policy was instituted four years ago of prion testing for all cattle destined for human consumption that are over 30 months of age. The 30-month cutoff point was chosen for surveillance by the Office International des Epizooties (OIE; also known as the World Organization for Animal Health), but it was never intended for food safety. Some European countries have arbitrarily adopted a 24-

month cutoff. It is irrational to believe that all cattle younger than 24 months of age are free of prions and that those older than 24 months are potentially infected. Initially, the Japanese government proposed adopting the European Union's testing protocol, but consumer advocates forced the government to change its policy and test every slaughtered animal.

Rapid prion tests used in Europe vary in their sensitivity and reliability. Until now, the tests have not been sufficiently sensitive. Whether or not one or more of the newer tests can provide the desired sensitivity is unclear. Further, confining testing to brain tissue may be imprudent because other tissues such as muscle and lymphoid cells can harbor substantial levels of prions.

Given that seemingly healthy animals can carry prions, I believe that testing all slaughtered animals is the only rational policy. But this policy needs to be accompanied by a systemic approach to reward food suppliers for identifying livestock harboring prions. To maximize the protection from ingesting prions, we must aim to eliminate prions from the food supply by using the most sensitive and reliable test. The current system of using the least sensitive of the government-approved tests to minimize the number of prion-positive livestock is an unacceptable, dangerous common practice that must be terminated immediately. Providing the most safe food supply is a critical responsibility of every government—it is not an optional, incidental activity.

Acknowledgments

This work was supported by grants from the National Institutes of Health (AG02132, AG10770, and AG021601) as well as by a gift from the G. Harold and Leila Y. Mathers Charitable Foundation. S. B. P. has financial interests in InPro Biotechnology, Inc.

Correspondence should be addressed to: Institute for Neurodegenerative Diseases, 513 Parnassus Ave, HSE-774, University of California, San Francisco, CA 94143-0518; Tel: (415) 476-4482; Fax: (415) 476-8386. E-mail: stanley@ind.ucsf.edu.

SURVEILLANCE AND PREVENTION OF vCJD AND BSE: THE AUSTRALIAN PERSPECTIVE

Steven Collins, M.D.[2]
University of Melbourne, Parkville, Australia

As an introduction to bovine spongiform encephalopathy (BSE) and its consequent zoonosis, variant Creutzfeldt-Jakob disease (vCJD), I will briefly review the first human TSE epidemic, kuru, which contains a number of important in-

[2]Australian National CJD Registry and Department of Pathology.

sights and lessons. Kuru occurred endemically among the Fore linguistic group of the eastern highlands of Papua New Guinea (PNG). The first cases of kuru came to the attention of Western medicine in the middle to late 1950s as Australian patrols were gradually reaching the more remote areas of PNG (Gajdusek and Zigas, 1957). Predominantly manifesting as an inexorably progressive cerebellar ataxia with later onset dementia (Gajdusek, 1962), the etiology and spread of the disease were eventually linked to cannibalistic rites of mourning for deceased relatives (Gajdusek, 1977). Not long after noting neuropathologic and other similarities between kuru and scrapie (Hadlow, 1959), kuru was proven to be a transmissible spongiform encephalopathy (Gajdusek et al., 1966). The predilection of kuru for women and children was related to their more usual consumption of the highly infectious central nervous system tissues. It is believed that ritualistic endocannibalism was successfully eradicated by the end of the 1950s.

Detailed epidemiologic studies of kuru suggested a mean incubation period of around 12 years, but ongoing contemporary field surveillance supports the likelihood that the most recent cases have incubation periods spanning up to 50 years (Collinge, 1999; Collinge et al., 2006). Consequently, based on these observations and those from various animal models of prion disease (Dickinson et al., 1975; Hill et al., 2000), there may not be a finite incubation period. Once exposed, the risk of developing a TSE may persist lifelong. Further, kuru indicated that despite the very low transmissibility of TSEs compared with many conventional microbes, high levels of disease can arise, including through an oral route of inoculation, if unique circumstances prevail to support "unnatural" intraspecies recycling of highly infectious tissues. At the height of the epidemic, annual mortality from the disease approached 50 percent in some Fore villages, with an annual incidence of approximately 10 percent in a number of Fore tribes (Gajdusek and Zigas, 1957).

Bovine Spongiform Encephalopathy and Variant Creutzfeldt-Jakob Disease

By the mid-1980s, United Kingdom veterinary authorities had confidently recognized BSE as a new form of cattle disease. In retrospect, the early years of the BSE epidemic evinced undue reassurance from the scrapie precedent. The lack of documented evidence of scrapie transmission to humans from farmed sheep and the generally low levels of endemic scrapie over the few hundred years that scrapie had been recognized in sheep flocks suggested BSE would perhaps behave similarly. In discomfiting contrast, the incidence of BSE rapidly escalated and by 1992 at the height of the UK epidemic, some 3,500 cases per month were confirmed; overall, an estimated 2 million contaminated cattle are believed to have entered the human food chain (Donnelly et al., 2002). Given the dramatic increase in BSE, in accordance with one of the recommendations of the Southwood enquiry, national surveillance for human prion diseases was prudently recommenced in the United Kingdom in 1990. Particular interest was to be given to ascertaining the occurrence of any new forms of disease that might have arisen zoonotically from BSE. In 1996, a new or variant form of CJD (vCJD) was reported by the National CJD Surveillance unit in Edinburgh, Scotland, with 10 younger adults and adolescents manifesting a phenotype hitherto not described (Will et al., 1996). A range of subsequent research has confirmed the likely causal link between vCJD and BSE (Hill et al., 1997).

A very recently reported case-control study of vCJD has highlighted diet as a principal risk factor, especially the consumption of greater amounts of products likely to contain bovine mechanically recovered meat (MRM) and bovine head meat (sausages, burgers, and pies) (Ward et al., 2006). These bovine meats are more prone to contamination by brain, spinal cord, and dorsal root ganglia, and the study results are therefore consistent with the hypothesis that people developing vCJD were exposed to greater amounts of those bovine meat products more likely to be contaminated by the highly infectious central nervous system tissue (summarized in Figure 6-1). One caveat concerning this data is the possibility of recall bias, suggested by the observation that the respondents for patients initially suspected to be manifesting vCJD but eventually proven to have a different illness also reported the same dietary associations.

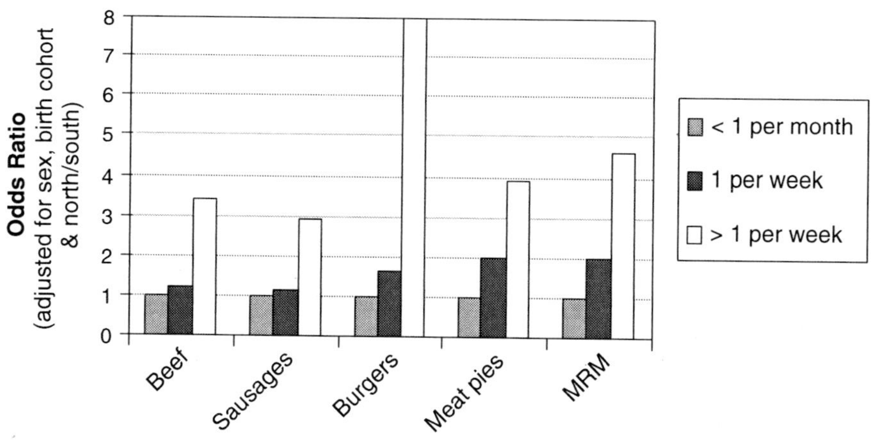

FIGURE 6-1 Reported frequency of food consumption, odds ratio of vCJD cases versus general population controls. Results of this case-controlled study suggest that people with vCJD consumed foods likely to contain bovine mechanically recovered meat (MRM) and bovine head meat (sausages, burgers, and pies) more frequently than as compared with the general population. Such meats are more prone to contamination with central nervous system tissue, and therefore—if the bovine source was infected with BSE—higher concentrations of prions. It should be noted, however, that because consumption rates were self-reported, they may reflect recall bias (see text).
SOURCE: Adapted from Ward et al. (2006).

As of July 2006, a total of 161 cases of vCJD have been diagnosed in the United Kingdom. Remarkable uniformity in the clinical illness has been maintained: it affects young people (the median age at onset is 26 years) with a median survival of 14 months. France has the second highest number of vCJD cases (18 in total), with case numbers and the temporal profile behaving as predicted from modeling based on transmissions through beef imported from the United Kingdom (Valleron et al., 2001). The primary United Kingdom vCJD epidemic is thought to be in decline, and most experts expect that the total number of cases will not exceed 200 (Valleron et al., 2001). However, the recent reports of three cases of vCJD related to transfusion of blood products and the higher than expected potential prevalence of subclinical or preclinical vCJD suggested by the retrospective study of archival appendix and tonsil specimens raises the sobering possibility of a secondary wave of iatrogenic vCJD (Hilton et al., 2004; Llewelyn et al., 2004). Based on animal transmission studies involving "species barriers" and subsequent strain adaptation, such human-to-human transmissions may prove far more efficient than the primary cross-species infections from cattle to humans through oral consumption of contaminated beef. Further, not only must we be alert to a possible secondary wave of vCJD, but given the unprecedented calamitous transmission of BSE to humans, we must also keep vigilant to the possibility of other cross-species transgressions from TSEs now apparently confined to animals, such as chronic wasting disease.

Australia's National CJD Registry

The Australian National CJD Registry (ANCJDR) is a federally funded surveillance unit that commenced operation in 1993, with the initial mission to ascertain further cases of human pituitary hormone-related CJD. At the inauguration of ANCJDR activities, five persons with pituitary hormone-related CJD were known, and no additional cases have been detected. The scope of ANCJDR human TSE monitoring has expanded with the passage of time, and as of 1996, following the discovery of vCJD, surveillance was broadened to include that disease (Collins et al., 2002). The ANCJDR has also participated in the European surveillance consortium (EUROCJD) since 1997. As of 2004, the Communicable Diseases Network Australia agreed to make human TSEs notifiable diseases in all Australian states and territories. Primary case review of suspect notified cases involves the ANCJDR, with evaluation outcomes a collaborative exercise between the appropriate state or territory and the registry.

Case definitions used by ANCJDR for classification purposes are those endorsed by EUROCJD. A range of standard surveillance methods are employed by the ANCJDR, including the use of semiannual surveys sent to all neurologists, neuropathologists and pathologists within Australia. Respondents are prompted to report any suspect, probable, or confirmed cases of CJD they have seen or been aware of in the preceding six months. Follow-up is undertaken for positive responses, and we also receive unprompted personal communications regarding suspect and confirmed CJD from these same medical practitioner groups. The ANCJDR annually reviews state and territory morbidity separation codings for citings of CJD or CJD-like illnesses, and conducts national death certificate searches as well. Since 1997, the most important mechanism of case notification has been through the national cerebrospinal fluid (CSF) 14-3-3 protein diagnostic testing service that the registry offers (Collins et al., 2000). For case confirmation, CSF 14-3-3 protein detection serves as a reasonably reliable and specific marker of sporadic CJD and is now an accepted component of case definitions for surveillance classification purposes (Zerr et al., 2000).

Neuropathologic examination of the brain remains necessary for confirmation and classification as a definite case of CJD (Collins et al., 2004), and given the problems frequently encountered with brain biopsies, postmortem examination is preferred and pursued in all patients with suspect CJD. Very occasionally routine autopsy will detect a completely unsuspected case of TSE. Unfortunately, however, postmortem rates in major teaching hospitals have declined dramatically throughout Australia over the past 10–15 years and are now running at around 12 percent. Further, fewer medical centers are willing to conduct autopsies on patients with suspected CJD. Over recent years the ANCJDR has maintained a postmortem rate of around 60 percent, but the aforementioned combination of factors is militating against our ability to obtain neuropathologic confirmation, which remains the gold standard for diagnosis.

Similar to all previous and ongoing human TSE surveillance, the vast majority of cases in the ANCJDR are sporadic; there are several familial cases and a small number of iatrogenic cases, but no cases of vCJD so far (see Table 6-1) (Collinge, 1999). Measures have been undertaken to try to ensure that vCJD has not been overlooked in Australia.

TABLE 6-1 Cases of Transmissible Spongiform Encephalopathies (TSE) Reported to the Australian National CJD Registry (ANCJDR), January 1, 1970 Through June 30, 2005

Classification	Sporadic CJD	Familial CJF/GSS	Iatrogenic CJD	Variant CJD	Unclassified	Total
Definite	265	29	5[a]	0	0	299
Probable	178	9	4	0	0	191
Possible	7	0	1	0	0	8
Incomplete	0	98[b]	98			98
Total	450	38	10	0	98	596

[a]Includes one definite iatrogenic case who received pituitary hormone treatment in Australia but disease onset and death occurred while a resident overseas. This case is not included in statistical analysis since morbidity and mortality did not occur within Australia.

[b]Includes 59 living cases.

SOURCE: Adapted from Klug et al. (2005).

Reaffirmation of Absence of vCJD in Australia

The likelihood of vCJD in a given country appears to reflect either the levels of endemic BSE, the amounts of imported contaminated United Kingdom beef products through 1980–1996, or—as in the experience of Canada, the United States, and perhaps Japan—its citizens' travel and migration patterns. Because the travel and migration profile of Australians appears similar to that of Canadians and Americans, the ANCJDR undertook a reexamination of the clinical files and neuropathologic reports of all cases referred to the registry who died between January 1, 1992, and June 30, 2003, and which had been classified as either sporadic CJD or non-CJD. None of the 365 reexamined cases fulfilled case definitions for possible, probable, or definite vCJD, and the molecular (PrP glycotyping) profile typical of vCJD was not seen in any of the 37 cases for which frozen tissues was available for Western blot analysis (Lewis et al., 2005).

Animal TSEs in Australia

To date, there have been no endogenous cases of either BSE or scrapie in Australia. Scrapie was inadvertently introduced in 1952 from the United Kingdom, but was quickly recognized and the affected flock slaughtered. There have been two cases of TSEs in felines in Australia: an imported cheetah and an Asiatic golden cat, both of which were believed to have contracted their disease through contaminated feed prior to their importation to Australia.

Protective Measures

For the protection of domestic commercial livestock, Australia has adopted a range of measures to lessen the risk of BSE and scrapie, which can be found at *www.aahc.com.au*. Since 1966, there has been a ban on the importation of meat and bone meal and any stock feed containing ruminant materials from anywhere in the world except New Zealand; this was initially imposed to avoid the risk of anthrax but was maintained thereafter. From 1988, live cattle from the United Kingdom and any other country reporting BSE cannot be imported into Australia. Owners of animals imported from countries in which BSE is subsequently discovered can choose to place the imported animals under lifelong quarantine or have them slaughtered.

A voluntary ban on ruminant-to-ruminant feeding of meat and bone meal was established in 1996 but became compulsory through Commonwealth legislation in October 1997. This was then expanded in June 1999 and again in March 2001, whereby vertebrate materials (except for milk, gelatin, and tallow and oils from fish and poultry) are prohibited from use in ruminant feeds (*www.aahc.com.au*). To ensure compliance with the feed bans, national audits are conducted. These include onsite visits to producers, animal feed manufacturers, and rendering plants, as well as PCR screening of meat and bone meal intended for feed. To date, three such audits have been completed.

Animal TSE Surveillance

Australia's National TSE Freedom Assurance program oversees and coordinates the National TSE Surveillance Program (NTSESP), education strategies, and enforcement of the ruminant feed ban (*www.aahc.com.au*). Prior to establishment of the national audits, more than 3,300 brains of cattle were examined histopathologically for BSE; no disease was found. In 1998, NTSESP was initiated to satisfy OIE requirements concerning the surveillance and monitoring of BSE and scrapie. Under this program, every animal (cow or sheep) showing signs of nervous system disease must be examined by designated veterinarians, who also take brain specimens for histopathologic examination. If disease is suspected, the samples are subjected to Western blot analysis. Approximately 450 sheep and 400 cattle per year with neurologic illness are examined through NTSESP. The program is designed to achieve a 99 percent confidence level, which means that it can detect one case of BSE per one million cattle. Following a change in the OIE terrestrial animal health code, an additional 400 sick animals (including downer animals, those that die on the farm, and those slaughtered to contain a disease outbreak) are now tested for BSE by Western blot of brain specimens.

Education

Education of stakeholders and the public is the final important component of Australia's effort to control BSE. Various media are used to introduce a broad understanding of legislation on this issue and its rationale with dissemination through agencies ranging from the Environmental Protection Agency, the State Farmer's Association, the Australian Veterinary Association, and Animal Health Australia, as well as through various state and territory education programs.

BSE AS A CASE STUDY OF PUBLIC HEALTH AND THE PUBLIC GOOD

Maura N. Ricketts, M.D., M.H.Sc., F.R.C.P.C.[3]
Health Canada

The case of BSE represents a special challenge for public health professionals because the initiative and the interventions necessary for the control of BSE

---

[3]Executive Director. Based upon a presentation made for the IOM's Forum on Microbial Threats, October 2005.

lie within the animal health sector. As a direct result of this, it is to be expected that debate, disagreements, and occasionally dispute will populate the arena when animal health experts and public health experts talk about BSE. Regardless, the last 20 years of experience with BSE have refined the analysis of risk, and there is increasingly large overlap in policy recommendations with a notable shift toward recognition of the importance of risk perception, ethics and societal values in shaping public policy, the implications for broader healthcare practice, and other aspects of public health. This paper will examine BSE from the perspective of public health in the expectation that the paradigm of public health might be seen to be one that is particularly sensible when the protection of human health is ultimately the goal of public policy.

What Is Public Health and What Does It Do?

The definition of public health has proven that it is, like other branches of medicine, both an art and a science. The examination of a definition of public health provides the foundation for understanding public health-based recommendations:

> Public health is one of the efforts organized by society to protect, promote, and restore the people's health. It is the combination of sciences, skills, and beliefs that are directed to the maintenance and improvement of the health of all the people through collective or social actions. . . . Public health activities change with changing technology and social values, but the goals remain the same: to reduce the amount of disease, premature death, and disease-produced discomfort and disability in the population. Public health is thus a social institution, a discipline and a practice (Last, 1983).

> The science and art of promoting health, preventing disease, prolonging life, and improving the quality of life through the organized efforts of society (Last, 2001).

A key component of the definition is the reference to "the organized efforts of society." In Table 6-2 are the functions of public health that have been nationally adopted in Canada. Even a superficial review of the functions will confirm the extent of societal commitment that is required.

The functions of public health map themselves into core program areas (see Table 6-3). These are the core programs that must be sustained by any functional public health organization.

When examined in matrix format (see Table 6-4), the public health decisions taken regarding vCJD become clearer.

What About vCJD?

How can public health principles be applied to the case of BSE? The first and foremost function of public health is health protection. Table 6-5 lays out a well-

TABLE 6-2 The Functions of Public Health

Population Health Assessment
• Understand the health of populations and the factors that underlie good health and that create health risks
Health Surveillance
• Early recognition of outbreaks, disease trends, health factors, and cases of illness
• Allows for earlier intervention and lessened impact
• Surveillance aids understanding of the impacts of efforts to improve health and reduce the impact of disease
Health Promotion
• Work with individuals, agencies, and communities to understand and improve health through healthy public policy, community-based interventions, and public participation
• Uses community development or policy advocacy and action regarding the environmental and socioeconomic determinants of health and illness
Disease and Injury Prevention
• As much as two-thirds of premature mortality is preventable through the application of available knowledge
• Includes investigation, contact tracing, and preventive measures targeted at reducing risks of outbreaks of infectious disease
Health Protection and Emergency Preparedness

SOURCE: National Advisory Committee on SARS and Public Health (2003).

accepted series of steps that are followed when an outbreak of an unknown disease is found among human populations.

It is to be noted that an "outbreak" could be a single case of a disease whenever that disease is sufficiently unusual, as is the case with vCJD or BSE. The reasoning for this is similar to the use of canaries in mines—as soon as the first canary dies, it is time to act before the first person dies. In the case of vCJD, the canary is the first case of BSE—as was so clearly illustrated in the United Kingdom (see Figure 6-2).

TABLE 6-3 Functions and Core Programs

Public Health Functions	Core Program Areas
• Population health assessment	• Communicable disease prevention and control
• Public health surveillance	• Prevention of chronic diseases and injuries
• Disease and injury prevention	• Health development through life cycle
• Health promotion	• Environmental health
• Health protection	• Emergency preparedness

SOURCE: National Advisory Committee on SARS and Public Health (2003).

TABLE 6-4 Activity Map for vCJD

	Public Health Functions				
Core Program Areas	Population Health Assessments	Public Health Surveillance	Disease and Injury Prevention	Health Promotion	Health Protection
Communicable disease prevention and control	X	X	X		X
Prevention of chronic diseases and injuries					
Health development through life cycle				X	
Environmental health	X	X	X	X	X
Emergency preparedness					

SOURCE: Ricketts (2005).

TABLE 6-5 Health Protection and the Management of an Outbreak

- ✓ Outbreak detection
- ✓ Epidemic investigation
- ✓ Establishment of case definition
- ✓ Establish etiology.
- ✓ Confirm cases.
  - ✓ Find cases.
  - ✓ Define scope of problem.
  - ✓ Descriptive epidemiology
  - ✓ Generate and test hypothesis.
- ✓ Report findings to peer review.
- ✓ Communications
- ✗ Control of epidemic through public health measures
  - ✗ Control and reduce exposure.
  - • Measures have been undertaken by animal health authorities, but do not result in complete avoidance of exposure.
  - ✗ Prevent exposure.
  - ✗ Prevent ongoing transmission among humans.
  - • Infection control, transplantation, blood safety measures partly address this need, but without screening and preclinical diagnostic testing, it is not possible to fully control exposure.
  - ✗ Eliminate or eradicate infection source.

NOTE: Checkmarks indicate functions that are within the scope of public health; Xs indicate activities that have not or cannot be accomplished with current interventions.

SOURCE: National Advisory Committee on SARS and Public Health (2003).

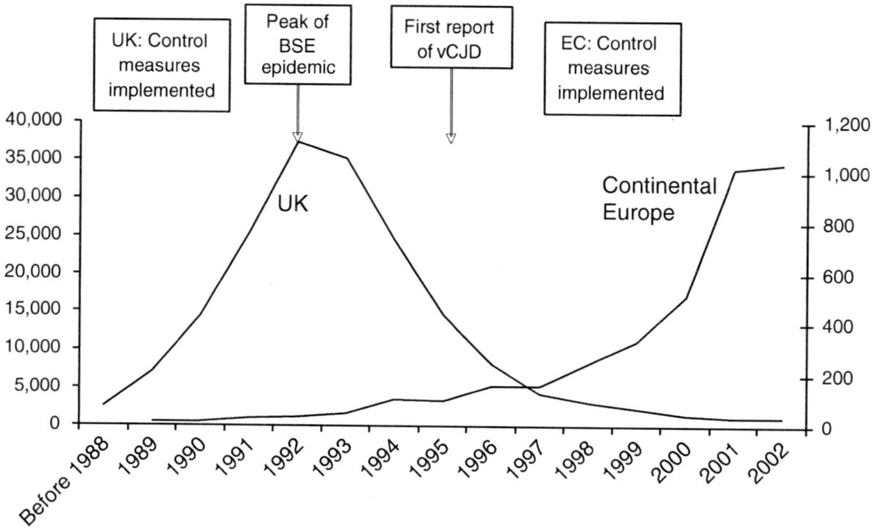

FIGURE 6-2 BSE and vCJD outbreak development in the UK; Epidemic curve of BSE in Europe (UK n = 180,845; continental Europe n = 3,286).
SOURCE: OIE (2006).

Population Health Assessment and Decision Making in Uncertainty

Since the first case of BSE and the subsequent first case report of vCJD some 10 years later, science and public policy have come a long way. Assumptions made early in the BSE epidemic, and even some made later, proved to be inaccurate or misplaced. It might have been said in the early years that those involved in developing policy to control BSE were, figuratively speaking, flying the plane while building it.

In public health, as in other arenas of public policy, it is necessary to make decisions even in the face of uncertainty. When uncertainty prevails, many other aspects of societal influence enter into the decision making, such as economic stability or principles such as risk avoidance or the precautionary principle. In the case of BSE, there were enormous economic and trade implications that directly impacted public policy.

At an entirely practical level, there are questions that will underlie the decisions finally taken by society. Where there are no answers, then it is required that assumptions are made. In an open society, the assumption should be stated. Based upon my experience in both public health and BSE, I propose the following core issues:

- How do people get vCJD?
- Is there any immunity? Treatment?
- Are there people at higher risk?
- Is there a test that can tell people they already are infected? Or will they get the disease?
- Are there ways to stop people from getting BSE? Or from getting sick?
- Do people die or recover?

How Do People Get vCJD?

The principal source of route and exposure for humans is through the consumption of food of bovine origin, just as for other animals. However, it can be seen that the risk must be very low because there are very few cases despite very large amounts of exposure. As of March 2006, 160 cases of vCJD (National CJD Surveillance Unit UK, 2006) had been reported in the United Kingdom—this in a country where it has been estimated that over 1 million infected cattle entered the human food chain (Ghani et al., 2000). It is now known that most of the BSE infectivity is found in particular parts of the infected cattle, and that the location of the infectivity shifts somewhat with age. Collectively, the contaminated tissues are referred to as specified bovine offals; those tissues that must be removed in order to protect human populations are the specified risk materials (SRM). Additionally, some kinds of mechanically recovered meat may become contaminated with neural tissue. The relative resistance of humans to BSE suggests that the removal of SRM and the modification of methods to mechanically recover meat would enormously reduce risks to human populations.

Human-to-human transmission is a possible secondary route of transmission of vCJD, but in this case, the risk must be very low because very few cases of human-to-human transmission have been recognized despite intense interest in this problem. All cases reported thus far are from the United Kingdom, and all involve transfusion of blood (Ward et al., 2003). In medical practice, it is anathema to cause disease during the course of treatment; despite the nearly immeasurable risk, extensive measures have been undertaken to protect against iatrogenic vCJD.

Is There Any Immunity? Treatment?

From the perspective of public health, the answer to both questions is no. Despite the possible advances in clinical medicine and proposed clinical trials, it is not possible to amend the public health risk assessment by making allowances for immune populations or for the potential impact of treatment.

Are There People at Higher Risk?

Clearly, there are. People residing in countries with a high incidence of BSE and where BSE control interventions have not completely removed the potential exposure of humans to high-risk tissues are at the highest risk. Additionally, it is recognized that people carrying the homozygous allele at codon 129 (Methionine/methionine) are overrepresented among vCJD cases. The number of people in the UK who have this gene combination and have not developed vCJD far exceeds the number of those who have. Finally, for the purposes of this paper, it must be noted that there is a risk based upon age; the age distribution is skewed toward younger adults. The reason for this remains obscure—could it be due to specific exposures? Is it because of particular physiologic characteristics of the age group? Could it be that everyone is at equal risk, but that the incubation period varies? These questions are asked, but not answered. Resultantly, if one was searching for a screening test that could identify high-risk populations, perhaps to offer them special interventions, these characteristics are not useful because very, very many more people with these patterns are not ill than are.

Is There a Test?

There is, to date, no test to detect the agent in food or by testing easily available biologic tissues of living animals, including humans. Testing in humans is completely limited to tests that are conducted after the appearance of symptoms.

In cattle, after slaughter, specific areas of cattle brains can be tested for BSE—these tests are being used more and more extensively globally. However, testing is comparatively expensive and requires special facilities and cannot be conducted on site at the time of slaughter. Detailed analysis of the impact of testing and other interventions can be found on the Canadian Food Inspection Web site, as on other Web sites (European Union, Switzerland, United Kingdom, France, and the United States for example).

Are There Ways to Prevent BSE Infection in Humans? Are There Ways to Prevent People Who Are Infected from Becoming Sick?

To both questions, the answer is no. None of the most time-tested interventions of public health (vaccination, prophylaxis) are useful. By implication, it is essential that humans must avoid exposure to the *source* of infection (e.g., contaminated cattle tissue).

Do People Die? Recover?

To date, no person with diagnosed vCJD has survived. It is not yet known if infection leads inevitably to disease, in part because there is no existing preclinical diagnostic test. Once the symptom complex is diagnosed, the disease leads, inevitably, to death. Preventing vCJD can only be accomplished, at this time, by preventing exposure to BSE.

Unlike many other population health issues, the principal tools for protecting the public are actually not in the control of either clinical or public health physicians. Animal and food security is the first line of defence. With the lessons of the past, it is possible to make good public policy decisions regarding vCJD and BSE. There is not a recipe for controlling or eradicating vCJD or BSE. Table 6-6 outlines the key activities to control BSE; thorough discussion is beyond the intended scope of this paper.

From the perspective of public health, a series of problems can be anticipated even in those areas where public health has established authority. Principal among them is the need for a highly sensitive and accurate surveillance system that can identify all cases of human TSE and accurately distinguish vCJD. Surveillance may be supported through legislative authorities where necessary and with the financial commitment of government where needed. Surveillance capacity will have to be centralized since the collection, analysis, and dissemination of information for action requires expertise in the disease complex as well as in handling pathogenic tissues. The very rarity of the disease and the implications of each

TABLE 6-6 Controlling BSE

Motivate reporting	
Control disease spread:	• Identify at-risk animals using scientifically based criteria, and destroy them; • Destroy the cohort (definition of cohort is important and ought to be based upon feed-cohorts); and • Feed safety requires identification of all sources of cross-contamination from slaughter to farmyard and removal of SBOs from the animal feed chain.
Reduce risk to humans from apparently healthy animals:	• Remove and destroy specified risk materials (SRMs are the tissues that might contain or be contaminated by the SBOs); • Control animal feed security; and • Test where necessary and where it will improve safety, and consider that testing every animal may not lead to improved safety if it diverts resources from prevention. Also consider whether the test is, in fact, insufficient to detect all contamination.

NOTE: SRM = specified risk materials; SBO = specified bovine offals.

SOURCE: Ricketts (2005).

case mean that a high, uniform standard must be set, without risk of duplication of case reports. In order that cases are identified, there is a need for specialized clinical knowledge. The awareness, interest, and participation of neurologists and neuropathologists through collaborative networking is essential. Additionally, there is a need for access to specific laboratory-based diagnostic capacity, including EKG, CSF testing, MRI, and neuropathology, all within a context of high autopsy rates.

The flow of accurate analysis to senior policy makers in government is required to ensure that a realistic and thorough BSE risk assessment is conducted and uses evidence from both human and animal health perspectives. The risk assessment model should examine modes of population exposure to the BSE agent and must do so with consideration of the scientific evidence and the multiple requirements of all stakeholders. There will be many interest groups and many different messages; by fostering trust and the honest prompt disclosure of information, nongovernmental organizations (NGOs) can support the overall public efforts and help prevent the dissemination of inaccurate or inflammatory messages. In all countries, one must consider that a trade-based economy is resistant to disclosure of risk and that competitive markets are affected by changes in import and export restrictions.

Finally, one must reflect upon the role of public opinion. vCJD is a highly dreaded disease accompanied by high levels of public outrage. People are outraged because they view the suffering and deaths as unnecessary; in fact, they may suggest that justice is not served because the death of a loved one is simply due to industry's interest in profiting over human health concerns. In Canada, public opinion supported the smaller and less industrialized practice of cattle ranching seen in some Canadian provinces.

Experience in public health has demonstrated that there are a number of strategies that work to prevent the spread of communicable disease. vCJD is a particular challenge because there are no opportunities to prevent vCJD short of preventing BSE infection. In no particular order, the following illustrates the range of activities that would be pursued:

- Healthy public policy should be implemented regarding exposure to BSE-contaminated tissues in all disciplines from occupational safety, infection control practices, biologics development and use, transplantation and transfusion safety, and food safety;
- Inform people about health issues so that they can make their own decisions in an informed manner;
- Prevent and respond to outbreaks and emergencies, with particular emphasis on the need to conduct surveillance for vCJD;
- Help people develop personal skills (resilience), particularly those directly impacted by BSE through sickness or business;

- Collaborate for intersectoral and community action, recognizing that the entire community is affected;
- Enforce laws and regulations, notably in feed and food safety;
- Reorient and assure the quality of health services, particularly recognizing that there will be confusion between other forms of human TSEs and vCJD. Additionally, given the experience in the United Kingdom, recognition that those who develop the disease are young;
- Create supportive environments for all stakeholders; and
- Evaluate the impact of interventions.

Many lessons were learned as a result of the outbreak of BSE in the United Kingdom and Europe. It is important to control the *risk* of BSE exposure; countries that have focused on the *rate* of BSE have been unable to prevent its importation and spread. As in a commonly used homily, a chain is only as strong as its weakest link. The key link for public health practitioners is that BSE and vCJD are the same agent. Simply put, if there were no further infections of cattle with BSE, there would be no further cases of vCJD.

INCENTIVES AND DISINCENTIVES FOR DISEASE SURVEILLANCE AND REPORTING: THE BSE CASE STUDY

Will Hueston, D.V.M., Ph.D.[4]
University of Minnesota

My contribution to this workshop comes in the form of seven lessons that I have learned from 16 years of involvement with bovine spongiform encephalopathy (BSE), followed by a brief list of recommendations derived from these lessons. The lessons and recommendations are drawn from my experience working as a private practice veterinarian, a resident veterinarian for an agribusiness enterprise, a university faculty member, a government animal health official, and an adviser and consultant to national and state government, national and international organizations, and food system companies from production to retail and food service.

Lesson 1: Detecting a New Animal Disease Is Extremely Difficult

Most individual animal diseases are treated on the farm following clinical diagnosis by the animal owner, farm manager, or in difficult cases, a private-practice veterinarian. If that clinical diagnosis is incorrect, and/or the animal does not recover, the animal is usually sold (culled), eaten, or buried. Most animal

[4]Professor and Director, Center for Animal Health and Food Safety.

diagnostic services accessible in such situations are provided on a fee-for-service basis. Only foreign animal disease investigations and diagnostics are provided free of charge by government veterinarians, as they are seen as a public good. Even then, however, the diagnostic workup is generally limited to ruling out a specific foreign animal disease (e.g., foot-and-mouth disease or BSE); there is no follow-up to determine the exact cause of illness if foreign animal diseases are ruled out. Consequently, it is very difficult to detect the signals of the emergence of a new animal disease.

Limited national monitoring and surveillance does occur, such as the National Animal Health Monitoring system and more recently the National Animal Health Laboratory Network. Creating inclusive national animal disease databases has been hampered by the lack of widely accepted standardized nomenclature for animal diseases and presenting signs. Unfortunately, most animal diagnostic laboratory and veterinary hospital record-keeping systems are designed to facilitate financial accounting and billing, not epidemiologic analysis.

By comparison with Europe, Canada, New Zealand, and Australia, the U.S. federal animal health laboratory system is quite limited. The federal government supports two national laboratories, one operated by the Department of Homeland Security on Plum Island, New York, and the other is operated by the USDA Animal and Plant Health Inspection Services Veterinary Services in Ames, Iowa. Research and diagnostics at these facilities focus on diseases for which there is a specific programmatic target, such as foreign animal diseases at Plum Island, and domestic program diseases such as brucellosis, tuberculosis, and BSE at Ames. These two laboratories provide reference services for state and private laboratories (confirmation of specific program diseases). The U.S. government does not have a national laboratory focused specifically on the detection or description of emerging animal diseases.

Animal disease diagnostics in the United States are performed by state, university, and private laboratories that vary greatly in terms of their quality and capacity. About 12 of the 50 state animal diagnostic laboratories are linked in a pilot version of a national animal health laboratory network. Limited funding has been provided to these laboratories to allow them to cooperate with the federal laboratories for foreign animal disease diagnostics but not for the identification and characterization of emerging diseases.

Lesson 2: Recognizing BSE in a Low-Incidence Country Is Difficult Even Under the Best Circumstances

BSE has no unique presenting clinical signs. Therefore, the disease can only be detected through specialized diagnostic testing of brain samples; it cannot be diagnosed by clinical evaluation of the live animal or by gross necropsy such as that carried out on a dead animal on the farm.

Most countries conduct passive surveillance for BSE and other animal diseases, providing diagnostic services for those animals voluntarily presented to the laboratory rather than actively searching for cattle demonstrating clinical signs compatible with BSE or dying of unknown causes. This focus on passive surveillance leads to confusion between the absence of evidence for a disease and the evidence of its absence. Countries with no "BSE suspects" presented for diagnostic workup claim that no BSE exists, even though the clinical signs associated with BSE (changes in mentation, sensation, and locomotion) are found in a number of commonly occurring cattle diseases that can only be differentiated from BSE by extensive diagnostic workup. In addition, adherence to the "disease present or absent" paradigm further reduces the effectiveness of passive surveillance by establishing a bias against detecting the disease so that a country can continue to represent themselves as "BSE-free."

There are huge disincentives for expanding national surveillance for BSE. BSE surveillance is expensive, with the total costs for collecting and testing each sample usually in excess of US$20. Furthermore, it is not in the national interest to discover BSE unless there is a plan in place for addressing it. Reporting BSE can have devastating economic and political consequences; whereas, historically a country's failure to detect the disease, or its lack of an adequate surveillance system, has been rewarded by continued trade.

Lesson 3: Most Farmers Are Honest, but Disincentives for Reporting BSE Greatly Outweigh the Incentives

Animal production has historically been measured by the number of animals produced, not the quantity and quality of food generated. Therefore, many producers see themselves as raising animals rather than as part of the food system. We are continuing to work to change that paradigm in order to foster a shared responsibility for the food system, from producer to consumer.

For years most countries in the world have pursued a cheap food policy, where the price of food has assumed paramount importance. Consequently, food producers throughout the food system (from the farm to the consumer's table) strive to keep costs as low as possible. Although animal diseases impose costs on farmers, they recognize that absence of disease (100 percent prevention and control) is not always the optimal economic strategy. Producers weigh the costs of disease diagnostics, prevention, and control against the potential benefits they may ensure. They seek diagnostic support if they believe that understanding and preventing economically important diseases can reduce the cost of production more than the marginal cost of the diagnostics and prevention strategies, or if their products can be accorded a higher health status and, hence, a higher value, as a result of negative results on diagnostic tests where the risk of positive tests is low.

One is hard pressed to find individual producer incentives for reporting suspected cases of BSE in the United States. There is no treatment for BSE, and government-mandated controls increase production costs. Feed is the single greatest contributor to cost of production, and government feed regulations have removed a low-cost protein supplement. Removal and destruction of specified risk materials (those tissues where BSE agent accumulates in affected cows) has increased the costs of processing and reduced the value of each animal slaughtered. Additionally, the government certifies the nation's BSE status, but not that of individual herds. Thus the individual producer gains no benefit from conscientious submission of suspect cattle where all the test results are negative.

At the same time, there are numerous disincentives for reporting BSE. Producers on whose farm a BSE cow is identified are ostracized by the rest of the industry, and their products are shunned by consumers and wholesale buyers. Their business (and personal life) is disrupted by the government, industry and media response. Finally, disposal of affected or suspect animals is difficult and often expensive, and government response to BSE diagnosis in a herd has all too often involved destruction of many more animals than epidemiologically necessary to control the disease.

Considering all the disincentives, a phrase uttered by the Prime Minister of Alberta was taken out of context as a new mantra for some cattle producers: "Shoot, shovel, and shut up" rather than report BSE suspects.

Lesson 4: Testing Can Become an End Unto Itself

Before implementing a widespread testing regime for disease surveillance or health monitoring, the purpose of the testing must be clarified. The purpose will change over the course of an epidemic, so it must always be clear why it is done, in order that appropriate sample size can be determined and the test results interpreted appropriately.

Testing alone cannot afford safety (defined by dictionaries as the "absence of risk"), and it is meaningless without the concurrent implementation of animal and public health measures. Testing the wrong populations can create a false sense of security that, while politically expedient, does not constitute a public health measure. For instance, controlled BSE challenge studies and accumulated BSE surveillance results demonstrate that young animals will test negative to all of our currently available tests even if exposed to BSE; this is because the disease takes years to create discernible damage to the central nervous system and for the disease agent, the prion protein, to accumulate to detectable levels. Consequently, testing only young cattle assures that all tests are negative but says nothing about the BSE status of a country. Similarly, testing *all* cattle in a country with BSE decreases the apparent prevalence of the disease because of all the young cattle testing negative regardless of the extent of BSE in the adult population.

Lesson 5: Focus on Risk, Not the Presence or Absence of Disease

The key for human and animal health protection is effective risk management, not the disease status of the country. Most countries have focused disproportionately on the reported presence or absence of disease rather than on the effectiveness of the risk management. Internally, the lack of positive diagnostic tests has propelled officials to proclaim disease freedom, thereby creating a false sense of security and reducing the imperative of prevention and control. Outside their borders, countries have tended toward implementation of total trade bans when a trading partner identifies BSE, a policy that ignores the fact that a variety of risk management measures exist that allow for the safe trade of animals and animal products from countries regardless of their disease status. Infectious diseases do not respect national borders, and yet we frequently hear the statement "we have sealed our borders," all too often followed by the false reassurance that the disease of concern will "never" occur here. Not only are these statements factually inaccurate, but also they represent the ultimate risk communication error—providing absolute guarantees. Above all else, we usually fail to consider most zoonoses in the context of ecosystem risk management, and we develop national public policy rather than a regional or global approach.

Lesson 6: Take Opportunity Costs into Account

Every dollar spent on BSE testing, prevention, or control is unavailable to address a different risk or challenge. The cost of BSE testing may be disproportionate to the resulting public health benefit, as compared with addressing other pressing issues in protecting the global food system. Similarly, taking a zero-risk approach forecasts ever increasing costs as the precautionary principle tends toward taking preemptive actions on every identified hazard, no matter how small the risk. Developing animal health and public health priorities must be conducting from a holistic perspective in which all hazards are considered and the opportunity costs of various initiatives weighed. Similarly, surveillance priorities should be established through broad-based considerations of risk management, not simply from a desire to impress the public or trading partners by more tests. I was struck by the concern voiced by one of my international colleagues caught in a massive (and expensive) government response to a few BSE cases. "What will we tell our grandchildren," he asked, "when we have spent all this money for a rare cattle disease with a relatively small human health impact, while at the same time we fail to take basic, proven public health measures for other diseases and conditions that impact the lives of millions because 'we have no money.'"

Lesson 7: High Health Status Is a Curse

Once high health status is attained, the impetus for maintaining an animal health and public health infrastructure fades. We celebrate the successful eradication of a whole string of animal diseases and successful risk management of zoonoses that plagued our grandparents such as bovine tuberculosis and undulant fever. Having achieved this unique high health status for the entire nation, then we turn around and ask why we are maintaining an infrastructure for something that no longer exists. Anchoring our animal and public health infrastructure on a limited number of "program" diseases undercuts the overall system as successes are celebrated. As a result of the resulting budget cuts and retrenchment, we have few resources to commit to investigating emerging disease threats and little surge capacity when a significant infectious disease outbreak occurs. Replacing experienced professionals with unseasoned new recruits saves money in the short run but costs the nation (and world) in the long term. That is where we find ourselves today as we struggle to manage emerging issues with limited resources. Cutting both physical and human resources provides a rapid means for decreasing budgets, but rebuilding an effective animal and public health infrastructure is a monumental undertaking in terms of resources *and* time.

Strategies for Managing This Dilemma

- Reframe surveillance discussions to focus on the purpose and the scientific basis for surveillance rather than the number of tests conducted;
- Consider the entire farm-to-table food system when designing surveillance systems to support effective risk management for the end consumer and the nation;
- Recognize that no one surveillance system fits all situations; the sampling design, sample size, and testing protocol must be adapted to the needs of each country in order to support optimal risk management;
- Create more incentives for reporting disease to pull in more samples, rather than simply demanding testing through regulatory initiatives and penalties;
- Develop a national animal identification system to support rapid response to disease outbreaks and long-term support for emerging disease detection;
- Strengthen the national animal health laboratory system and increase its capacity, perhaps by providing federal resources to states tied to performance requirements and reporting so that all states can meet a minimum level of proficiency and quality;
- Foster increased collaboration between biologic, medical, and social sciences in order to better understand the sociology and psychology of disease reporting and compliance. Biologic and medical sciences alone are not enough;
- Focus on risk management rather than disease eradication or "zero risk";
- Adopt and implement science-based regulations for BSE and other emerging diseases building on international standards;
- Build public-private partnerships to address emerging diseases on a global, rather than a national, scale;
- Recognize that all animal health issues are public health issues because of

their direct effects on human heath and their indirect effects on human well-being through their psychologic, economic, and ecologic consequences; and

- Break down the silos that separate various professions and different stages of the food system (agriculture, processing, distribution, retail, wholesale, and the consumer) in order to aggressively promote transdisciplinary approaches to animal and public health.

REFERENCES

Alper T, Cramp WA, Haig DA, Clarke MC. 1967. Does the agent of scrapie replicate without nucleic acid? *Nature* 214(90):764–766.

Alpers MP. 1968. Kuru: Implications of its transmissibility for the interpretation of its changing epidemiological pattern. In: Bailey OT, Smith DE, Eds. *The Central Nervous System: Some Experimental Models of Neurological Diseases.* Baltimore, MD: Williams and Wilkins Company. Pp. 234–251.

Alter M, Kahana E. 1976. Creutzfeldt-Jakob disease among Lybian Jews in Israel. *Science* 192 (4238):428.

Anderson RM, Donnelly CA, Ferguson NM, Woolhouse ME, Watt CJ, Udy HJ, MaWhinney S, Dunstan SP, Southwood TR, Wilesmith JW, Ryan JB, Hoinville LJ, Hillerton JE, Austin AR, Wells GA. 1996. Transmission dynamics and epidemiology of BSE in British cattle. *Nature* 382(6594):779–788.

Andreoletti O, Simon S, Lacroux C, Morel N, Tabouret G, Chabert A, Lugan S, Corbiere F, Ferre P, Foucras G, Laude H, Eychenne F, Grassi J, Schlecher F. 2004. PrPSc accumulation in myocytes from sheep incubating natural scrapie. *Nature Medicine* 10(6):591–593.

Baker HF, Ridley RM, Wells GAH. 1993. Experimental transmission of BSE and scrapie to the common marmoset. *Veterinary Record* 132(16):403–406.

Bartz JC, Kincaid AE, Bessen RA. 2003. Rapid prion neuroinvasion following tongue infection. *Journal of Virology* 77(1):583–591.

Bateman D, Hilton D, Love S, Zeidler M, Beck J, Collinge J. 1995. Sporadic Creutzfeldt-Jakob disease in a 18-year-old in the UK [Letter]. *Lancet* 346(8983):1155–1156.

Bellinger-Kawahara C, Cleaver JE, Diener TO, Prusiner SB. 1987a. Purified scrapie prions resist inactivation by UV irradiation. *Journal of Virology* 61(1):159–166.

Bellinger-Kawahara C, Diener TO, McKinley MP, Groth DF, Smith DR, Prusiner SB. 1987b. Purified scrapie prions resist inactivation by procedures that hydrolyze, modify, or shear nucleic acids. *Virology* 160(1):271–274.

Bosque PJ, Ryou C, Telling G, Peretz D, Legname G, DeArmond SJ, Prusiner SB. 2002. Prions in skeletal muscle. *Proceedings of the National Academy of Sciences* 99(6):3812–3817.

Brachmann A, Baxa U, Wickner RB. 2005. Prion generation *in vitro*: Amyloid of Ure2p is infectious. *EMBO Journal* 24(17):3082–3092.

Britton TC, Al-Sarraj S, Shaw C, Campbell T, Collinge J. 1995. Sporadic Creutzfeldt-Jakob disease in a 16-year-old in the UK [Letter]. *Lancet* 346(8983):1155.

Bruce ME, Dickinson AG. 1987. Biological evidence that the scrapie agent has an independent genome. *Journal of General Virology* 68(Pt. 1):79–89.

Bruce ME, Will RG, Ironside JW, McConnell I, Drummond D, Suttie A, McCardle L, Chree A, Hope J, Birkett C, Cousens S, Fraser H, Bostock CJ. 1997. Transmissions to mice indicate that 'new variant' CJD is caused by the BSE agent. *Nature* 389(6650):498–501.

Buschmann A, Groschup MH. 2005. Highly bovine spongiform encephalopathy-sensitive transgenic mice confirm the essential restriction of infectivity to the nervous system in clinically diseased cattle. *Journal of Infectious Diseases* 192(5):934–942.

Buschmann A, Pfaff E, Reifenberg K, Müller HM, Groschup MH. 2000. Detection of cattle-derived BSE prions using transgenic mice overexpressing bovine PrP(C). *Archives of Virology* 16(suppl): 75–86.

CDC (Centers for Disease Control and Prevention). 1996. Surveillance for Creutzfeldt-Jakob disease—United States. *Morbidity and Mortality Weekly Report* 45(31):665–668.

Chapman J, Ben-Israel J, Goldhammer Y, Korczyn AD. 1994. The risk of developing Creutzfeldt-Jakob disease in subjects with the *PRNP* gene codon 200 point mutation. *Neurology* 44(9):1683–1686.

Chesebro B. 2004. Biomedicine. A fresh look at BSE. *Science* 305(5692):1918–1921.

Collinge J. 1999. Variant Creutzfeldt-Jakob disease. *Lancet* 354(9175):317–323.

Collinge J, Sidle KCL, Meads J, Ironside J, Hill AF. 1996. Molecular analysis of prion strain variation and the aetiology of "new variant" CJD. *Nature* 383(6602):685–690.

Collinge J, Whitfield J, McKintosh E, Beck J, Mead S, Thomas DJ, Alpers MP. 2006. Kuru in the 21st century—an acquired human prion disease with very long incubation periods. *Lancet* 367(9528): 2068–2074.

Collins S, Boyd A, Fletcher A, Gonzales M, NcLean CA, Byron K, Masters CL. 2000. Creutzfeldt-Jakob disease: Diagnostic utility of 14-3-3 protein immunodetection in cerebrospinal fluid. *Journal of Clinical Neuroscience* 7(3):203–208.

Collins S, Boyd A, Lee JS, Lewis V, Fletcher A, McLean CA, Law M, Kaldor J, Smith MJ, Masters CL. 2002. Creutzfeldt-Jakob disease in Australia 1970–1999. *Neurology* 59(9):1365–1371.

Collins SJ, Lawson VA, Masters CL. 2004. Transmissible spongiform encephalopathies. *Lancet* 363(9402):51–61.

Dickinson AG, Fraser H, Outram GW. 1975. Scrapie incubation time can exceed natural lifespan. *Nature* 256(5520):732–733.

Donnelly CA, Ferguson NM, Ghani AC, Anderson RM. 2002. Implications of BSE infection screening data for the scale of the British BSE epidemic and current European infection levels. *Proceedings. Biological Sciences/The Royal Society* 269(1506):2179–2190.

Foster J, Goldmann W, Parnham D, Chong A, Hunter N. 2001. Partial dissociation of PrPSc deposition and vacuolation in the brains of scrapie and BSE experimentally affected goats. *Journal of General Virology* 82(Pt. 1):267–273.

Gajdusek DC. 1962. Kuru: An appraisal of five years of investigation. *Eugenics Quarterly* 9:69–74.

Gajdusek DC. 1977. Unconventional viruses and the origin and disappearance of kuru. *Science* 197(4307):943–960.

Gajdusek DC, Zigas V. 1957. Degenerative disease of the central nervous system in New Guinea. The endemic occurrence of "kuru" in the native population. *New England Journal of Medicine* 257(20):974–978.

Gajdusek DC, Gibbs CJ Jr, Alpers M. 1966. Experimental transmission of a kuru-like syndrome to chimpanzees. *Nature* 209(25):794–796.

GAO (Government Accountability Office). 2005 (February). *Mad Cow Disease: FDA's Management of the Feed Ban Has Improved, but Oversight Weaknesses Continue to Limit Program Effectiveness.* GAO-05-101. Washington, D.C.

Ghani AC, Ferguson NM, Donnelly CA, Anderson RM. 2000. Predicted vCJD mortality in Great Britain. *Nature* 406(6796):583–584.

Glasse RM. 1967. Cannibalism in the kuru region of New Guinea. *Transactions of the New York Academy of Sciences* 29(6):748–754.

Glatzel M, Abela E, Maissen M, Aguzzi A. 2003. Extraneural pathologic prion protein in sporadic Creutzfeldt-Jakob disease. *New England Journal of Medicine* 349(19):1812–1820.

Goldfarb LG, Brown P, Mitrova E, Cervenakova L, Goldin L, Korczyn AD, Chapman J, Galvez S, Cartier L, Rubenstein R, et al. 1991. Creutzfeldt-Jacob disease associated with the *PRNP* codon 200Lys mutation: An analysis of 45 families. *European Journal of Epidemiology* 7(5):477–486.

Goldmann W, Hunter N, Manson J, Hope J. 1990. The PrP gene of the sheep, a natural host of scrapie. *Proceedings of the VIIIth International Congress of Virology*. Berlin, August 26–31. P. 284.

Goldmann W, Hunter N, Martin T, Dawson M, Hope J. 1991. Different forms of the bovine PrP gene have five or six copies of a short, G-C-rich element within the protein-coding exon. *Journal of General Virology* 72(Pt. 1):201–204.

Grassi J, Comoy E, Simon S, Creminon C, Frobert Y, Trapmann S, Schimmel H, Hawkins SA, Moynagh J, Deslys JP, Wells GA. 2001. Rapid test for the preclinical postmortem diagnosis of BSE in central nervous system tissue. *Veterinary Record* 149(19):577–582.

Hadlow WJ. 1959. Scrapie and kuru [Letter]. *Lancet* 2:289–290.

Hill A, Desbruslais M, Joiner S, Sidle KC, Gowland I, Collinge J, Doey LJ, Lantos P. 1997. The same prion strain causes vCJD and BSE. *Nature* 389(6650):448–450.

Hill AF, Joiner S, Linehan J, Desbruslais M, Lantos PL, Collinge J. 2000. Species-barrier-independent prion replication in apparently resistant species. *Proceedings of the National Academy of Sciences* 97(18):10248–10253.

Hilton DA, Ghani AC, Conyers L, Edwards P, McCardle L, Ritchie D, Penney M, Hegazy D, Ironside JW. 2004. Prevalence of lymphoreticular prion protein accumulation in UK tissue samples. *Journal of Pathology* 203(3):733–739.

Hsiao KK, Scott M, Foster D, Groth DF, DeArmond SJ, Prusiner SB. 1990. Spontaneous neurodegeneration in transgenic mice with mutant prion protein. *Science* 250(4987):1587–1590.

Hsiao K, Meiner Z, Kahana E, Cass C, Kahana I, Avrahami D, Scarlato G, Abramsky O, Prusiner SB, Gabizon R. 1991. Mutation of the prion protein in Libyan Jews with Creutzfeldt-Jakob disease. *New England Journal of Medicine* 324(16):1091–1097.

Hsiao KK, Groth D, Scott M, Yang SL, Serban H, Rapp D, Foster D, Torchia M, DeArmond SJ, Prusiner SB. 1994. Serial transmission in rodents of neurodegeneration from transgenic mice expressing mutant prion protein. *Proceedings of the National Academy of Sciences* 91(19): 9126–9130.

Ironside JW. 1997. The new variant form of Creutzfeldt-Jakob disease: A novel prion protein amyloid disorder. *Amyloid: International Journal of Clinical and Experimental Investigation* 4:66–69.

Kaneko K, Ball HL, Wille H, Zhang H, Groth D, Torchia M, Tremblay P, Safar J, Prusiner SB, DeArmond SJ, Baldwin MA, Cohem FE. 2000. A synthetic peptide initiates Gerstmann-Sträussler-Scheinker (GSS) disease in transgenic mice. *Journal of Molecular Biology* 295(4): 997–1007.

Kimberlin RH. 1982. Scrapie agent: Prions or virinos? *Nature* 297(5862):107–108.

Klug GM, Boyd A, Lewis V, Kvasnicka M, Lee JS, Masters CL, Collins SJ. 2005. Creutzfeldt-Jakob disease: Australian surveillance update to 31 December 2004. *Communicable Diseases Intelligence* 29(3):269-271.

Kübler E, Oesch B, Raeber AJ. 2003. Diagnosis of prion diseases. *British Medical Bulletin* 66: 267–279.

Lasmézas CI, Deslys J-P, Demaimay R, Adjou KT, Lamoury F, Dormont D, Robain O, Ironside J, Hauw JJ. 1996. BSE transmission to macaques. *Nature* 381(6585):743–744.

Last JM, ed. 1983. *A Dictionary of Epidemiology*. Oxford: Oxford University Press.

Last JM, ed. 2001. *A Dictionary of Epidemiology*. Oxford: Oxford University Press.

Lee IS, Long JR, Prusiner SB, Safar JG. 2005. Selective precipitation of prions by polyoxometalate complexes. *Journal of the American Chemical Society* 127(40):13802–13803.

Legname G, Baskakov IV, Nguyen HO, Riesner D, Cohen FE, DeArmond SJ, Prusiner SB. 2004. Synthetic mammalian prions. *Science* 305(5684):673–676.

Legname G, Nguyen HO, Baskakov IV, Cohen FE, DeArmond SJ, Prusiner SB. 2005. Strain-specified characteristics of mouse synthetic prions. *Proceedings of the National Academy of Sciences* 102(6):2168–2173.

Lewis V, Hill AF, Klug GM, Boyd A, Masters CL, Collins SJ. 2005. Australian sporadic CJD analysis supports endogenous determinants of molecular-clinical profiles. *Neurology* 65(1):113–118.

Llewelyn CA, Hewitt PE, Knight RS, Amar K, Cousens S, Mackenzie J, Will RG. 2004. Possible transmission of variant Creutzfeldt-Jakob disease by blood transfusion. *Lancet* 363(9407): 417–421.

Maddelein ML, Dos Reis S, Duvezin-Caubet S, Coulary-Salin B, Saupe SJ. 2002. Amyloid aggregates of the HET-s prion protein are infectious. *Proceedings of the National Academy of Sciences* 99(11):7402–7407.

Minor P, Newham J, Jones N, Bergeron C, Gregori L, Asher D, van Engelenburg F, Stroebel T, Vey M, Barnard G, Head M; WHO Working Group on International Reference Materials for the Diagnosis and Study of Transmissible Spongiform Encephalopathies. 2004. Standards for the assay of Creutzfeldt-Jakob disease specimens. *Journal of General Virology* 85(Pt. 6):1777–1784.

National Advisory Committee on SARS and Public Health. 2003. *Learning from SARS—Renewal of Public Health in Canada.* Ottawa: Health Canada. [Online]. Available: http://www.phac-aspc.gc.ca/publicat/sars-sras/naylor/ [accessed July 25, 2006].

National CJD Surveillance Unit UK. 2006. *CJD Statistics.* [Online]. Available: http://www.cjd.ed.ac.uk/figures.htm [accessed March 17, 2006].

OIE (Office International des Epizooties). 2006. *Bovine Spongiform Encephalopathy (BSE).* [Online]. Available: http://www.oie.int/eng/info/en_esb.htm [accessed July 26, 2006].

Pan K, Baldwin M, Nguyen J, Gasset M, Serban A, Groth D, Mehlhorn I, Huang Z, Fletterick RJ, Cohen FE, Prusiner SB. 1993. Conversion of a-helices into b-sheets features in the formation of the scrapie prion proteins. *Proceedings of the National Academy of Sciences* 90(23):10962–10966.

Peden AH, Head MW, Ritchie DL, Bell JE, Ironside JW. 2004. Preclinical vCJD after blood transfusion in a *PRNP* codon 129 heterozygous patient. *Lancet* 364(9433):527–529.

Phillips NA, Bridgeman J, Ferguson-Smith M. 2000. *The BSE Inquiry.* Vol 2. London: Stationery Office.

Prusiner SB. 2004a. Detecting mad cow disease. *Scientific American* 291(1):86–93.

Prusiner SB. 2004b. *Prion Biology and Diseases.* 2nd ed. Cold Spring Harbor, NY: Cold Spring Harbor Laboratory Press.

Ricketts M. 2005 (October 26). *Session VI: What Are the Incentives and Disincentives Associated with Disease/Contamination Reporting? Impacts on Human Health and International Trade—BSE as a "Case Study."* Presentation at the Forum on Microbial Threats Workshop Meeting, Foodborne Threats to Health: The Policies and Practices of Surveillance, Prevention, Outbreak Investigations, and International Coordination, Washington, D.C., Institute of Medicine, Forum on Microbial Threats.

Roos R, Gajdusek DC, Gibbs CJ Jr. 1973. The clinical characteristics of transmissible Creutzfeldt-Jakob disease. *Brain* 96(1):1–20.

Safar J, Wille H, Itri V, Groth D, Serban H, Torchia M, Cohen FE, Prusiner SB. 1998. Eight prion strains have PrPSc molecules with different conformations. *Nature Medicine* 4(10):1157–1165.

Safar JG, Geschwind MD, Deering C, Didorenko S, Sattavat M, Sanchez H, Serban A, Vey M, Baron H, Giles K, Miller B, DeArmond SJ, Prusiner SB. 2005a. Diagnosis of human prion disease. *Proceedings of the National Academy of Sciences* 102(9):3501–3506.

Safar JG, Kellings K, Serban A, Groth D, Cleaver JE, Prusiner SB, Riesner D. 2005b. Search for a prion-specific nucleic acid. *Journal of Virology* 79(16):10796–10806.

Scott MR, Safar J, Telling G, Nguyen O, Groth D, Torchia M, Koehler R, Tremblay P, Walther D, Cohen FE, DeArmond SJ, Prusiner SB. 1997. Identification of a prion protein epitope modulating transmission of bovine spongiform encephalopathy prions to transgenic mice. *Proceedings of the National Academy of Sciences* 94(26):14279–14284.

Scott MR, Will R, Ironside J, Nguyen HO, Tremblay P, DeArmond SJ, Prusiner SB. 1999. Compelling transgenetic evidence for transmission of bovine spongiform encephalopathy prions to humans. *Proceedings of the National Academy of Sciences* 96(26):15137–15142.

Scott MR, Peretz D, Nguyen HO, DeArmond SJ, Prusiner SB. 2005. Transmission barriers for bovine, ovine, and human prions in transgenic mice. *Journal of Virology* 79(9):5259–5271.

Sparrer HE, Santoso A, Szoka FC Jr, Weissman JS. 2000. Evidence for the prion hypothesis: Induction of the yeast [*PSI*+] factor by in vitro-converted Sup35 protein. *Science* 289(5479):595–599.

Spencer MD, Knight RS, Will RG. 2002. First hundred cases of variant Creutzfeldt-Jakob disease: Retrospective case note review of early psychiatric and neurological features. *British Medical Journal* 324(7352):1479–1482.

Spudich S, Mastrianni JA, Wrensch M, Gabizon R, Meiner Z, Kahana I, Rosenmann H, Kahana E, Prusiner SB. 1995. Complete penetrance of Creutzfeldt-Jakob disease in Libyan Jews carrying the E200K mutation in the prion protein gene. *Molcular Medicine* 1(6):607–613.

Tanaka M, Chien P, Naber N, Cooke R, Weissman JS. 2004. Conformational variations in an infectious protein determine prion strain differences. *Nature* 428(6980):323–328.

Telling GC, Haga T, Torchia M, Tremblay P, DeArmond SJ, Prusiner SB. 1996. Interactions between wild-type and mutant prion proteins modulate neurodegeneration in transgenic mice. *Genes & Development* 10(14):1736–1750.

Thomzig A, Kratzel C, Lenz G, Kruger D, Beekes M. 2003. Widespread PrPSc accumulation in muscles of hamsters orally infected with scrapie. *EMBO Reports* 4(5):530–533.

Tremblay P, Ball HL, Kaneko K, Groth D, Hegde RS, Cohen FE, DeArmond SJ, Prusiner SB, Safar JG. 2004. Mutant PrPSc conformers induced by a synthetic peptide and several prion strains. *Journal of Virology* 78(4):2088–2099.

Valleron AJ, Boelle PY, Will R, Cesbron JY. 2001. Estimation of epidemic size and incubation time based on age characteristics of vCJD in the United Kingdom. *Science* 294(5547):1726–1728.

Wadsworth JD, Joiner S, Hill AF, Campbell TA, Desbruslais M, Luthert PJ, Collinge J. 2001. Tissue distribution of protease resistant prion protein in variant Creutzfeldt-Jakob disease using a highly sensitive immunoblotting assay. *Lancet* 358(9277):171–180.

Ward HJT, Everington D, Sanchez-Juan P, Smith A, Cooper S, Heath C, Knight RSG, Will RG. 2003 (October 8-10). *Secondary Transmission of Variant Creutzfeldt-Jakob Disease?* Presentation at the International Prion Conference, Munich.

Ward HJ, Everington D, Cousens SN, Smith-Bathgate B, Leitch M, Cooper S, Heath C, Knight RS, Smith PG, Will RG. 2006. Risk factors for variant Creutzfeldt-Jakob disease: A case-control study. *Annals of Neurology* 59(1):111–120.

Weissmann C. 1991. A "unified theory" of prion propagation. *Nature* 352(6337):679–683.

Wells GAH. 2002 (January 10–11). *Report on TSE Infectivity Distribution in Ruminant Tissues (State of Knowledge, December 2001).* Brussels: European Commission.

Will RG, Ironside JW, Zeidler M, Cousens S, Estibeiro K, Alperovitch A, Poser S, Pocchiari M, Hofman A, Smith PG. 1996. A new variant of Creutzfeldt-Jakob disease in the UK. *Lancet* 347(9006):921–925.

Will RG, Alpers MP, Dormont D, Schonberger LB. 2004. Infectious and sporadic prion diseases. In: Prusiner SB, Ed. *Prion Biology and Diseases.* 2nd ed. Cold Spring Harbor, NY: Cold Spring Harbor Laboratory Press. Pp. 629–671.

Yamakawa Y, Hagiwara K, Nohtomi K, Nakamura Y, Nishijima M, Higuchi Y, Sato Y, Sata T; Expert Committee for BSE Diagnosis, Ministry of Health, Labor and Welfare of Japan. 2003. Atypical proteinase K-resistant prion protein (PrPres) observed in an apparently healthy 23-month-old Holstein steer. *Japanese Journal of Infectious Diseases* 56(5-6):221–222.

Zerr I, Pocchiari M, Collins S, Brandel JP, de Pedro Cuesta J, Knight RS, Bernheimer H, Cardone F, Delasnerie-Laupretre N, Caudrado Corrales N, Ladogana A, Bodemer M, Fletcher A, Awan T, Ruiz Bremon A, Budka H, Laplanche JL, Will RG, Poser S. 2000. Analysis of EEG and CSF 14-3-3 proteins as aids to the diagnosis of Creutzfeldt-Jakob disease. *Neurology* 55(6):811–815.

7

Research and Policy Opportunities

OVERVIEW

Contributors to previous chapters have addressed research and policy opportunities in food safety oversight, surveillance, and disease reporting in protecting the food supply. Additional research and policy issues were raised in workshop presentations that focused on animal health, food defense, and food safety science.

Dr. Lonnie King, dean of the College of Veterinary Medicine at Michigan State University, presented key findings from the recently published report, *Animal Health at the Crossroads* (2005). This chapter begins with an excerpt from this report, which explored the critical linkage between animal and human health illustrated in case studies of key animal diseases. The study committee, assembled by the National Research Council (NRC), evaluated existing prevention and detection systems and identified opportunities and barriers to their improvement; many of their findings directly address the reduction of foodborne illness.

The chapter concludes with a paper by Dr. Francis Busta, director of the National Center for Food Protection and Defense (NCFPD), who describes research to protect the food supply from deliberate harm and to mitigate the effects of such an attack. Recognizing that many of the same tools and strategies could be used to guard against any incident of food adulteration, whether accidental or deliberate, Busta emphasizes techniques that address key questions raised by a foodborne attack: how it was staged, which threat agent was used, what decontamination and other public health measures should be taken, and how to inform the public about the incident.

The workshop concluded with a presentation by Dr. Sanford Miller, who noted the profound influence of such nonscientific issues on perceptions of risks to the food supply. Safety is not a biological property of food, Miller contended, but an intellectual concept influenced as much by the political, economic, and social factors that determine our perception of risk as by any quantifiable measure of hazard. Thus efforts to improve food safety must not only identify foodborne threats, but also translate these discoveries into regulation, communication, and legislation that accurately reflect the risks such threats pose to society. Meeting these challenges is the goal of the nascent field of food safety science, which integrates nutrition, microbiology, toxicology, molecular biology, genetics, functional biology, and conventional food science, and brings these disciplines to bear on the problem of ensuring a safe food supply through the practice of risk assessment.

"We all feel comfortable talking about science," Miller observed, "but the moment comes when science has to be translated into risk, and risk has to be translated into some kind of public policy action." The food safety scientist he envisions will use sophisticated, risk-based, scientifically sound models to determine how best to protect our food supply.

ANIMAL HEALTH AT THE CROSSROADS[1]

Committee on Assessing the Nation's Framework for Addressing Animal Diseases[2]
National Research Council

Synopsis

The national framework to safeguard animal health is of paramount importance to the U.S. economy, public health, and food supply. To strengthen the existing framework, the nation should establish a high-level, authoritative mechanism to coordinate interactions between the private sector and local, state, and federal agencies. New tools for detection, diagnosis, and risk analysis need to be developed now, and the capacity of the existing animal health laboratory network should be expanded for both routine and emergency diagnostic uses. Integrative animal health research programs, in which veterinary and medical scientists can work as collaborators, should be established. Colleges of veterinary medicine must lead an effort to develop a national animal health education plan to educate and train individuals from all sectors (from animal handlers to pathologists) in disease prevention and early detection, and to recruit veterinary students into careers in public health, food systems, biomedical research, diagnostic laboratory

[1]Reprinted from NRC (2005). *Animal Health at the Crossroads.* Washington, D.C.: The National Academies Press.

[2]Board on Agriculture and Natural Resources, Division on Earth and Life Studies.

investigation, pathology, epidemiology, ecosystem health, and food-animal practice. The United States must address the importation and health of exotic and wild-caught animals and commit itself to shared leadership roles with other countries and international organizations that address animal disease agents. Finally, a collective effort should be made to raise the level of public awareness about the importance of animal health and of the national investment in the framework to safeguard animal health.

Background

Animal health has broad implications, ranging from the health of individual animals and the well-being of human communities to issues of global security. Many people would be surprised by the assertion that our nation's highest priorities must include animal health, yet we must recognize and act on this reality to ensure a safe and healthy future. Among other things, animal diseases critically affect the adequacy of the food supply for a growing world population, and they have huge implications for global trade and commerce. Moreover, many animal disease agents are zoonotic—meaning that they are transmittable to humans—so they have dramatic implications for human health and safety, and for animal disease prevention. Animal disease prevention and control is crucial to improving public health on a global scale. Additionally, in an era of growing concern about the threat of terrorism, the potential impact of the intentional use of animal disease agents to cause morbidity and mortality, as well as economic damage, is enormous.

The U.S. animal health framework includes many federal, state, and local agencies that generally have differing mandates of law, and numerous other public and private entities and international organizations, each with its own goals and objectives, each responsible for maintaining animal health. In the past, this framework has been reasonably effective in responding to a range of demands and challenges. In recent years, however, animal health has been challenged in a manner not previously experienced.

Today animal health is at a crossroads. The risk of disease is coming from many directions, including the globalization of commerce, the restructuring and consolidation of global food and agriculture productions into larger commercial units, the interactions of humans and companion animals, human incursions into wildlife habitats, and the threat of bioterrorism. The impacts of these sources of risk are evident in recent disease events (Box 7-1).

Given the changing nature of the risks with which the framework must cope, it is unlikely that the current philosophy on how to protect animal health will be adequate in the future. The risks of animal disease must be dealt with not only in terms of protecting individual species of animals from specific pathogens, but also in a broader context that includes anticipating the emergence and spread of disease on local and global scales, and recognizing the relationships of animal

BOX 7-1
Impacts from Recent Disease Events

- In 2003, severe acute respiratory syndrome (SARS) sent a global shockwave, affecting countries with even few cases, such as the United States. Although SARS infected only 8,000 people globally, the disease spread to 30 countries and its effect on the global economy totaled $8 billion.
- The United Kingdom's economy has not yet recovered from a foot-and-mouth disease (FMD) outbreak in 2001, which also reverberated around the world, affecting both agricultural and nonagricultural interests (such as rural businesses and tourism/recreational use of the countryside).
- A single case of mad cow disease (bovine spongiform encephalopathy or BSE) in Washington State on December 23, 2003, had an immediate market impact and severe, sustained economic losses due to trade restrictions on U.S. cattle and their products. The infected animal was discovered as part of the government's policy to routinely test downer cattle for BSE, which has been linked to a new variant of Creutzfeldt-Jakob disease, a fatal neurological illness in humans. In June 2005, a second case of BSE was confirmed in the United States.
- In 2004, a new strain of highly pathogenic avian influenza (AI) spread through Southeast Asia, resulting in the loss of more than 100 million birds through mortality and control measures and dozens of human cases, highlighting the unpredictable and potentially catastrophic nature of emerging zoonotic disease. This new influenza strain was transmitted from birds to people, raising concern that it might be capable of evolving into the next pandemic influenza strain.
- In 1999, West Nile virus (WNV), an arbovirus similar to St. Louis encephalitis virus, emerged for the first time in the Western Hemisphere in New York from an unknown source. Over the next five years it swept across the continental United States, Canada, Mexico, Central America, and several Caribbean islands, carried by mosquito vectors infecting wild birds. In the United States in 2004, the virus was detected in approximately 2,250 humans (40 states), 1,250 horses (36 states), nearly 7,000 wild birds, mostly corvids (45 states), and in much smaller numbers in a few other animal species. While these numbers are substantially below those that occurred in the first wave of infection, WNV bodes to become endemic in wild birds and an ongoing source of infection transmitted to other species by mosquito vectors.

disease to human health and the environment. To address animal disease in that context, the animal health framework will have to be more flexible and inclusive of expertise available from research, medical, and public health communities, and from the fields of environmental sciences and public policy, among others. To respond comprehensively to new threats, the responsibilities of the framework's many actors will need to be clearly defined and their actions better coordinated. Admittedly, the process of transformation is difficult during periods when disease outbreaks consume all attention. However, *now* is the time to strengthen the structure of the current system and to instigate a change in its culture, so that it will be capable of responding effectively in the future.

This report explores the evolving challenges facing animal health, identifies vulnerabilities and gaps in the animal health framework, and recommends steps needed to fill gaps and improve the effectiveness of the framework.

Committee's Statement of Task

Recent animal and human health events have illustrated that the national system for protecting animal health is now facing a continuum of host-parasite relationships involving public health, wildlife, ecosystems, and food systems, operating in an increasingly complex global context (see Figure 7-1). Adapting the current framework to this new reality will be both a major challenge and a national imperative.

In recognition of the changing influences on animal health, the National Academies developed a concept for a three-phase analysis of the U.S. system for dealing with animal diseases and committed institutional funds to launch the first phase of the study. This report, which embodies the first phase of the study, presents an overview of the animal health framework and examines the framework's overall operation in the prevention, detection, and diagnosis of animal diseases. The proposed second phase of the study (pending supplemental external support) will focus on surveillance and monitoring capabilities, and the proposed third phase will focus on response and recovery from an animal disease epidemic. Although surveillance and monitoring play an important part in prevention, detection, and diagnosis, the second phase of the study, as currently envisioned, will analyze in greater depth the system's capacity and needs for surveillance and monitoring of animal diseases.

Relative to its respective focus, each phase of the study will: (1) review the state and quality of the current system for dealing with animal disease; (2) identify key opportunities and barriers to successfully preventing and controlling animal diseases; and (3) identify immediate courses of action for those on the front lines.

This first phase of the study did not attempt an in-depth review of the effectiveness of each individual component of the framework or of any specific agency involved in safeguarding animal health—a task well beyond the scope of this

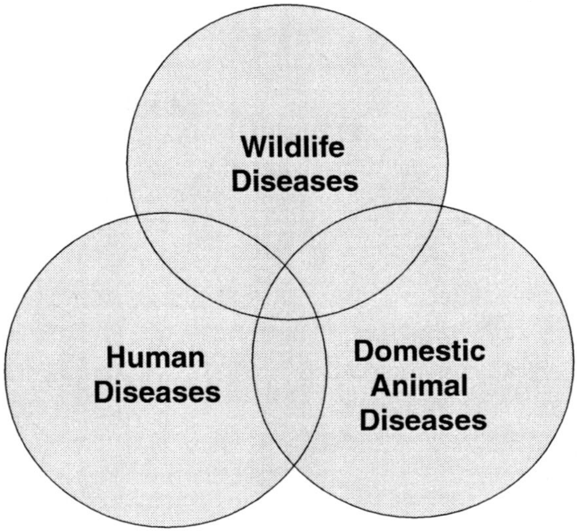

FIGURE 7-1 Interactions of emerging infectious diseases (EIDs) with a continuum that includes wildlife, domestic animal, and human populations. Few diseases affect exclusively one group, and the complex relations among host populations set the scene for disease emergence. Examples of EIDs that overlap these categories include Lyme disease (wildlife to domestic animals and humans); bovine tuberculosis (between domestic animals and wildlife); *Escherichia coli* O157:H7 (between domestic animals and humans); and Nipah virus and rabies (all three categories). Companion animals are categorized in the domestic animal section of the continuum.

effort—but did examine the effectiveness of the framework as a whole in relation to different animal disease scenarios. In doing so, it sought to identify ways to improve the framework.

Finally, although animals are subject to the same causes of disease as humans—that is, diseases with chemical, physical, microbial, or genetic causes—the study focuses primarily on infectious diseases, as directed by the Statement of Task (see Chapter 1, Box 1-1 from the NRC report *Animal Health at the Crossroads*, for the committee's Statement of Task). This focus arises from concern about the growing threat posed by the spread of emerging infectious disease associated with the increasing global interconnectedness of domestic animals, wildlife, and humans, and by the possibility of bioterrorism.

Overview of the Animal Health Framework

The essential components of the animal health framework include the following:

- People on the "front lines" of the animal production unit, animal habitat, or companion animal household (including ranch and farm workers, producers, feeders, breeders, park rangers, companion animal owners, wildlife rehabilitators, and zoo keepers);
- Veterinarians and other sources of professional advice and care for health-related issues (such as universities and diagnostic laboratories);
- Federal, state, and local animal health and public health agencies (consisting mainly of state departments of agriculture and state diagnostics laboratories within universities and elsewhere in state governments, and numerous bureaus and offices within over 10 federal departments, but primarily within the U.S. Departments of Agriculture, Homeland Security, and Health and Human Services);
- International collaborations among agencies, organizations, and governments (such as the World Organization for Animal Health and the World Health Organization); and
- Supporting institutions, industries, and organizations (including educators, researchers, and the public health and intelligence communities).

Because of the very large number of actors responsible in some way for safeguarding animal health, it is not surprising that effective coordination is a major challenge. In a retrospective analysis of numerous specific animal disease situations, the committee examined the collective capabilities and limitations of the framework with respect to its effectiveness in the prevention, detection, and diagnosis of animal diseases. Several weaknesses, needs, and gaps were consistently encountered in the framework's response to a broad spectrum of disease types including exotic Newcastle disease (END), foot-and-mouth disease (FMD), monkeypox, bovine spongiform encephalopathy (BSE), chronic wasting disease (CWD), West Nile virus (WNV), avian influenza (AI), and diseases caused by coronavirus. This examination led the committee to the following conclusions:

- The framework for animal health lacks adequate systems and tools for analyzing and managing risk, and planning for outbreaks.
- Efforts to develop and validate diagnostic assays and advanced vaccines of a recognized pathogen need to occur more rapidly.
- The workforce on the front lines of animal care is not adequately educated and trained to deal with animal disease issues, and there is a shortage of veterinarians in the workforce for animal disease prevention, detection, and diagnosis.
- Greater collaboration between public health and animal health officials can accelerate the detection and diagnosis of animal diseases.
- The broad capabilities that exist in universities, industry, state entities, veterinary diagnostic laboratories, and other local animal health infrastructure are underutilized.

- The lack of collaboration between the biomedical and veterinary communities is a lost opportunity that impedes the effectiveness of the framework.
- There is a need for state-of-the-art equipment and biocontainment facilities for both research and diagnostics. Federal, state, and private entities responsible for animal health have different authorities, and there are gaps in that authority, particularly in relation to wildlife disease.
- The past success of international collaboration in responding to animal disease demonstrates its importance in addressing animal diseases.

Recommendations for Strengthening the Animal Health Framework

Reflecting on the structure of the framework and based on the findings of its analysis of past animal health events, the committee offers the following 11 recommendations as potential opportunities for strengthening the framework's capabilities in the prevention, detection, and diagnosis of animal diseases.

Coordination of Framework Components

> *Recommendation 1:* **The nation should establish a high-level, centralized, authoritative, and accountable coordinating mechanism or focal point for engaging and enhancing partnerships among local, state, and federal agencies and the private sector.**

There is a need for a strategic focal point to enhance partnerships and to integrate all stakeholders into a cohesive whole. Many federal agencies are responsible for parts of animal health policy, with significant overlaps in the programmatic functions among them and also between federal agencies and programs directed through states or animal health organizations. On the other hand, there are also gaps in responsibility. Of particular concern is the paucity of federal oversight of the nonlivestock, animal-centered aspects of zoonotic diseases.

While there are several possible models for improved coordination in prevention, detection, and diagnosis, the committee did not recommend options for a specific system-wide mechanism, in part because it has only examined the animal health framework from the partial perspective of prevention, detection, and diagnosis.

Regardless of how a central coordinating mechanism or focal point is implemented, it will need to promote effective communication among various stakeholders and with the public during and outside episodes of animal disease outbreaks. Opportunities for information-sharing between agencies using electronic information systems should be developed. A methodic effort should be made to identify and link key databases and establish protocols for contributing data and generating alerts.

Technological Tools for Preventing, Detecting, and Diagnosing Animal Diseases

Recommendation 2: **Agencies and institutions—including the U.S. Department of Agriculture (USDA) and the Department of Homeland Security (DHS)—responsible for protecting animal industries, wildlife, and associated economies should encourage and support rapid development, validation, and adoption of new technologies and scientific tools for the detection, diagnosis, and prevention of animal diseases and zoonoses.**

The current animal health framework has been slow to evaluate, validate, and implement new scientific tools and technologies that could significantly enhance animal disease prevention, detection, and diagnostic capabilities for the United States. Despite a recent surge in activity related to post-September 11 homeland security efforts and associated focused funding, the active review and implementation of advancing technologies has been inadequate to protect and enhance the health of the country's animal populations and related economic systems. Technological advances—such as immune system modulators, animal-embedded monitoring (chips embedded underneath an animal's skin to monitor temperature and other physiological indices), and differential vaccines as prevention strategies, as well as a range of rapid, automated, sensitive, and portable sampling and assay systems for early warning and reliable diagnosis—have not been adequately exploited by the current animal health framework. Early biodefense warning systems, such as DHS' BioWatch or private industry's gene-based anthrax testing, are designed for rapid detection and identification of key pathogens by sampling air in public environments. These systems have been operating since early 2003 and are meant to assist public health experts in rapidly responding to the intentional release of a biologic agent (DHS, 2004a). Early warning technologies have not yet been adequately evaluated by the animal health infrastructure.

Scientific Preparedness for Diagnosing Animal Diseases: Laboratory Capacity and Capability

Recommendation 3: **The animal health laboratory network should be expanded and strengthened to ensure sufficient capability and capacity for both routine and emergency diagnostic needs and to ensure a robust linkage of all components (federal, state, university, and commercial laboratories) involved in the diagnosis of animal and zoonotic diseases.**

Laboratory diagnosis of animal diseases in the United States involves federal, state, university, and commercial entities. The committee focused its assessment on the condition of publicly funded laboratories and the current operational status of national laboratory networks. Funding and implementation of the pilot National Animal Health Laboratory Network (NAHLN) in June 2002 was an important and beneficial paradigm shift from an exclusive federal system to one with shared state and federal responsibility for foreign animal disease diagnosis. The pilot NAHLN involved 12 state/university diagnostic laboratories approved for disease testing using existing and newly developed assays. The NAHLN is no longer a pilot program and has since been redefined to include all laboratories performing contract work for the USDA on BSE, CWD, scrapie, AI, END, and classical swine fever (CSF). However, the current network lacks surge capacity and is not prepared for disease agents and toxins outside the narrow list of diseases that provided an initial focus for network development (for example, FMD or Rift Valley fever). In addition, implementing this recommendation will require the creation of formal linkages and operational relationships between the NAHLN, state and university veterinary diagnostic laboratories, and the Laboratory Response Network for Bioterrorism (LRN), established by the U.S. Centers for Disease Control and Prevention (CDC) in 1995 to improve the response capabilities of the nation's public health laboratory infrastructure. It will require development of additional biosafety level 3 (BSL-3) necropsy and laboratory capacity. Population-based diagnostic and detection systems also will need to be developed by diagnostic laboratories in order to provide the broad diagnostic outlook necessary for detection of new and emerging diseases.

Animal Health Research

> *Recommendation 4:* **Federal agencies involved in biomedical research (both human and veterinary) should establish a method to jointly fund new, competitive, comprehensive, and integrated animal health research programs; ensure that veterinary and medical scientists can work as collaborators; and enhance research, both domestically and internationally, on the detection, diagnosis, and prevention of animal and zoonotic disease encompassing both animal and human hosts.**

This process might be modeled on the National Institutes of Health (NIH)-administered Interagency Comparative Medicine Research Program, an interagency task force model, or some comparable process that promotes this type of cooperative research agenda.

This recommendation builds on the 2003 Institute of Medicine (IOM) report *Microbial Threats to Health: Emergence, Detection, and Response*, which states: "NIH should develop a comprehensive research agenda for infectious disease prevention and control in collaboration with other federal research institutions and laboratories (e.g., CDC, the U.S. Department of Defense, Department of Energy, the National Science Foundation), academia, and industry" (IOM, 2003). Currently, basic and translational research related to prevention, detection, and diagnosis of animal and zoonotic diseases is being conducted by a complex array of government, academic, and private institutions and there is minimal coordination, if any, in setting priorities to ensure that important research topics are not overlooked and to ensure the most effective use of scarce resources. A forthcoming National Research Council (NRC) report *Critical Needs for Research in Veterinary Science* will contain a more in-depth assessment of national needs for research in animal health.

Recommendation 5: **To strengthen the animal health and zoonotic disease research infrastructure, the committee recommends that competitive grants be made available to scientists to upgrade equipment for animal disease research and that the nation construct and maintain government and university biosafety level 3 (BSL-3 and BSL-3 Ag)[3] facilities for livestock (including large animals), poultry, and wildlife.**

Access to state-of-the-art equipment and technological tools is essential to successfully conduct the research needed to understand, prevent, and control emerging or exotic infectious agents. When a new infectious agent is suspected, efforts must be made to first rapidly define and characterize the agent, under strict biocontainment conditions. At present, few BSL-3 or BSL-3 Ag facilities are available strategically throughout the United States or are equipped and prepared for research on diseases of livestock, poultry, or wildlife, including zoonoses that require BSL-3 biocontainment. Additional BSL-3 facilities are needed for research and surge capacity (in case of outbreaks) for detection, diagnosis, and prevention of many zoonotic and all exotic animal pathogens.

International Interdependence and Collaboration

Recommendation 6: **The United States should commit resources and develop new shared leadership roles with other countries and international organizations in creating global systems for preventing, detecting, and diagnosing known and emerging diseases, disease agents, and disease threats as they relate to animal and public health.**

As the United States and the rest of the world become increasingly interdependent, it is essential to identify animal disease risk factors as they emerge and to focus more attention on the sources and precursors of infections. Taken collectively, the recent experience with SARS, West Nile virus, and monkeypox leads to the inescapable conclusion that globalization, population growth, and expansion of human activity into previously unoccupied habitats has essentially connected the United States to potential zoonotic and nonzoonotic pathogens residing throughout the world. This necessitates coordinated international collabo-

---

[3]Containment facilities are classified as Biosafety Levels 1 through 4, with 4 being the most restrictive. Biosafety level 3 (BSL-3 or BSL-3 Ag) provides the high degree of containment that is needed when studying a variety of organisms with a recognized potential for significant detrimental impact on animal or human health or on natural ecosystems.

ration efforts directed at identifying potential risks worldwide, including regulatory mechanisms that minimize the threat of introducing emerging infectious agents into the United States or other unaffected countries.

For potential and emerging infectious agents in other countries, assistance from the United States is more ad hoc or piecemeal than strategic and wide-ranging. By adopting a more comprehensive approach to helping countries strengthen their prevention, detection, and diagnostic capabilities, the United States will enhance its own animal health framework and security. Means to accomplish this include transferring technology between nations and providing training opportunities to international students and veterinarians to ensure self-sufficiency and sustainable surveillance. The United States can also encourage and support the enhancement of critical competencies within the national services, which includes active participation in the formulation of international standards and the timely reporting of zoonotic and exotic diseases. The charge to the committee explicitly states that it will "review the U.S. system and approach for dealing with animal diseases," and the committee regards the international dimension as an extremely critical component of the U.S. animal health framework. With increased globalization and movement of diseases, people, products, pathogens, and vectors, the United States cannot continue to impose a line between domestic and international issues, but should instead adopt an animal health system that identifies and responds to animal disease threats without regard to national boundaries.

Importation, Sale, and Transport of Animals

> *Recommendation 7:* **Integrated and standardized regulations should be developed and implemented nationally to address the import, sale, movement, and health of exotic, nondomesticated, and wild-caught animals.**

Such a policy development needs to include health professionals and laboratory-based analysis because wild-caught and exotic animals may carry pathogens and pose a risk of transmitting disease without demonstrating clinical signs. The monkeypox outbreak of 2003 highlighted a number of weaknesses in the animal health framework for addressing a newly emergent zoonotic disease. In particular, while several federal agencies (including the USDA, U.S. Department of the Interior's Fish and Wildlife Service, and the Department of Health and Human Services) have roles in preventing, detecting, and diagnosing zoonotic and other diseases transmitted by exotic animals, there is a lack of coordinated federal oversight of the animal-centered aspects of diseases transmitted by exotic animals. Prior to the interim final rule banning the import, sale, or distribution of prairie dogs and some African rodents (responsible for the monkeypox outbreak in 2003), import and movement of exotic animals was largely uncontrolled (and most exotic animal movement is still uncontrolled). Tracking of these animals in the

United States is inconsistent and ineffective, and there is a disturbing lack of standardized testing of the health status of exotic animals at the point of origin and in companion animal shops, trade fairs, and other venues. Considering that the emergence of new disease agents occurs most frequently at species interfaces, monkeypox is not likely to be the last zoonotic agent to emerge from an exotic animal in the United States.

Addressing Future Animal Disease Risks

> *Recommendation 8:* **The USDA, DHS, Department of Health and Human Services, and state animal and public health agencies and laboratories should improve, expand, and formalize the use of predictive, risk-based tools and models to develop prevention, detection, diagnostic, and biosecurity systems and strategies for indigenous, exotic, and emerging animal diseases.**

There has been increased recognition and use of well-structured and scientifically based mathematical, epidemiological, and risk analysis models and tools to define acceptable risks and mitigation strategies that can assist in policy and science-based decision making. Examples include models of the spread of FMD during the UK epidemic, and an assessment of the risk of BSE to U.S. agriculture, developed by Harvard University's Center for Risk Analysis for the USDA (Cohen et al., 2003; Haydon et al., 2004). Risk analysis and modeling have been criticized, mainly on the basis of insufficient scientific data or inappropriate assumptions. Therefore, efforts to develop scientific data on disease transmission, effectiveness of control programs, economic evaluation, and quantitative assessment of all factors involved in making policies and regulations should be a priority of the animal health infrastructure, working in collaboration with academia, industry, and global trade partners.

Threats from bioterrorism, emerging diseases, and foreign animal disease introductions add urgency to preventing or minimizing catastrophic consequences to the United States, other nations, and the global economy. Education and training of professionals to assess, manage, and communicate risk of animal disease and improved information available to stakeholders, including producers and the public, are important aspects of effective infrastructure that supports risk-based approaches.

Education and Training

> *Recommendation 9:* **Industry, producers, the American Veterinary Medical Association (AVMA), government agencies, and colleges of veterinary medicine should build veterinary capacity through both recruitment and preparation of additional veterinary graduates into careers in**

public health, food systems, biomedical research, diagnostic laboratory investigation, pathology, epidemiology, ecosystem health, and food animal practice.

There are insufficient graduates to meet the needs in a number of major and distinct fields of veterinary medicine dealing with various species of food-animals, rural practice (mixed domestic animals), ecosystem health (including wildlife disease and conservation biology), public health, the many dimensions of the food system, and biomedical science. In addition, veterinary graduates are not adequately prepared to deal with foreign animal diseases, public health, and ecosystem health, without further postgraduate studies. According to the Association of American Veterinary Medical Colleges (AAVMC), the 28 veterinary colleges in the United States graduate approximately 2,300 veterinarians per year and are currently unable to keep up with societal needs in private or public practice.

There has been a steady decline in the number of rural practitioners and of veterinarians employed in regulatory agencies. The USDA, underserved at present, predicts a shortfall of 584 veterinarians on its staff by 2007. Fifty percent of U.S. Public Health Service veterinarians are currently eligible for retirement.

Too few veterinary students are choosing to specialize in basic biomedical science or pathology, as noted in the recently published NRC report *National Need and Priorities for Veterinarians in Biomedical Research*, which suggests a strategy for recruiting and preparing more veterinarians for careers in laboratory animal medicine, comparative medicine, and comparative pathology (NRC, 2004). This committee endorses the recommendations of that report.

One strategy for building veterinary capacity is to design and implement training and educational curricula to better address these underserved areas of animal health. The Veterinary Medical Education and Workforce Development Act of 2004, which amends the Public Health Service Act, will be a useful first step that establishes a competitive grants program to build capacity in veterinary medical education and expands the workforce of veterinarians engaged in public health practice and biomedical research.

***Recommendation 10:* The USDA, state animal health agencies, the AVMA, and colleges and schools of veterinary medicine and departments of animal science should develop a national animal health education plan focusing on education and training of individuals from all sectors involved in disease prevention and early detection through day-to-day oversight of animals.**

Responsibility for implementing the educational plan would fall on those at the local level. Strong and well-functioning front-line detection is provided by animal handlers and personnel working with animals on a day-to-day basis. This backbone for effectively preventing animal disease outbreaks requires education and training to include awareness and recognition of clinical signs, as well as an elementary understanding of disease transmission and prevention. In addition, those with day-to-day oversight of animals need to understand the methods and responsibilities for reporting the signs of foreign and exotic animal diseases. Basic multilingual education and training are necessary for those with such direct oversight of animals, whereas more in-depth education to promote a greater depth and breadth of understanding of transmission and prevention is required for managers and owners.

Improving Public Awareness of the Economic, Social, and Human Health Effects of Animal Diseases

> ***Recommendation 11:*** **The government, private sector, and professional and industry associations should collectively educate and raise the level of awareness of the general public about the importance of public and private investment to strengthen the animal health framework.**

Increased public awareness is critical in supporting and implementing transformations needed to strengthen the framework against animal disease risks. The lack of cohesive national advocacy for public health issues generally creates a much more difficult environment in which to increase attention and investment in the framework for preventing, detecting, and diagnosing animal diseases.

The recent outbreaks of FMD, SARS, AI, and BSE are all reminders of the threats such diseases pose to the U.S. food supply, global economy, public health, and confidence in the safety of the food supply. The entire food and fiber system—including farm inputs, processing, manufacturing, exporting, and related services—is one of the largest sectors of the U.S. economy and accounts for output of over $2 trillion dollars, generating $1.24 trillion in added value, and 12.3 percent of total gross domestic product in 2001 (USDA, 2003). Nearly 17 percent of all U.S. workers are employed by the food and fiber system (USDA, 2003). Producers, companion animal owners, and others on the front line have a direct personal and private interest in detecting, diagnosing, and preventing animal diseases to avoid losses associated with reduced productivity, animal mortality, or potential effects on personal health and welfare. Although these losses can be significant, adverse social, economic, and human health impacts associated with animal diseases extend beyond producers or household animal owners.

Increased investment in educating the public about animal health will help to reduce disease and transmission; enhance public and animal health; ensure a secure, economical, and viable food supply; and improve trade and competitiveness. These educational efforts should include information about diseases of food-animals, wildlife, and companion animals.

PRIORITIES FOR RESEARCH IN FOOD DEFENSE

Francis F. Busta, Ph.D.,[4] *Shaun Kennedy, B.S.E.,*[5] *and Julie Ostrowsky, M.Sc.*[6]
University of Minnesota–Twin Cities Campus

Food defense, dealing with the threat of intentional acts of contamination at any point in the food system, is distinct from *food safety*, even though the two areas are closely linked. Food safety efforts target unintentional problems, such as "natural" or accidental contamination with microbial (e.g., *E. coli* or *Salmonella*) or chemical agents, with some degree of predictability regarding agents, processes, and products of concern. Food defense, by contrast, responds to the threat of sporadic manmade (terrorist) activity, involving high concentrations of contaminants that would not occur naturally or accidentally in the food supply (e.g., *B. anthracis*, biologically engineered organisms, or chemical toxins). Further, food defense involves dealing with hoaxes or threats sufficient to cause widespread disruption, fear, and panic, and, ultimately, the potential for large-scale, coordinated attacks with catastrophic results. Food defense, unlike food safety, is thereby integral to homeland security, particularly regarding efforts to strengthen critical infrastructure protection, threat assessment, and emergency preparedness and response.

The vulnerability of the nation's food system to terrorist attack (described in the Summary and Assessment and by several workshop contributors, e.g., Osterholm and Henry in Chapter 1; Acheson in Chapter 4) stems from several major factors. The farm-to-table food system encompasses a wide range of interdependent elements, from farm inputs, such as seeds and fertilizers, to production, manufacturing and processing, wholesale, distribution, through to the consumer via retail sales and food service. Both domestic and imported ingredients and products move throughout the system. This complexity offers a vast array of potential sites—accessible targets—for intentional contamination to occur. In addition, the degree to which foodborne illness occurs annually (due to "natural" or accidental contamination), despite extensive systems in place to protect the safety of the food supply, underscores the limitations of available food safety efforts. Although necessary to minimize the burden of foodborne illness, those efforts also provide the very information that could be misused deliberately as a roadmap for targeting an attack on the food system. Another major factor is the potentially high impact of a food-related terrorism incident or even an announced threat without an actual attack, given the likelihood of widespread fear and panic in the population and economic devastation to the private sector.

---

[4]Director, National Center for Food Protection and Defense.

[5]Deputy Director, National Center for Food Protection and Defense.

[6]Senior Program Analyst, National Center for Food Protection and Defense.

The federal government coordinates food defense activities under the umbrella of the DHS, with sector-specific responsibilities residing jointly with the DHHS and the USDA. Homeland Security Presidential Directive 7 (HSPD-7) issued in 2003 first identified the agriculture and food sector among the nation's critical infrastructures/key resources singled out for special protection under homeland security initiatives (White House, 2003). In 2004, the Homeland Security Presidential Directive 9 (HSPD-9) established a national policy to protect the food and agriculture system from terrorist attack (White House, 2004). DHS's National Infrastructure Protection Plan, currently under development, incorporates food and agriculture sector protection among its initiatives to protect the nation's critical infrastructures and key assets (DHS, 2005a,b; SEMP, 2005).

Addressing these critical issues surrounding the potential for food to be exploited as a vehicle for catastrophic attack requires a broad-based, comprehensive approach. Food defense, as a recently defined concept, creates new links among previously unrelated fields. This leads to a diverse, multidisciplinary agenda for food defense research, education, and training. On an operational level, collaborative initiatives across academia, industry, and government are necessary to develop and maintain new channels of communication, leverage resources, and coordinate responsibilities. The effectiveness of food defense efforts will depend on the quality of research outcomes as well as on the successful integration of newly developed technologies, programs, tools, and expertise into public- and private-sector stakeholder communities.

This discussion focuses on identifying high-priority areas for research that address two central issues in food defense: preventing major attacks on the food system and responding effectively if such an attack (or credible threats of an attack) were to occur. This research effort is central to the mission of the National Center for Food Protection and Defense (NCFPD), whose program is aimed at reducing the potential for contamination at any point along the food supply chain and mitigating potentially catastrophic public health and economic effects.[7]

NCFPD Programs

NCFPD (2006), led by the University of Minnesota, is one of six academic Centers of Excellence funded through grants from the DHS with the specific

[7]Investing in food defense research may well carry significant collateral benefits, beyond its primary value to homeland security, in terms of health and economic effects. Much of what we are learning about preventing and responding to potentially catastrophic attacks on the food system can be applied to ongoing efforts to reduce the burden of foodborne illness caused by more common sources of contamination (natural and accidental). Such advances can also be applied to enhancing routine security operations, such as reduction in the incidence of theft of food products, which commonly occurs all along the supply chain.

mandate for a food protection and defense center coming from HSPD-9 (DHS, 2004a). Other Homeland Security Centers of Excellence include: Center for Risk and Economic Analysis of Terrorism Events, led by the University of Southern California; National Center for Foreign Animal and Zoonotic Disease Defense, led by Texas A&M University; National Center for the Study of Terrorism and Responses to Terrorism, led by the University of Maryland; Center for the Study of Preparedness and Catastrophic Event Response, led by Johns Hopkins University; and Center for Advancing Microbial Risk Assessment, led by Michigan State University, in collaboration with the U.S. Environmental Protection Agency (EPA) (DHS, 2006).

Developed as a multidisciplinary and mission-focused research consortium, NCFPD addresses the vulnerability of the nation's food system to attack through intentional contamination with biological, chemical or radiological agents. NCFPD takes a comprehensive, farm-to-table view of the food system, encompassing all aspects from primary production through transportation and food processing to retail and food service. In delivering on its mission to defend the safety and security of the food system through research and education, NCFPD places a high priority on threats to the food system that could lead to catastrophic damage to public health or the economy.

Academic collaborators in NCFPD's research consortium include the University of Minnesota, Michigan State University, University of Wisconsin–Madison, North Dakota State University, Georgia Institute of Technology, University of Tennessee–Knoxville, and individual investigators from 21 other universities. Additional research partners are drawn from private-sector research organizations, professional organizations, and food and agriculture agencies. Over 30 industry experts serve as unpaid advisors, providing technical advice, critical end-user feedback, and strategic oversight. To leverage expertise and resources programmatically, close collaboration is maintained with federal and state regulatory agencies, other Homeland Security Centers of Excellence, the national laboratories, and private-sector stakeholders.

NCFPD's program incorporates cutting-edge research aimed at food defense from a variety of disciplines, including supply chain management, logistics, epidemiology, public health, risk assessment, economics, molecular biology, food microbiology, biomedical engineering, toxicology, and risk communication. More than 140 experts in these areas were selected to participate in NCFPD's research consortium, based on approval of peer-reviewed research proposals submitted by teams of investigators. Thirty-four collaborative research and education projects are currently in progress. A summary of NCFPD initiatives appears in Table 7-1.

NCFPD's program provides a comprehensive framework for identifying priorities and unmet needs in food defense research. Based on the fundamental issues outlined in DHS's Broad Agency Announcement (DHS, 2004b) calling for proposals for a university Center of Excellence in food protection and defense, NCFPD's program is organized thematically into three primary areas: systems,

TABLE 7-1 National Center for Food Protection and Defense Research Initiatives

- Strategies for hardening the supply chain
- Improved outbreak surveillance/investigation approaches for rapid event identification and traceback
- Realistic models to guide investments and intervention strategy selection for cost-effective preparedness, response, and recovery
- Detection technologies to rapidly identify contamination to accelerate containment, recall, response, and recovery
- Inactivation approaches to enable facility recovery now, with preferred options for the future
- Food handling and processing approaches to reduce the probability of harm
- Risk communication tools, standards and training to maximize appropriate actions while minimizing fear
- Educational programs to train the next generation of food system professionals
- Integrative, transdisciplinary effort spanning the food chain from field to fork
- Strategic partnerships with all key food system stakeholder groups:
  - Significantly leveraging opportunities
  - Connected to the users to ensure relevance
  - Technology transfer options and multiuse opportunities identified up front
- Focused on realistic vulnerabilities and real-world solutions; new technologies, tools and approaches

SOURCE: Busta (2005).

agents, and training. Priorities for research in each of these areas are outlined below.

Research Needs: Systems

Supply chain security encompasses policies and practices within industry and its regulators to reduce vulnerabilities, minimize disruptions caused by threats or contamination incidents, and maximize the system's resiliency through effective response plans. Major research needs include the following:

- Characterizing and benchmarking supply chain security practices, such as basic security processes (e.g., protecting employees), incident management, logistics and transportation security, and companies' supply chain relationships.
- Assessing those practices that have the greatest impact on efforts to enhance supply chain security.
- Developing a common standard for security guidelines within the food industry.
- Providing strategies for secure communication and information management among federal, state, and industry officials during a potential attack on the food system.

An effective public health response to incidents of contamination can directly limit the scope of an incident, reduce the risk of foodborne illness, mitigate economic damage, and possibly help deter future attempts. Priorities for research include the following:

- Develop predictive models and tools to assess the nature, scope, and impact of intentional contamination incidents and responses to those incidents.
- Improve strategies for coordinating preparedness and response activities across local, state, and federal public health, laboratory, and regulatory jurisdictions.

Given the nature of the food system and its interdependency with other sectors of the economy, a deliberate attack on the food system could have broad impacts on the national economy. Estimates of the potential national cost of such attacks are relevant to policy decisions involving the allocation of scarce resources. Research needs include the following:

- Assess the potential economic impact of a major food system attack on the national economy and on the private sector.
- Analyze the cost-effectiveness of public, nongovernmental, and industry investment in strategies to enhance supply chain security (e.g., use of "smart seals" or radio frequency identification (RFID) tags to track products through shipment).
- Evaluate the public's willingness to support greater public investment in measures to protect the food system from deliberate contamination.
- Assess the probability of future attacks on the food system.

Research Needs: Agents

To better recognize foodborne attacks and identify the contaminating agent involved, technologies are needed to sample and detect contaminants in food and to trace contaminated food products (or their ingredients) through the supply chain. Detection of food contaminants is complicated by the food matrix—the chemical and molecular nature of individual foods and the effects of food viscosity, homogeneity, conductivity, and pH on a given agent. Chemical agents present an especially daunting problem because they are difficult to detect and many of them resist food processing designed to safeguard against biological contamination. Existing toxicological tests for chemical agents are limited. Current research aims to take advantage of such properties as chemical class, molecular weight, and solubility as a means to detection. Overall needs for detection include the following:

- Develop rapid, accurate, and reliable methods to detect select agents and chemical toxins in the food supply.
- Enable efficient monitoring and testing in a range of food production, processing, distribution, and retail settings.
- Enhance preanalytical effective preparation of samples for rapid analysis by separation, concentration, and/or purification of select agents from food matrices, recognizing that the complex environments of foods place a premium on preanalytical processes to enable effective detection.
- Facilitate the rapid translation and integration of newly developed diagnostic research methods into the national laboratory infrastructure, for example by assuring that new methodologies are appropriately validated and by coordinating surge capacity among laboratories during a food contamination incident.

Protecting public health in the event of a foodborne attack will involve the decontamination of affected products, people, and physical environments, as well as the safe disposal of contaminated foods. Such processes are managed at the federal level by the EPA and regulated by EPA restrictions on disinfectant use (state level variations are also important). Priorities for research in this area include the following:

- Develop effective large-scale means of disposing of contaminated food and decontaminating individuals, facilities, or sites.
- Develop safe and practical methods for neutralizing selected biological agents in food processing facilities and in consumer households.
- Develop effective protocols for managing disposal, containment, remediation, and recovery processes following a contamination incident.
- Develop methods to isolate or inactivate potential contaminants, including spores, toxins, and chemical agents, to facilitate detection in the food matrix and to provide a routine level of protection against contamination.

Research Needs: Training

Preparedness for dealing effectively with a food system attack goes beyond appropriate technical preparation of the first responder groups to include capabilities for rapidly mobilizing and delivering appropriate and credible risk communication messages to the public, as well as prior training of key spokespersons in the public and private sectors. Research needs include the following:

- Education and training strategies from undergraduate programs through to specialized graduate and professional training to prepare all relevant food system stakeholders with the knowledge and skills to prevent, minimize the consequences of, and recover from a food system attack.

- Develop guidelines and best practices for active engagement of multiple audiences in effective risk communications prior to, during, and after an intentional food contamination event or hoax.
- Develop methods to enhance the training of key spokespersons and subject matter experts to improve their risk communication expertise.

Effective engagement in food defense efforts at all levels depends critically on the development of a cadre of professionals equipped to deal with this wide array of issues. High-quality education and training programs are needed to expand the pool of available personnel with expertise in food defense. This includes developing just-in-time training materials, advanced course content, virtual training programs, and interdisciplinary degree options for undergraduates, graduates, and professionals.

Conclusion

Many researchers, including NCFPD collaborators, have broken ground on issues essential to protecting the U.S. food supply and defending it from deliberate contamination. Preventing intentional contamination of the food system requires a shift in mindset: traditional food safety efforts must move from minimizing the possibility of contamination events that can normally happen to preventing those that cannot be permitted to occur. Not only must these efforts be continued and expanded, but to be most effective, their results also need to be shared. Several workshop participants have advocated the creation of a multidimensional database of accumulated knowledge regarding foodborne attack agents, food targets, and detection and decontamination under various conditions. Such a resource could reduce the considerable duplication of research on food defense that occurs in the absence of scientific exchange, and it may also provide a springboard for innovation in the field.

REFERENCES

Busta F. 2005 (October 26). *Session VII: Threat Reduction Research and Policy Opportunities.* Presentation at the Forum on Microbial Threats Workshop Meeting, Foodborne Threats to Health: The Policies and Practices of Surveillance, Prevention, Outbreak Investigations, and International Coordination, Washington, D.C., Institute of Medicine, Forum on Microbial Threats.

Cohen, JT, Duggar K, Gray GM, Kreindel S, Abdelrahman H, HabteMariam T, Oryang D, and Tameru B. 2003. *Revised Risk Assessment: Evaluation of the Potential for Bovine Spongiform Encephalopathy in the United States.* Harvard Center for Risk Analysis, Harvard School of Public Health. Prepared for the U.S. Department of Agriculture. November 26, 2001, revised October 2003. [Online]. Available: http://www.hcra.harvard.edu/pdf/madcow.pdf [accessed June 27, 2006].

DHS (U.S. Department of Homeland Security). 2004a (January 29). *President's Budget Includes $254 Million to Further Improve Nation's Bio-Surveillance Capabilities.* [Online]. Available: http://www.dhs.gov/dhspublic/display?content=3092 [accessed June 27, 2006].

DHS. 2004b. *Homeland Security Presidential Directive/HSPD-9, Defense of U.S. Agriculture and Food.* [Online]. Available: http://www.whitehouse.gov/news/releases/2004/02/20040203-2.html [accessed April 17, 2006].

DHS. 2004c. *Broad Agency Announcement.* [Online]. Available: http://www.dhs.gov/interweb/assetlibrary/BAA_Agro.doc [accessed April 17, 2006].

DHS. 2005a. *Draft National Infrastructure Protection Plan.* [Online]. Available: http://www.fas.org/irp/agency/dhs/nipp110205.pdf [accessed April 17, 2006].

DHS. 2005b. *Interim National Infrastructure Protection Plan.* [Online]. Available: http://www.newsecurityconcepts.com/DataFiles/interim-nipp.pdf [accessed April 17, 2006].

DHS. 2006. *Homeland Security Centers of Excellence.* [Online]. Available: http://www.dhs.gov/dhspublic/interapp/editorial/ editorial_0498.xml [accessed April 17, 2006].

Haydon DT, Kao RR, and Kitching PK. 2004. The UK foot and mouth disease outbreak—the aftermath. *Nature Reviews* 2(8):675–681.

IOM (Institute of Medicine). 2003. *Microbial Threats to Health: Emergence, Detection, and Response.* Washington, D.C.: The National Academies Press.

NCFPD (National Center for Food Protection and Defense). 2006. *NCFPD Homepage.* [Online]. Available: http://www.ncfpd.umn.edu/ [accessed April 17, 2006].

NRC (National Research Council). 2004. *National Need and Priorities for Veterinarians in Biomedical Research.* Washington, D.C.: The National Academies Press.

NRC. 2005. *Animal Health at the Crossroads.* Washington, D.C.: The National Academies Press.

SEMP (Suburban Emergency Management Project). 2005. *What Is the Interim National Infrastructure Protection Plan?* [Online]. Available: http://www.semp.us/biots/biot_200.html [accessed April 17, 2006].

USDA (U.S. Department of Agriculture). 2003 (October 16). *Food Market Structures: The U.S. Food and Fiber System.* [Online]. Available: http://ers.usda.gov/briefing/foodmarketstructures/foodandfiber.htm [accessed June 27, 2006].

White House. 2003. *Homeland Security Presidential Directive HSPD-7.* [Online]. Available: http://www.whitehouse.gov/news/releases/2003/12/20031217-5.html [accessed April 17, 2006].

White House. 2004. *Homeland Security Presidential Directive HSPD-9.* [Online]. Available: http://www.whitehouse.gov/news/releases/2004/02/print/20040203-2.html [accessed April 17, 2006].

APPENDIX

A

Forum on Microbial Threats

Board on Global Health

Institute of Medicine

The National Academies

Foodborne Threats to Health: The Practice and Policies of Surveillance, Prevention, Outbreak Investigations, and International Coordination

October 25 and 26, 2005
KECK 100
National Academies
500 Fifth Street, N.W.
Washington, D.C. 20001

AGENDA

Tuesday, October 25, 2005

8:30–9:00: **Continental Breakfast**

9:00: **Welcome and Opening Remarks**
Stanley Lemon, The University of Texas Medical Branch, Galveston
Chair, Forum on Microbial Threats
Margaret A. (Peggy) Hamburg, Nuclear Threat Initiative

Vice-chair, Forum on Microbial Threats

Session I: The Current U.S. Food Supply—*Ruth Berkelman*, Moderator

9:20: **Globalization of the food supply**—Discussion to address the "inputs" to the U.S. food supply—locally, regionally, and globally—and how the percentage of those inputs has changed over time.

- **Craig Henry**, Vice president, FPA

9:50: Discussion

10:15: Break

Session II: The Food Supply "Threat Spectrum"—*Michael Osterholm*, Moderator

9:00: **Welcome and Opening Remarks**

10:30: **Overview of the threat spectrum—Unintentional vs. intentional**

- **Michael Osterholm**, University of Minnesota

11:00: Discussion

11:15: **Burden of illness associated with foodborne threats to health**

- **Rob Tauxe**, CDC, Atlanta, GA

11:45: Discussion

12:00–12:45: Lunch

Session III: The Food Supply "Threat Spectrum": Case Studies—*David Acheson*, Moderator

12:45: **Cyclosporiasis in imported fresh basil**

- **Barbara Herwaldt**, CDC, Atlanta, GA
- **Dean Bodager**, Florida Department of Public Health

1:15: **Hepatitis A from imported green onions**

- **Beth Bell**, CDC, Atlanta, GA

1:45–2:15: Discussion

2:15–2:30: Break

2:30–3:30: **Botulinum toxin—David Acheson, presenter**
Discussants:
- **Milton Leitenberg**, University of Maryland
- **Clay Detlefsen**, Vice president for Regulatory Affairs, International Dairy Foods Association

3:30–3:50: Discussion

Session IV: What are the Tools and Technologies for Real-Time Surveillance of the Food Supply for Conventional and Unconventional Adulterants? Local/Regional/National/Global—*Dr. Pat Fitch*, Moderator

3:50–5:00:
- **John Besser**, Minnesota Department of Health
- **Bob (Robert L.) Buchanan**, Director, Office of Science, CFSAN
- **Kimberly Elenberg**, USDA, FSIS, Office of Food Safety and Emergency Preparedness

5:00–5:45: Open Discussion of Day 1/Adjournment of the first day

6:00: Reception

7:15: **Dinner Meeting of the Forum on Microbial Threats**
[location: The Atrium, 3rd Floor; KECK Center]

Wednesday, October 26, 2005

8:00–8:30: Continental Breakfast

8:30: **Opening Remarks/Summary of Day 1**
P. Frederick Sparling, UNC, Vice-chair, Forum on Microbial Threats

Session V: Who Is Responsible for Ensuring the Wholesomeness of the Food Supply? Domestic and International Perspectives—*Dr. Jim Hughes*, Moderator

8:45: **The U.S. Food Safety System**
- **John Bailar, III**, University of Chicago (Chair, NRC Report: *Ensuring Safe Food: From Production to Consumption*)

9:15: **The International Food Safety System—WHO perspective**

- **Jørgen Schlundt**, Director of the Food Safety Program (WHO)

9:45: Discussion

10:15–10:30: Break

Session VI: What Are the Incentives and Disincentives Associated with Disease/Contamination Reporting? Impacts on Human Health and International Trade—BSE as a "Case Study"—*Dr. Lonnie King*, Moderator

10:30–12:00: **Case study of BSE**—Human illness associated with BSE-tainted meat and meat products; surveillance tools and technologies; impacts on international trade associated with reporting a "positive"

Overview: Stanley Prusiner, UC San Francisco

- **Steven Collins**, Department of Pathology, University of Melbourne, Parkville, Australia
- **Maura Ricketts**, Executive Director, Health Canada
- **Wil Hueston**, University of Minnesota

12:00–12:15: Discussion

12:15–12:45: Discussion of Morning Sessions

12:45–1:30: Lunch

Session VII: Threat Reduction Research and Policy Opportunities—*Dr. George Korch*, Moderator

1:30–2:45: Panelists

- **Lonnie King**, Chair, NRC Report: *Animal Health at the Crossroads*
- **Sanford Miller**, Food Policy Institute
- **Frank Busta**, University of Minnesota

2:45–3:15: Discussion

3:15–4:00: **Next Steps**

4:15: Adjourn

APPENDIX B

Acronyms[1]

AAVMC	Association of American Veterinary Medical Colleges
AEI	American Enterprise Institute
AI	avian influenza
AMS	Agricultural Marketing Service
ANCJDR	Australian National CJD Registry
APHIS	Animal and Plant Health Inspection Service
APHL	Association of Public Health Laboratories
ARS	Agriculture Research Service
ASM	American Society for Microbiology
AVMA	American Veterinary Medical Association
BIDS	Border Infectious Disease Surveillance
BRC	Biologic Regulatory Commission
BSE	bovine spongiform encephalopathy
BSL	biosafety level
BW	biological weapons
CAMR	Center for Applied Microbiological Research
CBW	chemical and biological weapons
CCMS	Consumer Complaint Monitoring System
CDC	Centers for Disease Control and Prevention
CDI	Conformation Dependent Immunoassay

[1]Also, see P. 179 in Chapter 5, Table 5-1: Networks and Resources in Food Safety.

CFSAN	Center for Food Safety and Applied Nutrition
CISSM	Center for International Security Studies at Maryland
CRS	Congressional Research Service
CSF	classic swine fever
CSPI	Center for Science in the Public Interest
CSREES	Cooperative State Research, Education, and Extension Service
CSTE	Council for State and Territorial Epidemiologists
CVM	Center for Veterinary Medicine
CW	chemical weapons
CWD	chronic wasting disease
DHS	Department of Homeland Security
DPVS	due process vetting system
EID	emerging infectious disease
END	exotic Newcastle disease
EPA	Environmental Protection Agency
EPFC	Emerging Patterns in Food Complaints
ERS	Economic Research Service
EUROCJD	European and Allied Countries CJD Group
FAO	Food and Agriculture Organization of the United Nations
FBI	Federal Bureau of Investigation
fCJD	familial Creutzfeldt-Jakob disease
FDA	Food and Drug Administration
FEMA	Federal Emergency Management Agency
FMD	foot-and-mouth disease
FMI	Food Marketing Institute
FOUO	For Official Use Only
FSIS	Food Safety and Inspection Service
FSSA	FDA Security Surveillance Assignment
GAO	Government Accountability Office
GFAP	glial fibrillary acidic protein
GIPSA	Grain Inspection, Packers and Stockyards Administration
HACCP	Hazard Analysis and Critical Control Point
HAV	hepatitis A virus
HGH	human growth hormone
HHS	Department of Health and Human Services
HSPD	Homeland Security Presidential Directive
IDFA	International Dairy Foods Association

IHC	immunohistochemistry
IHR	international health regulations
IOM	Institute of Medicine
LRC	Least Restrictive Classification
LRN	Laboratory Response Network
MBM	meat-and-bone meal
MRM	mechanically recovered meat
NAHLN	National Animal Health Laboratory Network
NASS	National Agricultural Statistics Service
NATO	North Atlantic Treaty Organization
NCFPD	National Center for Food Protection and Defense
NCTR	National Center for Toxicological Research
NGO	nongovernmental organization
NIH	National Institutes of Health
NMFS	National Marine Fisheries Service
NOAA	National Oceanic and Atmospheric Administration
NRC	National Research Council
NRDC	Nature Resources Defense Council
OECA	Office of Enforcement and Compliance Assurance
OIE	Office International des Epizooties
OPPTS	Office of Prevention, Pesticides and Toxic Substances
ORA	Office of Regulatory Affairs
ORACBA	Office of Risk Assessment and Cost-Benefit Analysis
ORM	operational risk management
OTA	Organic Trade Association
PFGE	pulsed-field gel electrophoresis
PH	public health
PHL	public health laboratories
PNG	Papua New Guinea
RFID	radio frequency identification
RT-PCR	reverse transcriptase polymerase chain reaction
SARS	severe acute respiratory syndrome
SBO	specified bovine offal
sCJD	sporadic Creutzfeldt-Jakob disease
SPPA	Strategic Partnership Program Agroterrorism
SRM	specified risk materials

TSE	transmissible spongiform encephalopathy
UNMOVIC	United Nations Monitoring, Verification, and Inspection Commission
UNSCOM	United Nations Special Commission
USAMRIID	United States Army Medical Research Institute for Infectious Diseases
USDA	U.S. Department of Agriculture
vCJD	variant Creutzfeldt-Jakob disease
WHO	World Health Organization
WNV	West Nile virus

APPENDIX

C

Forum Member Biographies

Stanley M. Lemon, M.D. (*Chair*), is the John Sealy Distinguished University Chair and director of the Institute for Human Infections and Immunity at the University of Texas Medical Branch (UTMB) at Galveston. He received his undergraduate A.B. degree in biochemical sciences from Princeton University summa cum laude, and his M.D. with honors from the University of Rochester. He completed postgraduate training in internal medicine and infectious diseases at the University of North Carolina at Chapel Hill, and is board certified in both. From 1977 to 1983, he served with the U.S. Army Medical Research and Development Command, followed by a 14-year period on the faculty of the University of North Carolina School of Medicine. He moved to UTMB in 1997, serving first as chair of the Department of Microbiology and Immunology, then as dean of the School of Medicine from 1999 to 2004. Dr. Lemon's research interests relate to the molecular virology and pathogenesis of the positive-stranded RNA viruses responsible for hepatitis. He has had a long-standing interest in antiviral and vaccine development, and has served previously as chair of the Anti-Infective Drugs Advisory Committee of the U.S. Food and Drug Administration (FDA). He is the past chair of the Steering Committee on Hepatitis and Poliomyelitis of the World Health Organization (WHO) Programme on Vaccine Development. He presently serves as a member of the U.S. Delegation of the U.S.–Japan Cooperative Medical Sciences Program, and chairs the Board of Scientific Councilors of the National Center for Infectious Diseases (NCID) of the Centers for Disease Control and Prevention (CDC). He was co-chair of the Committee on Advances in Technology and the Prevention of their Application to Next Generation Biowarfare Threats for the National Academy of Sciences (NAS) and recently chaired an Institute of Medicine (IOM) study committee related to vaccines for the protection of the military against naturally occurring infectious disease threats.

P. Frederick Sparling, M.D. (*Vice-chair*), is the J. Herbert Bate Professor Emeritus of Medicine, Microbiology, and Immunology at the University of North Carolina (UNC) at Chapel Hill and is director of the North Carolina Sexually Transmitted Infections Research Center. Previously, he served as chair of the Department of Medicine and chair of the Department of Microbiology and Immunology at UNC. He was president of the Infectious Disease Society of America from 1996–1997. He was also a member of the IOM's Committee on Microbial Threats to Health (1991–1992). Dr. Sparling's laboratory research is in the molecular biology of bacterial outer membrane proteins involved in pathogenesis, with a major emphasis on *gonococci* and *meningococci*. His current studies focus on the biochemistry and genetics of iron-scavenging mechanisms used by gonococci and *meningococci* and the structure and function of the *gonococcal porin* proteins. He is pursuing the goal of a vaccine for gonorrhea.

Margaret A. Hamburg, M.D. (*Vice-chair*), is vice president for Biological Programs at the Nuclear Threat Initiative, a charitable organization working to reduce the global threat from nuclear, biological, and chemical weapons. She is in charge of the biological program area. She completed her internship and residency in internal medicine at the New York Hospital/Cornell University Medical Center and is certified by the American Board of Internal Medicine. Dr. Hamburg is a graduate of Harvard College and Harvard Medical School. Before taking on her current position, she was the Assistant Secretary for Planning and Evaluation, U.S. Department of Health and Human Services (DHHS), serving as a principal policy advisor to the Secretary of Health and Human Services with responsibilities including policy formulation and analysis, the development and review of regulations and/or legislation, budget analysis, strategic planning, and the conduct and coordination of policy research and program evaluation. Prior to this, she served for almost six years as the Commissioner of Health for the City of New York. As chief health officer in the nation's largest city, her many accomplishments included the design and implementation of an internationally recognized tuberculosis control program that produced dramatic declines in tuberculosis cases, the development of initiatives that raised childhood immunization rates to record levels, and the creation of the first public health bioterrorism preparedness program in the nation. She currently serves on the Harvard University Board of Overseers. She has been elected to membership in the IOM, the New York Academy of Medicine, and the Council on Foreign Relations, and is a fellow of the American Association for the Advancement of Science and the American College of Physicians.

David W. K. Acheson, M.D., is chief medical officer at the FDA's Center for Food Safety and Applied Nutrition. He received his medical degree at the University of London. After completing internships in general surgery and medicine, he continued his postdoctoral training in Manchester, England, as a Wellcome Trust research fellow. He subsequently was a Wellcome Trust training fellow in Infectious Diseases at the New England Medical Center and at the Wellcome Research Unit in Vellore, India. He was associate professor of medicine, Division of Geographic Medicine and Infectious Diseases, New England Medical Center, until 2001. He then joined the faculties of the Department of Epidemiology and Preventive Medicine and Department of Microbiology and Immunology at the University of Maryland Medical School. Currently at the FDA, his research concentration is on foodborne pathogens and encompasses a mixture of molecular pathogenesis, cell biology, and epidemiology. Specifically, his research focuses on Shiga toxin-producing *E. coli* and understanding toxin interaction with intestinal epithelial cells using tissue culture models. His laboratory has also undertaken a study to examine Shiga toxin-producing *E. coli* in food animals in relation to virulence factors and antimicrobial resistance patterns. More recently, Dr. Acheson initiated a project to understand the molecular pathogenesis of *Campylobacter jejuni*. Other studies have undertaken surveillance of diarrheal disease in the community to determine causes, outcomes, and risk factors of unexplained diarrhea. Dr. Acheson has authored or coauthored more than 72 journal articles, and 42 book chapters and reviews, and is coauthor of the book *Safe Eating* (Dell Health, 1998). He is reviewer of more than 10 journals and is on the editorial board of *Infection and Immunity* and *Clinical Infectious Diseases*. He is a fellow of the Royal College of Physicians, and the Infectious Disease Society of America, and holds several patents.

Ruth L. Berkelman, M.D., is the Rollins Professor and director of the Center for Public Health Preparedness and Research at the Rollins School of Public Health, Emory University in Atlanta. She received her A.B. from Princeton University and her M.D. from Harvard Medical School. Board certified in pediatrics and internal medicine, she began her career at the CDC in 1980, and later became deputy director of the NCID. She also served as a senior advisor to the director, CDC, and Assistant Surgeon General in the U.S. Public Health Service. In 2001, she came to her current position at Emory University, directing a center focused on emerging infectious disease and other urgent threats to health, including terrorism. She has also consulted with the biologic program of the Nuclear Threat Initiative and is most recognized for her work in infectious diseases and disease surveillance. She was elected to the IOM in 2004. Currently a member of the IOM's Forum on Microbial Threats and the Board on Life Sciences of the National Academy of Science, she also chairs the Board of Public and Scientific Affairs at the American Society of Microbiology.

Enriqueta C. Bond, Ph.D., is president of the Burroughs Wellcome Fund. She received her undergraduate degree from Wellesley College, her M.A. from the University of Virginia, and her Ph.D. in molecular biology and biochemical genetics from Georgetown University. She is a member of the Institute of Medicine, the American Association for the Advancement of Science, the American Society for Microbiology, and the American Public Health Association. Dr. Bond serves on the council of the IOM as its vice-chair; she chairs the Board of Scientific Counselors for the NCID at the CDC, and she chairs the IOM's Clinical Research Roundtable. She serves on the board and executive committee of the Research Triangle Park Foundation and on the board of the Medicines for Malaria Venture. Prior to being named president of the Burroughs Wellcome Fund in 1994, she served on the staff of the IOM since 1979, becoming the IOM's executive officer in 1989.

Roger G. Breeze, Ph.D., received his veterinary degree (1968) and Ph.D. degree in veterinary pathology (1973) at the University of Glasgow, Scotland. He was engaged in teaching, diagnostic pathology, and research on respiratory and cardiovascular diseases at the University of Glasgow Veterinary School from 1968 to 1977 and at Washington State University College of Veterinary Medicine, where he was professor and chair of the Department of Microbiology and Pathology from 1977 to 1987. From 1984 to 1987 he was deputy director of the Washington Technology Center, the state's high-technology sciences initiative, based in the College of Engineering at the University of Washington. In 1987, he was appointed director of the USDA's Plum Island Animal Disease Center, a biosafety level 3 facility for research and diagnosis of the world's most dangerous livestock diseases. In that role, he initiated research into the genomic and functional genomic basis of disease pathogenesis, diagnosis, and control of livestock RNA and DNA virus infections. This work became the basis of U.S. defense against natural and deliberate infection with these agents and led to his involvement in the early 1990s in biological weapons defense and proliferation prevention. From 1995 to 1998 he directed research programs in 20 laboratories in the southeast for the USDA Agricultural Research Service before going to Washington, D.C., to establish biological weapons defense research programs for the USDA. He received the Distinguished Executive Award from President Clinton in 1998 for his work at Plum Island and in biodefense. Since 2004, he has been CEO of Centaur Science Group, which provides consulting services in biodefense. His main commitment is to the Defense Threat Reduction Agency's Biological Weapons Proliferation Prevention program in Europe, the Caucasus, and Central Asia.

Steven J. Brickner, Ph.D., is research advisor, antibacterials chemistry, at Pfizer Global Research and Development. He received his Ph.D. in organic chemistry from Cornell University and was a National Institutes of Health (NIH) postdoctoral research fellow at the University of Wisconsin–Madison. He is a medicinal chemist with nearly 20 years of research experience in the pharmaceutical industry, all focused on the discovery and development of novel antibacterial agents. He is an inventor or coinventor on 21 U.S. patents and has published numerous scientific papers, primarily within the area of the oxazolidinones. Prior to joining Pfizer in 1996, he led a team at Pharmacia and Upjohn that discovered and developed linezolid, the first member of a new class of antibiotics to be approved in the last 35 years.

Nancy Carter-Foster, M.S.T.M., is senior advisor for health affairs for the U.S. Department of State, Assistant Secretary for Science and Health, and the Secretary's Representative on HIV/AIDS. She is responsible for identifying emerging health issues and making policy recommendations for the United States foreign policy concerns regarding international health, and coordinates the department's interactions with the nongovernmental community. She is a member of the IOM's Forum on Microbial Threats, the Infectious Diseases Society of America (IDSA), and the American Association of the Advancement of Science (AAAS). She has helped bring focus to global health issues in U.S. foreign policy and brought a national security focus to global health. In prior positions as director for congressional and legislative affairs for the Economic and Business Affairs Bureau of the U.S. Department of State, Foreign Policy Advisory to the majority whip U.S. House of Representatives, trade specialist advisor to the House of Representatives Ways and Means Trade Subcommittee, and consultant to the World Bank, Asia Technical Environment Division, Ms. Carter-Foster has worked on a wide variety of health, trade, and environmental issues, amassing in-depth knowledge and experience in policy development and program implementation.

Gail H. Cassell, Ph.D., is vice president of Scientific Affairs, Distinguished Lilly Research Scholar for Infectious Diseases, Eli Lilly & Company. Previously, she was the Charles H. McCauley Professor and (since 1987) chair of the Department of Microbiology, University of Alabama Schools of Medicine and Dentistry at Birmingham, a department which, under her leadership, has ranked first in research funding from the NIH since 1989. She is a member of the Director's Advisory Committee of the CDC. Dr. Cassell is past president of the American Society for Microbiology (ASM) and is serving her third three-year term as chair of the Public and Scientific Affairs Board of the ASM. She is a former member of the NIH Director's Advisory Committee and a former member of the Advisory Council of the National Institute of Allergy and Infectious Diseases (NIAID). She has also served as an advisor on infectious diseases and indirect costs of research to the White House Office on Science and Technology and was previously chair of the Board of Scientific Counselors of the NCID at the CDC. She served eight years on the Bacteriology-Mycology-II Study Section and served as its chair for three years. She serves on the editorial boards of several prestigious scientific journals and has authored over 275 articles and book chapters. She has been intimately involved in the establishment of science policy and legislation related to biomedical research and public health. Dr. Cassell has received several national and international awards and an honorary degree for her research on infectious diseases.

COL Ralph (Loren) Erickson, M.D., Dr.P.H., M.P.H., is the Director of the Department of Defense Global Emerging Infections Surveillance and Response System (DoD-GEIS) headquartered in Silver Spring, Maryland. He holds degrees in Chemistry (B.S., University of Washington), Medicine (M.D., Uniformed Services University of the Health Sciences), and Public Health (M.P.H., Harvard; Dr.P.H., Johns Hopkins). Residency trained and board certified in Preventive Medicine, Dr. Erickson has held a number of leadership positions within the Army Medical Department to include: Director of the General Preventive Medicine Residency Program, Walter Reed Army Institute of Research; Director of Epidemiology and Disease Surveillance, U.S. Army Center for Health Promotion and Preventive Medicine; Commander of the U.S. Army Center for Health Promotion and Preventive Medicine (Europe); and Specialty Leader for all U.S. Army Preventive Medicine physicians.

Mark B. Feinberg, M.D., Ph.D., is vice president for Policy, Public Health, and Medical Affairs in the Merck Vaccine Division of Merck & Co., Inc. He received his bachelor's degree magna cum laude from the University of Pennsylvania in 1978, and his M.D. and Ph.D. degrees from Stanford University School of Medicine in 1987. From 1985–1986, Dr. Feinberg served as a project officer for the Committee on a National Strategy for AIDS of the IOM and the National Academy of Sciences (NAS). Following receipt of his M.D. and Ph.D. degrees, he pursued postgraduate residency training in internal medicine at the Brigham and Women's Hospital of Harvard Medical School and postdoctoral fellowship research in the laboratory of Dr. David Baltimore at the Whitehead Institute for Biomedical Research. From 1991 to 1995, Dr. Feinberg was an assistant professor of medicine and microbiology and immunology at the University of California, San Francisco (UCSF), where he also served as an attending physician in the AIDS/Oncology Division and as director of the Virology Research Laboratory at San Francisco General Hospital. From 1995 to 1997, he was a medical officer in the Office of AIDS Research in the office of the director of the NIH, and chair of the NIH Coordinating Committee on AIDS Etiology and Pathogenesis Research. During this period, he also served as executive secretary of the NIH Panel to Define Principles of Therapy of HIV Infection. Prior to joining Merck in 2004, Dr. Feinberg served as professor of medicine and microbiology and immunology at the Emory University School of Medicine and as an investigator at the Emory Vaccine Center. He also founded and served as the medical director of the Hope Clinic—a clinical research facility devoted to the clinical evaluation of novel vaccines and to translational research studies of human immune system biology. At UCSF and Emory, Dr. Feinberg and colleagues were engaged in the preclinical development and evaluation of novel vaccines for HIV and other infectious diseases and in basic research studies focused on revealing fundamental aspects of host-virus relationships that underlie the pathogenesis of HIV and simian immunodeficiency virus (SIV) infections. In addition to his other professional roles, he has also served as a consultant to, and member of, several committees of the IOM and the NAS.

J. Patrick Fitch, Ph.D., joined Battelle in 2006 as vice president for Biodefense Programs, after more than 20 years of experience leading multidisciplinary applied science teams as large as 250 staff members (including biologists, veterinarians, physicians, engineers, physicists, chemists, and computer scientists) as well as a $75 million per year program at the Lawrence Livermore National Laboratory (LLNL). From 2001 to 2006, he led LLNL's Chemical and Biological National Security Program (CBNP), which ranges from basic pathogen biology and material science to deployed systems and has had many accomplishments including performing more than one million assays on national security samples, stand-up and operation of 24/7 reachback capabilities, stand-up of a nationwide bio-alert system, three R&D 100 awards, and design of signatures for validated assays in the CDC Laboratory Response Network. Under Dr. Fitch's leadership, BASIS was designed, demonstrated, and deployed, leading to the nationwide system, BioWatch. He has authored several books and book chapters including *An Engineering Introduction to Biotechnology*. He has chaired and served on several panels of the National Academies. His advisory board activities have included the U.S. Animal Health Association, the Texas A&M University DHS Center of Excellence, Central Florida University (College Engineering), Colorado State University (College of Engineering), the California State Breast Cancer Research Program, and *Biomolecular Engineering*. Dr. Fitch was a fellow of the American Society for Laser Medicine and Surgery and an associate editor of *Circuits, Systems and Signal Processing*. He has received two national awards for medical devices, a technical writing award for an article in *Science*, and an international best paper award from the IEEE. He also co-invented the technology, developed the initial business plan, and successfully raised venture investments for a spin-out high tech medical device start-up company. Dr. Fitch received his Ph.D. from Purdue University and B.S. degrees from Loyola College.

Capt. Darrell R. Galloway, MSC, Ph.D., is chief of Medical S&T Division for the Chemical & Biological Defense Directorate at the Defense Threat Reduction Agency. He received his baccalaureate degree in microbiology from the California State University in Los Angeles in 1973. After completing military service in the U.S. Army as a medical corpsman from 1969–1972, Captain Galloway entered graduate school and completed a doctoral degree in biochemistry in 1978 from the University of California, followed by two years of postgraduate training in immunochemistry as a Fellow of the National Cancer Institute at the Scripps Clinic and Research Foundation in La Jolla, CA. Captain Galloway began his

Navy career at the Naval Medical Research Institute in Bethesda, MD, where he served as a research scientist from 1980–1984 working on vaccine development. In late 1984 Captain Galloway left active service to pursue an academic appointment at The Ohio State University where he is a tenured faculty member in the Department of Microbiology. He also holds appointments at the University of Maryland Biotechnology Institute and the Uniformed Services University of Health Sciences. He has an international reputation in the area of bacterial toxin research and has published more than 50 research papers on various studies of bacterial toxins. In recent years Captain Galloway's research has concentrated on anthrax and the development of DNA-based vaccine technology. His laboratory has contributed substantially to the development of a new DNA-based vaccine against anthrax which has completed the first phase of clinical trials. Captain Galloway is a member of the American Society for Microbiology and has served as past president of the Ohio Branch of that organization. He received an NIH Research Career Development Award. In 2005 Captain Galloway was awarded the Joel M. Dalrymple Award for significant contributions to biodefense vaccine development.

S. Elizabeth George, Ph.D., is deputy director, Biological Countermeasures Portfolio Science and Technology Directorate, Department of Homeland Security (DHS). Until merging into the new department in 2003, she was the program manager of the Chemical and Biological National Security Program in the Department of Energy's National Nuclear Security Administration's Office of Nonproliferation Research & Engineering. Significant accomplishments include the design and deployment of BioWatch, the nation's first civilian biological threat agent-monitoring system and PROTECT, the first civilian operational chemical detection and response capability deployed in the Washington subway system. Previously, she spent 16 years at the U.S. Environmental Protection Agency (EPA), Office of Research and Development, National Health and Ecological Effects Research Laboratory, Environmental Carcinogenesis Division, where she was branch chief of the Molecular and Cellular Toxicology Branch. She received her B.S. in biology (1977) from Virginia Polytechnic Institute and State University and M.S. and Ph.D. in microbiology (1979 and 1984) from North Carolina State University. She was an NRC fellow (1984–1986) in the laboratory of Dr. Larry Claxton at the U.S. EPA. Dr. George is the 2005 chair of the Chemical and Biological Terrorism Defense Gordon Research Conference. She has served as councilor for the Environmental Mutagen Society and president and secretary of the Genotoxicity and Environmental Mutagen Society. She holds memberships in the American Society for Microbiology and the American Association for the Advancement of Science and is an adjunct faculty member in the School of Rural Public Health, Texas A&M University. She is a recipient of the EPA Bronze Medal and Scientific and Technological Achievement Awards and DHS Under

Secretary's Award for Science and Technology. She is author of numerous journal articles and has presented her research at national and international meetings.

Jesse L. Goodman, M.D., M.P.H., was professor of medicine and chief of infectious diseases at the University of Minnesota, and is now serving as deputy director for the FDA's Center for Biologics Evaluation and Research, where he is active in a broad range of scientific, public health, and policy issues. After joining the FDA commissioner's office, he has worked closely with several centers and helped coordinate the FDA's response to the antimicrobial resistance problem. He was cochair of a recently formed federal interagency task force that developed the national Public Health Action Plan on antimicrobial resistance. He graduated from Harvard College and attended the Albert Einstein College of Medicine followed by internal medicine, hematology, oncology, and infectious diseases training at the University of Pennsylvania and University of California–Los Angeles, where he was also chief medical resident. He received his master's of public health from the University of Minnesota. He has been active in community public health activities, including creating an environmental health partnership in St. Paul, Minnesota. In recent years, his laboratory's research has focused on the molecular pathogenesis of tick-borne diseases. His laboratory isolated the etiological intracellular agent of the emerging tick-borne infection, human granulocytic ehrlichiosis, and identified its leukocyte receptor. He has also been an active clinician and teacher and has directed or participated in major multicenter clinical studies. He is a fellow of the Infectious Diseases Society of America and, among several honors, has been elected to the American Society for Clinical Investigation.

Eduardo Gotuzzo, M.D., is principal professor and director at the Instituto de Medicina Tropical "Alexander von Humbolt," Universidad Peruana Cayetan Heredia (UPCH), in Lima, Peru, as well as chief of the Department of Infectious and Tropical Diseases at the Cayetano Heredia Hospital. He is also an adjunct professor of medicine at the University of Alabama–Birmingham School of Medicine. Dr. Gotuzzo is an active member in numerous international societies, and has been president of the Latin America Society of Tropical Disease (2000–2003), the Scientific Program of Infectious Diseases Society of America (2000–2003), the International Organizing Committee of the International Congress of Infectious Diseases (1994–present), president elect of the International Society for Infectious Diseases (1996–1998), and president of the Peruvian Society of Internal Medicine (1991–1992). He has published over 230 articles and chapters as well as 6 manuals and 1 book. Recent honors and awards include being named an honorary member of American Society of Tropical Medicine and Hygiene (since 2002), associate member of the National Academy of Medicine (since 2002), honorary member of the Society of Internal Medicine (since 2000), distinguished visitor at the Faculty of Medical Sciences, University of Cordoba, Argentina (since 1999), and received the Golden Medal for Outstanding Contribution in the Field of Infectious Diseases awarded by the Trnava University, Slovakia (1998), among many others.

Jo Handelsman, Ph.D., received her Ph.D. in molecular biology from the University of Wisconsin (UW)–Madison in 1984 and joined the faculty of the UW–Madison Department of Plant Pathology in 1985 where she is currently a Howard Hughes Medical Institute (HHMI) Professor. Her research focuses on the genetic and functional diversity of microorganisms in soil and insect gut communities. The Handelsman lab has concentrated on discovery and biological activity of novel antibiotics from cultured and uncultured bacteria and has contributed to the pioneering of a new technique, called metagenomics, that facilitates the genomic analysis of assemblages of uncultured microorganisms. Handelsman is studying the midgut of the gypsy moth to understand the basis for resistance and susceptibility of microbial communities to invasion, developing it as a model for the microbial community in the human gut. In addition to her passion for understanding the secret lives of bacteria, Dr. Handelsman is dedicated to improving science education and the advancement of women in research universities. She is director of the Howard Hughes Medical Institute New Generation Program for Scientific Teaching, which is dedicated to teaching graduate students and postdoctoral students the principles and practices of teaching and mentoring. She is codirector of the National Academies Summer Institute for Undergraduate Education in Biology, which is a collaborative venture between HHMI and the National Academies that aims to train a nationwide network of faculty who are outstanding teachers and mentors. Dr. Handelsman is codirector of the Women in Science and Engineering Leadership Institute, at the University of Wisconsin–Madison, whose mission is to understand the impediments to the successful recruitment and advancement of women faculty in the sciences and to develop and study interventions intended to reduce the barriers.

Carole A. Heilman, Ph.D., is director of the Division of Microbiology and Infectious Diseases (DMID) of the NIAID. She received her bachelor's degree in biology from Boston University in 1972, and earned her master's degree and doctorate in microbiology from Rutgers University in 1976 and 1979, respectively. Dr. Heilman began her career at the NIH as a postdoctoral research associate with the National Cancer Institute where she carried out research on the regulation of gene expression during cancer development. In 1986, she came to NIAID as the influenza and viral respiratory diseases program officer in DMID and, in 1988, she was appointed chief of the respiratory diseases branch where she coordinated the development of acellular pertussis vaccines. She joined the Division of AIDS as deputy director in 1997 and was responsible for developing the Innovation Grant Program for Approaches in HIV Vaccine Research. She is the recipient of several notable awards for outstanding achievement. Throughout her extramural career, Dr. Heilman has contributed articles on vaccine design and development to many scientific journals and has served as a consultant to the World Bank and WHO in this area. She is also a member of several professional societies, including the Infectious Diseases Society of America, the American Society for Microbiology, and the American Society of Virology.

David L. Heymann, M.D., is currently the executive director of the WHO Communicable Diseases Cluster. From October 1995 to July 1998 he was director of the WHO Programme on Emerging and Other Communicable Diseases Surveillance and Control. Prior to becoming director of this program, he was the chief of research activities in the Global Programme on AIDS. From 1976 to 1989, prior to joining WHO, Dr. Heymann spent 13 years working as a medical epidemiologist in sub-Saharan Africa (Cameroon, Ivory Coast, the former Zaire, and Malawi) on assignment from the CDC in CDC-supported activities aimed at strengthening capacity in surveillance of infectious diseases and their control, with special emphasis on the childhood immunizable diseases, African hemorrhagic fevers, pox viruses, and malaria. While based in Africa, he participated in the investigation of the first outbreak of Ebola in Yambuku (former Zaire) in 1976, then again investigated the second outbreak of Ebola in 1977 in Tandala, and in 1995 directed the international response to the Ebola outbreak in Kikwit. Prior to 1976, Dr. Heymann spent two years in India as a medical officer in the WHO Smallpox Eradication Programme. He holds a B.A. from the Pennsylvania State University, an M.D. from Wake Forest University, and a Diploma in Tropical Medicine and Hygiene from the London School of Hygiene and Tropical Medicine. He has also completed practical epidemiology training in the Epidemic Intelligence Service (EIS) training program of the CDC. He has published 131 scientific articles on infectious diseases in peer-reviewed medical and scientific journals.

Phil Hosbach, Ph.D., is vice president of New Products and Immunization Policy at Sanofi Pasteur. The departments under his supervision are new product marketing, state and federal government policy, business intelligence, bids and contracts, medical communications, public health sales, and public health marketing. His current responsibilities include oversight of immunization policy development. He acts as Sanofi Pasteur's principle liaison with the CDC. Mr. Hosbach graduated from Lafayette College in 1984 with a degree in biology. He has 20 years of pharmaceutical industry experience, including the last 17 years focused solely on vaccines. He began his career at American Home Products in Clinical Research in 1984. He joined Aventis Pasteur (then Connaught Labs) in 1987 as clinical research coordinator and has held research and development positions of increasing responsibility, including clinical research manager and director of clinical operations. Mr. Hosbach also served as project manager for the development and licensure of Tripedia, the first diphtheria, tetanus, and acellular pertussis

(DTaP) vaccine approved by the FDA for use in U.S. infants. During his clinical research career at Aventis Pasteur, he contributed to the development and licensure of seven vaccines and has authored or coauthored several clinical research articles. From 2000 through 2002, Mr. Hosbach served on the board of directors for Pocono Medical Center, in East Stroudsburg, Pennsylvania. Since 2003 he has actively served on the board of directors of Pocono Health Systems, which includes Pocono Medical Center.

James M. Hughes, M.D., received his B.A. in 1966 and M.D. in 1971 from Stanford University. He completed a residency in internal medicine at the University of Washington and a fellowship in infectious diseases at the University of Virginia. He is board certified in internal medicine, infectious diseases, and preventive medicine. He first joined the CDC as an epidemic intelligence service officer in 1973. During his CDC career, he has worked primarily in the areas of foodborne disease and infection control in healthcare settings. He became director of the NCID in 1992. The center is currently working to address domestic and global challenges posed by emerging infectious diseases and the threat of bioterrorism. He is a member of the IOM and a fellow of the American College of Physicians, the Infectious Diseases Society of America, and the American Association for the Advancement of Science. He is an Assistant Surgeon General in the Public Health Service.

Stephen A. Johnston, Ph.D., is a professor and director at the University of Texas Southwestern Medical Center. A major focus of his lab has been technology development. His interest of late has been especially in the area of vaccine development. He was coinventor with Dr. John Sanford of the hand-held, helium gene gun, and he and Dr. Sanford used the gene gun to first demonstrate gene (DNA) immunization. Genetic vaccines have revolutionized approaches to delivering and developing vaccines. In this regard, Johnston's group first published on a method, expression library immunization, that offers a systematic approach to searching genomic information for new vaccines. His group has also developed techniques for discovering peptides that target specific cells and is employing this to create more effective, targeted vaccines. Through the Center for Biomedical Inventions, his group with collaborators in immunology, instrumentation, genomics, and chemistry is attempting to forge a fully integrated approach to developing the best methods for delivery and discovering vaccines.

Gerald T. Keusch, M.D., is provost and dean for Global Health at Boston University and Boston University School of Public Health. He is a graduate of Columbia College (1958) and Harvard Medical School (1963). After completing a residency in internal medicine, fellowship training in infectious diseases, and two years as an NIH research associate at the SEATO Medical Research Laboratory in Bangkok, Thailand, Dr. Keusch joined the faculty of Mt. Sinai School of Medicine in 1970, where he established a laboratory to study the pathogenesis of bacillary dysentery and the biology and biochemistry of Shiga toxin. In 1979, he moved to Tufts Medical School and New England Medical Center in Boston to found the Division of Geographic Medicine, which focused on the molecular and cellular biology of tropical infectious disease. In 1986, he integrated the clinical infectious diseases program into the Division of Geographic Medicine and Infectious Diseases, continuing as division chief until 1998. He has worked in the laboratory and in the field in Latin America, Africa, and Asia on basic and clinical infectious diseases and HIV/AIDS research. From 1998 to 2003, he was associate director for international research and director of the Fogarty International Center at the NIH. Dr. Keusch is a member of the American Society for Clinical Investigation, the Association of American Physicians, the American Society for Microbiology, and the Infectious Diseases Society of America. He is the recipient of the Squibb (1981), Finland (1997), and Bristol (2002) Awards of the Infectious Diseases Society of America. In 2002, he was elected to the IOM.

Rima F. Khabbaz, M.D., is director of the NCID at the CDC. She received her B.S. in 1975 and her M.D. in 1979 from the American University of Beirut in Beirut, Lebanon. She trained in internal medicine and completed a fellowship in infectious diseases at the University of Maryland in Baltimore. She is board certified in internal medicine. She first joined the CDC as an epidemic intelligence service officer in 1980. During her CDC career, she worked primarily in the areas of healthcare-associated infections and viral diseases. She is a fellow of the Infectious Diseases Society of America and an elected member of the American Epidemiologic Society. She served on the Blood Product Advisory Committee of the FDA, on the FDA's Transmissible Spongiform Encephalopathy Advisory Committee, and on the Infectious Diseases Society of America's Annual Meeting Scientific Program Committee. She played a leading role in developing the CDC's programs related to blood safety and food safety and in the CDC's responses to outbreaks of new and reemerging diseases.

Lonnie J. King, D.V.M., is dean of the College of Veterinary Medicine, Michigan State University. His previous positions include both associate administrator and administrator of the USDA Animal and Plant Health Inspection Service (APHIS) and deputy administrator for USDA/APHIS/Veterinary Services. Before his government career, Dr. King was in private practice. He also has experience as a field veterinary medical officer, station epidemiologist, and staff assignments involving emergency programs and animal health information. He has also directed the American Veterinary Medical Association's Office of Governmental Relations and is certified in the American College of Veterinary Preventive Medicine. He has served as president of the Association of American Veterinary Medicine Colleges and currently serves as cochair of the National Commission on Veterinary Economic Issues, is the lead dean at Michigan State University for food safety with responsibility for the National Food Safety and Toxicology Center, and also serves at the Institute for Environmental Toxicology and the Center for Emerging Infectious Diseases. He is codeveloper and course leader for science, politics, and animal health policy. He received his B.S. and D.V.M degrees from Ohio State University and his M.S. degree in epidemiology from the University of Minnesota. He has also completed the Senior Executive Program at Harvard University, and received an M.P.A. from American University. Dr. King previously served on the Committee for Opportunities in Agriculture, the Steering Committee for a Workshop on the Control and Prevention of Animal Diseases, and the Committee to Ensure Safe Food from Production to Consumption.

COL George W. Korch, Ph.D., is commander, United States Army Medical Research Institute for Infectious Diseases, Ft. Detrick, Maryland. Dr. Korch attended Boston University and earned a B.S. in biology in 1974, followed by postgraduate study in mammalian ecology at the University of Kansas from 1975 to 1978. He earned his Ph.D. from the Johns Hopkins School of Hygiene and Public Health in immunology and infectious diseases in 1985, followed by postdoctoral experience at Johns Hopkins from 1985 to 1986. His area of training and specialty is the study of the epidemiology of zoonotic viral pathogens and in medical entomology. For the past 15 years, he has also engaged in research and program management for medical defense against biological pathogens used in terrorism or warfare.

Joshua Lederberg, Ph.D., is professor emeritus of molecular genetics and informatics and Sackler Foundation Scholar at the Rockefeller University in New York City. His lifelong research, for which he received the Nobel Prize in 1958, has been in genetic structure and function in microorganisms. He has a keen interest in international health and was cochair of a previous IOM Committee on Emerging Microbial Threats to Health (1990–1992) and currently is cochair of the Committee on Emerging Microbial Threats to Health in the 21st Century. He has been a member of the NAS since 1957 and is a charter member of the IOM.

Lynn G. Marks, M.D., is board certified in internal medicine and infectious diseases. He was on faculty at the University of South Alabama College of Medicine in the Infectious Diseases Department focusing on patient care, teaching, and research. His academic research interest was on the molecular genetics of bacterial pathogenicity. He subsequently joined SmithKline Beecham's (now GlaxoSmithKline) anti-infectives clinical group and later progressed to global head of the Consumer Healthcare Division Medical and Regulatory Group. He then returned to pharmaceutical research and development as global head of the Infectious Diseases Therapeutic Area Strategy Team for GlaxoSmithKline.

Mary McBride, Ph.D., is the Deputy Program Leader for Science and Technology within the Chemical and Biological National Security Program (CBNP) at Lawrence Livermore National Laboratory. The Program's primary mission is to develop and field advanced strategies that dramatically improve the nation's capabilities to prevent, prepare for, detect and respond to chemical or biological terrorism. Dr. McBride directs and manages the research efforts of more than 65 multidisciplinary professional and technical staff in a program of integrated research that leverages investments across all sectors (academic to industrial). She plans, coordinates, evaluates, and manages the transition from basic research, to proof of principle, to demonstration and pilots, to operational systems with hand-off to end-users and commercialization for numerous projects. She conceived and developed a research program to develop diagnostic assays and instrumentation for infectious diseases intended for use at point-of-care. Recently, Dr. McBride also initiated a research program to rapidly prototype a chip-based system for detection and identification of microbial antibiotic resistance and virulence factors with intended hand-off to industry for commercialization within 18 months. Dr. McBride is also especially interested and active in a variety of interagency activities. She is the technical lead for a project designed to establish assay equivalency and interoperability between DoD, USPS, and HHS biomonitoring systems, and she is developing an integrated plan intended to enable private sector, academia, and USG performers to establish detection/identification assays as "public health actionable". She recently completed four month assignment at Department of Homeland Security serving as an advisor to S&T Biological Countermeasures. Dr. McBride earned a Ph.D. from the University of California, Davis in analytical chemistry in 1998. She joined LLNL as a postdoctoral research associate in 1999. She has published over 30 peer-reviewed publications, holds five patents related to biodetection instrumentation/assays, and has received an R&D 100 award and LLNL's highest scientific achievement award, the Laboratory S&T award.

Edward McSweegan, Ph.D., is a program officer at NIAID. He graduated from Boston College in 1978 (B.S.) and has degrees in microbiology from the University of New Hampshire (M.S.) and the University of Rhode Island (Ph.D.). He was an NRC Associate from 1984 to 1986 and did postdoctoral research at the Naval Medical Research Institute in Bethesda, Maryland. Dr. McSweegan served as an American Association for the Advancement of Science Diplomacy fellow in the U.S. State Department from 1986 to 1988 and negotiated science and technology agreements with Poland, Hungary, and the former Soviet Union. After moving to the NIH, he continued to work on international health and science projects in Egypt, Israel, India, and Russia. Currently, he manages NIAID's bilateral program with India, the Indo–U.S. Vaccine Action Program, and represents NIAID in the DHHS Biotechnology Engagement Program (BTEP) with Russia and related countries. He is a member of the American Association for the Advancement of Science, the American Society for Microbiology, and the D.C. Science Writers Association. He is the author of numerous journal articles and science articles.

Stephen S. Morse, Ph.D., is director of the Center for Public Health Preparedness at the Mailman School of Public Health of Columbia University and is a faculty member in the epidemiology department. He recently returned to Columbia from four years in government service as program manager at the Defense Advanced Research Projects Agency (DARPA), where he codirected the Pathogen Countermeasures Program and subsequently directed the Advanced Diagnostics Program. Before coming to Columbia, he was assistant professor of virology at the Rockefeller University in New York, where he remains an adjunct faculty member. He is the editor of two books, *Emerging Viruses* (Oxford University Press, 1993; paperback, 1996) (selected by *American Scientist* for its list of 100 Top Science Books of the 20th Century), and *The Evolutionary Biology of Viruses* (Raven Press, 1994). He currently serves as a section editor of the CDC journal, *Emerging Infectious Diseases,* and was formerly an editor-in-chief of the Pasteur Institute's journal, *Research in Virology*. Dr. Morse was chair and principal organizer of the 1989 NIAID/NIH Conference on Emerging Viruses (for which he originated the term and concept of *emerging viruses/infections*); served as a member of the IOM-NAS Committee on Emerging Microbial Threats to Health (and chaired its Task Force on Viruses), and was a contributor to its report, *Emerging Infections* (1992); was a member of the IOM's Committee on Xenograft Transplantation; currently serves on the Steering Committee of the IOM's Forum on Emerging Infections, and has served as an adviser to WHO, the Pan-American Health Organization, the FDA, the Defense Threat Reduction Agency, and other agencies. He is a fellow of the New York Academy of Sciences and a past chair of its microbiology section. He was the founding chair of ProMED (the nonprofit international Program to Monitor Emerging Diseases) and was one of the originators of ProMED-mail, an international network inaugurated by ProMED in 1994 for outbreak reporting and disease monitoring using the Internet. Dr. Morse received his Ph.D. from the University of Wisconsin–Madison.

Michael T. Osterholm, Ph.D., M.P.H., is director of the Center for Infectious Disease Research and Policy at the University of Minnesota where he is also professor at the School of Public Health. Previously, Dr. Osterholm was the state epidemiologist and chief of the acute disease epidemiology section for the Minnesota Department of Health. He has received numerous research awards from the NIAID and the CDC. He served as principal investigator for the CDC-sponsored Emerging Infections Program in Minnesota. He has published more than 240 articles and abstracts on various emerging infectious disease problems and is the author of the best selling book, *Living Terrors: What America Needs to Know to Survive the Coming Bioterrorist Catastrophe*. He is past president of the Council of State and Territorial Epidemiologists. He currently serves on the NAS-IOM Forum on Emerging Infections. He has also served on the IOM Committee to Ensure Safe Food from Production to Consumption, the IOM Committee on the Department of Defense Persian Gulf Syndrome Comprehensive Clinical Evaluation Program, and as a reviewer for the IOM report on chemical and biological terrorism.

George Poste, Ph.D., D.V.M., is director of the Arizona Biodesign Institute and Dell E. Webb Distinguished Professor of Biology at Arizona State University. From 1992 to 1999, he was chief science and technology officer and president, Research and Development of SmithKline Beecham (SB). During his tenure at SB, he was associated with the successful registration of 29 drug, vaccine, and diagnostic products. He is chairman of diaDexus and Structural GenomiX in California and Orchid Biosciences in Princeton. He serves on the board of directors of AdvancePCS and Monsanto. He is an advisor on biotechnology to several venture capital funds and investment banks. In May 2003, he was appointed as director of the Arizona Biodesign Institute at Arizona State University. This is a major new initiative combining research groups in biotechnology, nanotechnology, materials science, advanced computing, and neuromorphic engineering. He is a fellow of Pembroke College at Cambridge and distinguished fellow at the Hoover Institution and Stanford University. He is a member of the Defense Science Board of the U.S. Department of Defense, and in this capacity he chairs the Task Force on Bioterrorism. He is also a member of the NAS Working Group on Defense Against Bioweapons. Dr. Poste is a board-certified pathologist, a fellow of the Royal Society, and a fellow of the Academy of Medical Sciences. He was awarded the rank of Commander of the British Empire by Queen Elizabeth II in 1999 for services to medicine and for the advancement of biotechnology. He has published over 350 scientific papers; coedited 15 books on cancer, biotechnology, and infectious diseases; and serves on the editorial board of multiple technical journals. He is invited routinely to be the keynote speaker at a wide variety of academic, corporate, investment, and government meetings to discuss the impact of biotechnology and genetics on healthcare and the challenges posed by bioterrorism.

David A. Relman, M.D., Ph.D., is an associate professor of medicine (infectious diseases and geographic medicine) and of microbiology and immunology at Stanford University School of Medicine, Stanford, CA, and chief of the infectious disease section at the Veterans Affairs (VA) Palo Alto Health Care System, Palo Alto, CA. Dr. Relman received his B.S. in biology from Massachusetts Institute of Technology, Cambridge, Massachusetts, and his M.D. from Harvard Medical School. He completed his residency in internal medicine and a clinical fellowship in infectious diseases at Massachusetts General Hospital, Boston, after which he moved to Stanford in 1994. His major focus is laboratory research directed toward characterizing the human endogenous microbial flora, host-microbe interactions, and identifying previously unrecognized microbial pathogens using molecular and genomic approaches. He has described a number of new human microbial pathogens. Dr. Relman's lab (*http://relman.stanford.edu*) is currently exploring human oral and intestinal microbial ecology, sources of variation in host genomewide expression responses to infection and during states of health, and how *Bordetella* species (including the agent of whooping cough) cause disease. He has published over 150 peer-reviewed articles, reviews, editorials, and book chapters on pathogen discovery and bacterial pathogenesis. He has served on scientific program committees for the American Society of Microbiology; the Infectious Diseases Society of America (IDSA); advisory panels for the NIH, CDC, the Departments of Energy and Defense, and the National Aeronautics and Space Administration. He was cochair of the Committee on Advances in Technology and the Prevention of their Application to Next Generation Biowarefare Threats for the NAS. He is a member of the board of directors of the IDSA and the Board of Scientific Counselors at the National Institute of Dental and Craniofacial Research at the NIH. He received the Squibb Award from the IDSA in 2001, the Senior Scholar Award in Global Infectious Diseases from the Ellison Medical Foundation in 2002, and is a fellow of the American Academy of Microbiology.

Gary A. Roselle, M.D., received his M.D. from Ohio State University School of Medicine in 1973. He served his residency at Northwestern University School of Medicine and his infectious diseases fellowship at the University of Cincinnati School of Medicine. He is the program director for infectious diseases for the VA Central Office in Washington, D.C., as well as the chief of the medical service at the Cincinnati VA Medical Center. He is a professor of medicine in the Department of Internal Medicine, Division of Infectious Diseases at the University of Cincinnati College of Medicine. Dr. Roselle serves on several national advisory committees. In addition, he is currently heading the Emerging Pathogens Initiative for the Department of Veterans Affairs. He has received commendations from the Cincinnati Medical Center Director, the Under Secretary for Health for the Department of Veterans Affairs, and the Secretary of Veterans Affairs for his work in the infectious diseases program for the Department of Veterans Affairs. He has been an invited speaker at several national and international meetings and has published over 80 papers and several book chapters.

Janet Shoemaker is director of the American Society for Microbiology's Public Affairs Office, a position she has held since 1989. She is responsible for managing the legislative and regulatory affairs of this 42,000-member organization, the largest single biological science society in the world. She has served as principal investigator for a project funded by the National Science Foundation (NSF) to collect and disseminate data on the job market for recent doctorates in microbiology and has played a key role in American Society for Microbiology (ASM) projects, including the production of the ASM *Employment Outlook in the Microbiological Sciences* and *The Impact of Managed Care and Health System Change on Clinical Microbiology*. Previously, she held positions as assistant director of public affairs for the ASM, as ASM coordinator of the U.S./U.S.S.R. Exchange Program in Microbiology, a program sponsored and coordinated by the NSF and the U.S. Department of State, and as a freelance editor and writer. She received her baccalaureate, cum laude, from the University of Massachusetts, and is a graduate of the George Washington University programs in public policy and in editing and publications. She has served as commissioner to the Commission on Professionals in Science and Technology, and as the ASM representative to the ad hoc Group for Medical Research Funding, and is a member of Women in Government Relations, the American Society of Association Executives, and the American Association for the Advancement of Science. She has coauthored published articles on research funding, biotechnology, biological weapons control, and public policy issues related to microbiology.

Brian J. Staskawicz, Ph.D., is professor and chair, Department of Plant and Microbial Biology, University of California, Berkeley. Dr. Staskawicz received his B.A. in biology from Bates College in 1974 and his Ph.D. from the University of California, Berkeley in 1980. Dr. Staskawicz's work has greatly contributed to understanding the molecular interactions between plants and their pathogens. He was elected to the NAS in 1998 for elucidating the mechanisms of disease resistance, as his lab was the first to clone a bacterial effector gene from a pathogen and among the first to clone and characterize plant disease resistance genes. Dr. Staskawicz's research focuses on the interaction of the bacteria, Pseudomonas and Xanthomonas, with Arabidopsis, tomato and pepper. He has published extensively in this area and is a one of the leading scientists in the world working on elucidating the molecular basis of plant innate immunity.

Terence Taylor is president and director of the International Council for the Life Sciences (ICLS). He is responsible for the overall direction of the ICLS and its programs, which have the goal of enhancing global biosafety and biosecurity. Previously he was assistant director of the International Institute for Strategic Studies (IISS) (1995 to 2005), a leading independent international institute and president and executive director of its U.S. office (2001 to 2005). He studies international security policy; risk analysis, scientific and technological developments and their impact on political and economic stability worldwide. At IISS he was one of the Institute's leading experts on issues associated with nuclear, biological, and chemical weapons and their means of delivery. In his previous appointments he has had particular responsibilities for issues affecting public safety and security in relation to biological risks and advances in the life sciences. He was one of the commissioners to the UN Special Commission on Iraq for which he also conducted missions as a chief inspector. He was a research fellow on the Science Program at the Center for International Security and Co-operation at Stanford University where he carried out, among other subjects, studies of the implications for government and industry of the weapons of mass destruction treaties and agreements. He has also carried out consultancy work for the International Committee of the Red Cross on the implementation and development of the laws of armed conflict. He has served as chairman of the World Federation of Scientists' Permanent Monitoring Panel on Risk Analysis. He served as a career officer in the British Army on operations in many parts of the world including counterterrorist operations and UN peacekeeping. His publications include monographs, book chapters and articles for, among others, Stanford University, the World Economic Forum, the Stockholm International Peace Research Institute (SIPRI), the Crimes of War Project, the *International Herald Tribune*, the *Wall Street Journal*, the *International Defence Review*, the *Independent* (London), *Tiempo* (Madrid), the *International and Comparative Law Quarterly*, *The Washington Quarterly*, and other scholarly journals including unsigned contributions to IISS publications.